Chronic Pain and HIV
A practical approach

Chronic Pain and HIV

A practical approach

EDITED BY

Jessica S. Merlin
Peter A. Selwyn
Glenn J. Treisman
Angela G. Giovanniello

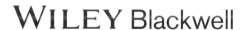

This edition first published 2016 © 2016 by Blackwell Publishing Ltd

Registered office: John Wiley & Sons, Ltd, The Atrium, Southern Gate, Chichester, West Sussex, PO19 8SQ, UK

Editorial offices: 9600 Garsington Road, Oxford, OX4 2DQ, UK

The Atrium, Southern Gate, Chichester, West Sussex, PO19 8SQ, UK

111 River Street, Hoboken, NJ 07030-5774, USA

For details of our global editorial offices, for customer services and for information about how to apply for permission to reuse the copyright material in this book please see our website at www.wiley.com/wiley-blackwell

Library of Congress Cataloging-in-Publication Data

Names: Merlin, Jessica, editor. | Selwyn, Peter A., editor. | Treisman, Glenn
   J., 1956- , editor. | Giovanniello, Angela, editor.
Title: Chronic pain and HIV : a practical approach / edited by Jessica
   Merlin, Peter A Selwyn, Glenn Treisman, Angela Giovanniello.
Description: Chichester, West Sussex ; Hoboken, NJ : John Wiley & Sons Inc.,
   2016. | Includes bibliographical references and index.
Identifiers: LCCN 2015040507 | ISBN 9781118777411 (cloth)
Subjects: | MESH: Chronic Pain. | HIV Infections. | Comorbidity.
Classification: LCC RC607.A26 | NLM WC 503 | DDC 616.97/920472–dc23 LC record available at
http://lccn.loc.gov/2015040507

A catalogue record for this book is available from the British Library.

Wiley also publishes its books in a variety of electronic formats. Some content that appears in print may not be available in electronic books.

Cover image: Getty/Piotr Raczak/EyeEm

Typset in 8.5/11pt, MeridienLTStd by SPi Global, Chennai, India.
Printed and bound in Malaysia by Vivar Printing Sdn Bhd

1   2016

Contents

Foreword

Chronic pain is defined as pain lasting longer than 3–6 months, beyond the period of normal tissue healing.[1] "Relieving Pain in America," a 2011 Report from the Institute of Medicine of the National Academy of Sciences, identified chronic pain as a serious public health concern and offered a "blueprint for transforming prevalence, care, education, and research."[2] A follow-up National Pain Strategy (2015) is currently being developed. Internationally, the World Health Organization recognizes chronic pain as both a public health and human rights issue, and the 2014 World Health Assembly has passed Resolution 67 calling on member states to integrate pain treatment and palliative care services for patients with chronic diseases such as cancer and HIV/AIDS into their national health strategies.[3]

This increased national and international attention to prioritize chronic pain as a public health issue makes this book a timely and valuable reference text to guide policymakers and clinicians as they develop comprehensive strategies to address chronic pain among individuals with HIV.

In the early years of the AIDS epidemic, before disease-specific treatment was even available, clinicians learned to treat pain and suffering even as they could not alter the natural history of the disease. Few conditions in recent history have represented such an extreme example of the concept of "total pain" as AIDS in the preantiretroviral era.[4] Patients at that time often experienced an often overwhelming succession of opportunistic infections, some of which caused or aggravated physical pain; emotional, social, and spiritual pain were also often intense, pervasive, and for some, unrelenting.

In less than two decades, the clinical landscape of AIDS has been completely transformed; remarkably, in the current HIV treatment era, rapid advances in disease treatment have provided the patient with HIV the potential for a normal or near-normal life span. However, the experience of chronic pain interferes with a patient's quality of life and physical functioning, impacts adherence to antiretroviral therapy and HIV primary care, and is associated with significant psychological and social distress and substance use disorders. Ironically, even as the incidence of opportunistic infections has decreased sharply, the incidence of chronic comorbidities in long-surviving patients with HIV has just as dramatically increased. Chronic inflammation, end-organ failure, systemic metabolic abnormalities, psychosocial, and other challenges of an aging and increasingly frail and disabled population, all have added to the complexity and necessity of having a new understanding of pain and its treatment in the antiretroviral era. Multifactorial health disparities further impact care and treatment for many HIV-infected patients, particularly those from vulnerable or disenfranchised populations. This specialized textbook addresses these complex issues that can influence pain care for the patient with HIV. It is both a primer and a comprehensive review defining the field of chronic pain management for patients with HIV.

Edited by Drs Merlin, Giovanniello, Treisman, and Selwyn – all of whom have had extensive experience with HIV/AIDS and pain/palliative care – each chapter is written by experts who provide a review of the relevant literature. Taken together, this book outlines a biopsychosocial model of care for the patient with HIV and chronic pain.

Yet this book does more than define the field – it offers front-line clinicians practical advice. It teaches healthcare professionals how to communicate with patients with chronic pain; provides the specific assessment tools that may help to routinize assessment of pain and psychological distress; models shared decision-making in therapeutic planning; and describes the current effective pharmacologic and nonpharmacologic approaches to achieve rehabilitation, functioning, and health. Emphasis on psychiatric assessment and knowledge about substance use disorders as well as the discussions on the safe use of opioids in pain treatment for those with abuse histories are particularly valuable sections for all healthcare professionals to know and learn. Clinicians will find consolation in the chapter on the difficult patient that provides strategies for addressing these challenging patients in a professional manner and also helps them manage their own distress.

A unique feature of this text is its tone, which is evident in each of the chapters. Individuals with HIV are a vulnerable population with a high prevalence of mental illness, incarceration, homelessness, and injection drug use. Chronic pain is also a highly stigmatized disease; these dual stigmas often present a barrier to patient care. The authors articulate the need for positive regard for individuals with both HIV and chronic pain, who are stigmatized and marginalized in our healthcare system. The professionalism and compassion presented in a nonjudgmental format infuses the discourse about assessment and treatment options.

As a group, the authors support the integration of chronic pain treatment into routine HIV care but call out the current challenges and barriers – patient-related, provider-related, and systems-related – that are faced in accessing or implementing a care strategy. In this aspect, the book is aspirational in defining a quality standard of care that should become the norm for individuals with HIV and chronic pain.

While defining the field of chronic pain care in HIV, the book also serves to expose the dearth of detailed studies that limit definitive guideline development and encourage inadequate assessment and treatment. This issue is not specific to HIV pain research but is common to the field of chronic pain care in general, where the lack of a robust research agenda and funding stream thwarts the development of innovative therapies.

In his reflections on medical care, Anatole Broyard encourages physicians to "take the sick man into his heart."[5] This book helps us to do so with the specific skills necessary to provide humane, competent, and compassionate care for the individual with HIV and chronic pain.

Kathleen Foley, MD and Peter Selwyn, MD

References

1 Merskey, H., et al. (1994) "Part III: pain terms, a current list with definitions and notes on usage" *Classification of Chronic Pain*, 2nd ed., IASP Task Force on Taxonomy, edited by H. Merskey and N. Bogduk, IASP Press.

2 Institute of Medicine (2011) *Relieving Pain in America: A Blueprint for Transforming Prevention, Care, Education, and Research*. The National Academies Press, Washington, DC.

3 Burki, T.K. (2014) WHO resolution on access to palliative care. *Lancet Oncology*, **15** (3), e109.

4 Clark, D. (2000) 'Total pain': the work of Cicely Saunders and the Hospice movement. *Bulletin of the American Physical Society*, **10** (4), 13–15.

5 Broyard, A. (1992) Intoxicated by my illness. In: Broyard, A. (ed), *Fawcett Columbine Book*. Ballantyne Books.

About the editors

Jessica S. Merlin, MD, MBA

Dr Merlin is an Assistant Professor of Medicine in the divisions of Infectious Diseases and Gerontology, Geriatrics, and Palliative Care at the University of Alabama at Birmingham. She received her MD and MBA degrees, as well as her training in internal medicine and infectious diseases, at the University of Pennsylvania, and her palliative care training at the Mount Sinai School of Medicine. She runs one of a handful of HIV-focused chronic pain clinics in the United States. Her NIH-funded research focuses on the clinical epidemiology of chronic pain in individuals with HIV, developing behavioral interventions for chronic pain in this population, and addressing concerning behaviors that arise in individuals on long-term opioid therapy. She is the recipient of several national awards and was named an Inspirational Leader under 40 by the American Academy of Hospice and Palliative Medicine, and won the organization's Young Investigator award for her HIV/chronic pain research.

Peter A. Selwyn, MD, MPH

Dr Peter Selwyn received his MD degree from Harvard Medical School, his MPH degree from the Columbia University School of Public Health, and completed his residency training at Montefiore Medical Center, Bronx, NY. He is currently the Chairman of the Department of Family and Social Medicine, the Director of the Palliative Care Program, and the Professor of Family Medicine, Internal Medicine, and Epidemiology and Population Health at Montefiore Medical Center and Albert Einstein College of Medicine. He has been involved in clinical care, research, and education in the field of HIV and palliative care since the early AIDS epidemic.

Glenn J. Treisman, MD, PhD

Glenn Jordan Treisman is the Eugene Meyer III Professor of Psychiatry and Behavioral Sciences and Internal Medicine at the Johns Hopkins University School of Medicine. He is the Director of the AIDS Psychiatry Program and the Co-director of the Pain Treatment Program at Johns Hopkins Hospital. He is best known for his groundbreaking work in the field of HIV, where he has been described as "the father of AIDS psychiatry." He has cared for patients with HIV since early in the epidemic and described the role of mental illness in the HIV epidemic. He is the author of The Psychiatry of AIDS, the first comprehensive textbook on the subject, as well as numerous articles on related subjects. He was recognized for this work by the American College of Physicians with the presentation of the William C. Menninger Memorial Award for Distinguished Contribution to the Science of Mental Health in 2006.

Angela G. Giovanniello, PharmD, AAHIVP

Angela Giovanniello received both her undergraduate and graduate pharmacy degrees from St John's University and completed her fellowship in HIV pharmacotherapy at the University at Buffalo. For over a decade, she has been an integral part of providing HIV care and resident education at a number of community health centers associated with Montefiore Medical Group and Albert Einstein College of Medicine. In addition to currently being the clinical coordinator of the office-based Buprenorphine Program that is continually expanding, she is pursuing a degree in acupuncture to provide alternative treatment options for pain management. She has written, edited, and reviewed a number of publications during her career including for the New York State Department of Health, peer reviewed journals, and patient education publications.

List of contributors

J. H. Atkinson, MD
Professor, Psychiatry Service, VA San Diego
Healthcare System, San Diego, CA 92161, USA
Professor, Department of Psychiatry, University of
California, San Diego, CA 92093, USA
Professor, HIV Neurobehavioral Research Program,
University of California, San Diego, CA 92093, USA

Antje M. Barreveld, MD
Assistant Professor of Anesthesiology, Tufts University
School of Medicine, Newton-Wellesley Hospital,
Newton, MA 02462, USA

William C. Becker, MD
Assistant Professor, Department of Internal Medicine,
Yale University School of Medicine, New Haven,
CT 06510, USA

R. Douglas Bruce, MD, MA, MS
Chief of Medicine, Cornell Scott-Hill Health Center,
Department of Medicine, Yale University, New Haven,
CT 06520, USA

Nu C. Chai, MD
Chief Resident, Department of Neurology, Johns
Hopkins University, Baltimore, MD 21218, USA

C. Brendan Clark, PhD
Assistant Professor, Department of Psychiatry,
University of Alabama at Birmingham, Birmingham,
AL 35233, USA

Michael R. Clark, MD, MPH, MBA
Professor, Department of Psychiatry and Behavioral
Sciences, Johns Hopkins University, Baltimore, MD
21218, USA

Catherine Deamant, MD
Division of General Internal Medicine and Primary
Care, Cook County Health and Hospitals System,
Chicago, IL 60612, USA

E. Jennifer Edelman, MD, MHS
Assistant Professor, Department of Internal Medicine,
Yale University School of Medicine, New Haven,
CT 06510, USA

Olga Fermo, MD
Resident, Department of Neurology, Johns Hopkins
University, Baltimore, MD 21218, USA

Kathleen Foley, MD
Professor, Department of Neurology, Memorial Sloan
Kettering Cancer Center, New York, NY, USA

Angela G. Giovanniello, PharmD, AAHIVP
Department of Family and Social Medicine, Albert
Einstein College of Medicine, Bronx, NY 10461, USA

Burel R. Goodin, PhD
Assistant Professor, Department of Psychology,
University of Alabama at Birmingham, Birmingham,
AL 35233, USA
Assistant Professor, Department of Anesthesiology
and Perioperative Medicine, University of Alabama at
Birmingham, Birmingham, AL 35233, USA

Liz Gwyther, MD
Lecturer in Palliative Care, School of Public Health
and Family Medicine, University of Cape Town, Chair,
World Hospice and Palliative Care Alliance, Anzio
Road, Observatory, Cape Town 7925, South Africa

Richard Harding, PhD
Reader in Palliative Care, Department of Palliative
Care, Policy, & Rehabilitation, Cicely Saunders
Institute, King's College London, London, United
Kingdom

Christopher A. Hess, MD
Clinical Instructor, Harvard Medical School, Pain
Medicine Fellow, Brigham and Women's Hospital,
Boston, MA 02115, USA

Irene J. Higginson, MD, PhD
Professor of Palliative Care and Policy, Department of
Palliative Care, Policy, & Rehabilitation, Cicely
Saunders Institute, King's College London, London,
United Kingdom

John R. Keltner, MD, PhD
Assistant Professor, Psychiatry Service, VA San Diego
Healthcare System, 3350 La Jolla Village Drive,
San Diego, CA 92161, USA

Assistant Professor, Department of Psychiatry, University of California, San Diego, CA, USA
Assistant Professor, HIV Neurobehavioral Research Program, University of California, 9500 Gilman Drive, La Jolla, San Diego, CA 92093, USA

David J. Kim, MD
University of Alabama at Birmingham, Birmingham, AL 35233, USA

Paula J. Lum, MD, MPH
Professor, Department of Medicine, University of California, San Francisco, San Francisco, CA 94143, USA

Justin C. McArthur, MBBS, MPH, FAAN, FANA
Professor of Neurology, Pathology, Medicine, and Epidemiology, Director, Department of Neurology, Johns Hopkins University School of Medicine, Baltimore, MD 21205, USA

Jennifer McNeely, MD, MS
Assistant Professor, Department of Population Health, Division of General Internal Medicine, New York University School of Medicine, New York, NY 10016, USA
Assistant Professor, Department of Medicine, Division of General Internal Medicine, New York University School of Medicine, New York, NY 10016, USA

Jessica S. Merlin, MD, MBA
Assistant Professor, Department of Medicine, Division of Infectious Diseases, Division of Gerontology, Geriatrics, and Palliative Care, University of Alabama at Birmingham, Birmingham, AL 35233, USA

Susan Nathan, MD
Assistant Professor, Department of Internal Medicine, Division of Geriatrics, Section of Palliative Medicine, Rush University Medical Center, Chicago, IL 60612, USA

Michael A. Owens, BS
Doctoral Student, Department of Psychology, University of Alabama at Birmingham, Birmingham, AL 35233, USA

Meera Pahuja, MD, MSc
Assistant Professor, Department of Internal Medicine, Division of Hematology, Oncology, and Palliative Care, Virginia Commonwealth University, Richmond, VA 23284, USA

Shetal Patel, PhD
VA San Diego Healthcare System, San Diego, CA 92161, USA

Christine Ritchie, MD, MSPH
Professor, Division of Geriatrics, Department of Medicine, University of California, San Francisco, San Francisco, CA 94143, USA

Jessica Robinson-Papp, MD
Assistant Professor, Department of Neurology, Icahn School of Medicine at Mount Sinai, New York, NY 10029, USA

Jason D. Rosenberg, MD
Assistant Professor, Department of Neurology, Johns Hopkins University, Baltimore, MD 21218, USA

Durga Roy, MD, MS
Assistant Professor, Department of Psychiatry and Behavioral Sciences, Johns Hopkins University, Baltimore, MD 21218, USA

Peter Selwyn, MD, MPH
Professor, Department of Family and Social Medicine, Albert Einstein College of Medicine, Bronx, NY 10461, USA

Joanna L. Starrels, MD, MS
Associate Professor, Department of Medicine, Albert Einstein College of Medicine, Bronx, NY 10461, USA

Glenn Treisman, MD, PhD
Professor, Department of Psychiatry and Behavioral Sciences, Department of Internal Medicine, Johns Hopkins University School of Medicine, Baltimore, MD 21205, USA

Alen Voskanian, MD, MBA
Assistant Clinical Professor of Medicine, David Geffen School of Medicine, University of California, Los Angeles, CA, USA
Regional Medical Director, VITAS Healthcare, Los Angeles, CA, USA

CHAPTER 1

Epidemiology of chronic pain in HIV-infected individuals

Meera Pahuja

Department of Internal Medicine, Division of Hematology, Oncology, and Palliative Care, Virginia Commonwealth University, Richmond, VA, USA

Introduction

Chronic pain is increasingly recognized as an important comorbidity of HIV-infected patients. In the current treatment era, HIV-infected patients who adhere to highly active antiretroviral therapy (HAART) and are engaged and retained in HIV primary care can achieve near-normal life expectancy [1]. Although patients with HIV can lead long lives, they often suffer from high rates of medical and psychiatric comorbidities. Due to a myriad of factors, chronic pain has also emerged as an important chronic condition in HIV-infected patients. This chapter focuses on the prevalence, etiology, and impact of comorbid chronic pain in HIV-infected individuals.

A changing HIV epidemic

Early in the epidemic, HIV infection inevitably progressed to AIDS, often shortly after diagnosis. Pain and other physical symptoms were largely related to sequelae or opportunistic infections, uncontrolled HIV replication [2], and early antiretroviral therapies such as the "d-drugs," which cause peripheral neuropathy [3]. Although there is no data on the prevalence of chronic pain in this early era, given the relatively rapid progression of disease, much of the pain experienced was acute. Like other forms of acute pain, it was managed by treating the underlying cause when possible, and symptomatically using opioids [4].

In 1996, the discovery of effective, well-tolerated antiretroviral therapy changed HIV infection from an inevitably fatal disease to a complex, chronic infection. The key steps in maintaining HIV as a chronic infection involve timely HIV diagnosis, linkage to care, adherence to treatment, and ultimately viral suppression. These steps are otherwise known as the "HIV treatment cascade" and navigation through the cascade is key to successful treatment [5]. As HIV becomes a chronic infection, studies have found that life expectancy of infected patients has increased. A study of US national HIV surveillance data from 25 states including 220,646 people from 1996 to 2005 found that life expectancy at diagnosis had increased from 10.5 to 22.5 years [6]. This increase in life expectancy has contributed to a surge in the number of people living with HIV and to shift the age distribution of the epidemic. By 2015, half of the HIV-infected population in the United States will be older than 50 [7]. The interaction of HIV disease with the aging process can cause accentuated aging and earlier development of comorbid conditions frequently seen in older adults [7].

With decreasing mortality, increased life expectancy, and consequent increasing comorbid illnesses, pain syndromes have emerged as a chronic condition with HIV infection. Chronic pain is defined as pain lasting longer than 3–6 months, beyond the period of normal

Chronic Pain and HIV: A Practical Approach, First Edition.
Edited by Jessica S. Merlin, Peter A. Selwyn, Glenn J. Treisman and Angela G. Giovanniello.
© 2016 John Wiley & Sons, Ltd. Published 2016 by John Wiley & Sons, Ltd.

healing [8]. Chronic pain is a major health problem in the United States, affecting about 100 million adults [9]. Pain is the most common symptom for which patients seek care [10], and costs the nation up to $635 billion each year in medical treatment and lost productivity [9]. A recent cross-sectional Internet-based survey in the United States found that about a third of adults experienced chronic pain, most commonly lower back pain and osteoarthritis pain [11].

Chronic pain in the HAART era

Though there are no studies designed to directly compare the prevalence of chronic pain in HIV-infected patients versus the general population, the range of chronic pain observed in HIV-infected patients tends to be higher than that in the general population. Studies from the HIV treatment era document high levels of pain in HIV-infected patients with prevalence estimates of anywhere from 39% to as high as 85% [12–20]. Studies also show that patients' pain is often underdiagnosed and inadequately treated. A study of 34 HIV treatment facilities found that 30% of outpatients and 62% of inpatients reported pain due to HIV disease and the pain severity significantly decreased patients' quality of life. They also found that doctors underestimated pain severity in 52% of patients. Of the patients reported moderate-to-severe pain, 57% did not receive any treatment and 22% received weak opioids. Doctors were more likely to give an opiate prescription if they estimated the pain to be severe or if they thought the patients were sicker [2].

Compounding this underdiagnoses suboptimal treatment of chronic pain are the racial disparities associated with the domestic HIV epidemic. HIV infection disproportionately affects vulnerable populations such as racial/ethnic minorities, women, and people of low socioeconomic status [21]. In 2009, the rate of new HIV infections was eight times higher for blacks and three times higher for Hispanics than whites. In addition to this, HIV/AIDS mortality was nine times higher for blacks than whites. Also, in 2009, 280,000 women were estimated to be living with HIV in the United States, with 15 times higher rates of new infections in black women and three times higher rates in Hispanic women [22]. Studies suggest that these vulnerable groups have higher rates of pain and more likely to be undertreated for their pain [23–26]. A recent telephone survey found that race, ethnicity, and socioeconomic factors influenced access to care for chronic pain [27]. Studies have also suggested in other chronic disease states that opioids were less likely to be prescribed for Black and Hispanic patients than White patients [28,29]. A recent study looking at the indigent HIV-infected population found chronic pain prevalence as high as 90% and 92% of these patients were found to have moderate-to-severe pain [20].

Pain is seen with increasing frequency in HIV-infected patients who have comorbid substance use and psychological disorders [30]. A recent study of 156 ambulatory HIV-infected patients in the United States found that 48.7% reported pain, of whom 51.3% had moderate-to-severe pain intensity and 57.3% of participants felt that their pain caused moderate-to-severe interference with their lives. This study further found that patients with psychiatric illness were 40% more likely to have pain and patients with a history of IV drug use who had pain were more likely to have severe or moderate pain than patients without a history of IV drug use. The authors suggested that comorbid IV drug use and psychiatric illness need to be addressed when treating pain and symptoms [12]. In fact, studies suggest that psychiatric illness can be more difficult to treat without concurrent pain treatment [31].

Etiology of chronic pain in HIV

The etiology of chronic pain in the current treatment era is multifactorial and likely related to direct effects of HIV or HAART, opportunistic infections, increasing number of chronic comorbid conditions, the aging HIV-infected population, and other conditions unrelated to HIV [32]. HIV infection and HAART can cause pain by direct toxicity to the nervous system. Neuropathic pain is an important component of

HIV-infected patients' pain in the pre-HAART and current treatment era. Distal sensory polyneuropathy, the most common cause of neuropathic pain in HIV-infected patients, can be related to exposure to older ART regimens including stavudine, didonosine, and zalcitabine, or current protease inhibitor therapy and simple HIV infection [33] and prevalence estimates in the current treatment era range from 4.3% to 21.8% [34–36]. Headaches are also a common symptom of HIV-infected patients and in a recent cross-sectional study of 200 HIV-infected patients in an outpatient setting, 53.5% of patients reported headache symptoms, of which 85% met criteria for migraine and 14.5% met criteria for tension headaches. Severity of HIV was associated with headache severity, frequency, and disability [37]. In addition, as in the general population, low back pain is a common complaint in HIV-infected patients. In a recent study of 124 patients followed at an ambulatory palliative care clinic in the United States found that pain was the most common reason for referral and 21% of patients complained of low back pain [38] (see Chapter 4, Musculoskeletal pain in individuals with HIV and Chapter 2, Pathophysiology of chronic pain in individuals with HIV).

Medical comorbidities such as cardiovascular disease [39], metabolic bone disease [40], diabetes [40], non-AIDS defining malignancies [41], and frailty [7] occur with increasing prevalence in HIV-infected populations. There are many theories as to why these non-AIDS events are occurring in greater numbers and at an earlier age than a noninfected population. First, among the HIV-infected community, traditional modifiable risk factors such as smoking, alcohol abuse, and substance use are more prevalent than in the noninfected population [42]. Direct toxic effects of ART or metabolic changes related to exposure to ART have also been shown to increase the risk for non-AIDS events. Finally, there is a rapidly growing body of evidence that HIV infection itself is a proinflammatory state and can contribute to the early development of many of these non-AIDS events [43] (see Chapter 7, Common medical comorbid conditions and chronic pain in HIV).

It is likely that aging and high burden of medical comorbidities contribute to chronic pain in HIV-infected patients. A recent telephone survey of HIV-infected patients older than 50 years assessing quality of life and chronic illness burden found that pain-related syndromes were second only to hypertension and 45% of the participants noted chronic pain other than back pain and headache, 35% had arthritis, 33% had chronic back pain, and 17% had chronic headaches [44]. Lower health-related quality of life (HRQOL) [45] and faster decline of physical functioning [46] have been shown to be associated with older age in HIV-infected patients.

Impact of chronic pain on HIV health behavior

Given recent recognition of comorbid chronic pain in HIV-infected patients, several studies have investigated the relationship between chronic pain and HIV health behaviors such as adherence to HAART and retention in care. One study of 70 HIV-infected outpatients on methadone maintenance found that 57% of participants reported pain and that participants with pain were 87% less likely to be adherent to ART compared to those without pain [47].

Another important indicator of successful management of HIV infection along the treatment cascade is retention in care, and a recent study of 2811 patients in the United States found that patients with greater than one missed visit in the first year following diagnosis had a 71% increased mortality risk [48]. Another study in the United States of 1521 HIV-infected patients found that the presence of pain increased the odds of a no-show visit in participants without substance abuse and pain conversely reduced the odds of a no-show visit in participants with substance abuse. The authors suggest that the presence of pain negatively affected retention in care because patients may have felt too sick to come to their office or they prioritized pain relief over HIV management. They also suggest that patients with substance abuse maybe have been more likely to attend their appointments because of increasing pain management needs. The authors conclude that further research is necessary into evidence-based approaches to pain management in HIV-infected patients [13].

Chronic pain in HIV-infected patients can also impact physical function. Physical function is an important component of HRQOL and one of the most important clinical outcomes in chronic pain care (see Chapter 10, Pharmacologic and Nonpharmacologic Treatment of Chronic Pain). A recent study of 1903 HIV-infected outpatients found that 37% of patients had pain, 27% of patients had mood disorders, and 8% were substance abusers. Pain was independently associated with up to 10 times greater odds of impaired physical function [49]. The authors suggest that appropriate management of pain is paramount to HIV disease management given that impaired physical function has been linked to increased mortality in HIV-infected patients [50].

Pain is also associated with increased healthcare utilization in the general population. A recent study at a large US academic health center, evaluating healthcare utilization, compared HIV-infected patients with chronic pain on opiates versus similar patients not on opiates. They used emergency room visits and hospitalizations as a measure of utilization and found that there was trend to increased emergency room visits and hospitalization in patients on opiates [51].

Conclusion

Here one can start to see the framework of how chronic pain has emerged as a frequent and important chronic condition in HIV-infected patients in the current treatment era. Unique to our HIV patients suffering from chronic pain, pain can negatively impact adherence to lifesaving medications and decrease retention in care – both vital components of the HIV treatment cascade. Treating pain while taking into account comorbid psychiatric disease and substance abuse is of utmost importance to successfully caring for our HIV-infected community. The rest of the book will delve deeper into mechanisms of chronic pain, specific and common pain syndromes, comorbid conditions additive effect to chronic pain,

special populations of HIV-infected patients with concurrent substance abuse or psychiatric disorders, and finally pharmacologic and nonpharmacologic treatment of chronic pain. In addition, the book will touch on opioid risk mitigation strategies, approaches to "difficult" patients and further tools for educating providers about chronic pain.

References

1 Samji, H. *et al.* (2013) Closing the gap: increases in life expectancy among treated HIV-positive individuals in the United States and Canada. *PLoS One*, **8** (12), e81355.

2 Larue F., Fontaine A., Colleau S.M. (1997) Underestimation and undertreatment of pain in HIV disease: multicentre study. *British Medical Journal*, **314** (7073), 23–28.

3 Pahuja, M. *et al.* (2012) Effects of a reduced dose of stavudine on the incidence and severity of peripheral neuropathy in HIV-infected adults in South Africa. *Antiviral Therapy*, **17** (4), 737–743.

4 Hewitt, D.J. *et al.* (1997) Pain syndromes and etiologies in ambulatory AIDS patients. *Pain*, **70** (2–3), 117–123.

5 De Cock, K.M. (2014) Plus ca change … antiretroviral therapy, HIV prevention, and the HIV treatment cascade. *Clinical Infectious Diseases*, **58** (7), 1012–1014.

6 Harrison, K.M., Song, R. & Zhang, X. (2010) Life expectancy after HIV diagnosis based on national HIV surveillance data from 25 states, United States. *Journal of Acquired Immune Deficiency Syndromes*, **53** (1), 124–130.

7 Onen, N.F. & Overton, E.T. (2011) A review of premature frailty in HIV-infected persons; another manifestation of HIV-related accelerated aging. *Current Aging Science*, **4** (1), 33–41.

8 International Association for the Study of Pain, Subcommittee on Taxonomy (1986) Classification of chronic pain. Descriptions of chronic pain syndromes and definitions of pain terms. *Pain Supplement*, **3**, S1–226.

9 Institute of Medicine (2011) *Relieving Pain in America: A blueprint for Transforming Prevention, Care, Education and Research*. The National Academies Press, Washington, DC.

10 Cherry, D.K., Burt, C.W. & Woodwell, D.A. (2003) National ambulatory medical care

survey: 2001 summary. *Advance Data*, (337), 1–44.

11 Johannes, C.B. *et al.* (2010) The prevalence of chronic pain in United States adults: results of an Internet-based survey. *The Journal of Pain*, **11** (11), 1230–1239.

12 Merlin, J.S. *et al.* (2012) Pain and physical and psychological symptoms in ambulatory HIV patients in the current treatment era. *Journal of Pain and Symptom Management*, **43** (3), 638–645.

13 Merlin, J.S. *et al.* (2012) Pain, mood, and substance abuse in HIV: implications for clinic visit utilization, ART adherence, and virologic failure. *Journal of Acquired Immune Deficiency Syndromes*, **61** (2), 164–170.

14 Newshan, G., Bennett, J. & Holman, S. (2002) Pain and other symptoms in ambulatory HIV patients in the age of highly active antiretroviral therapy. *Journal of the Association of Nurses in AIDS Care*, **13** (4), 78–83.

15 Harding, R. *et al.* (2010) Symptoms are highly prevalent among HIV outpatients and associated with poor adherence and unprotected sexual intercourse. *Sexually Transmitted Infections*, **86** (7), 520–524.

16 Lee, K.A. *et al.* (2009) Symptom experience in HIV-infected adults: a function of demographic and clinical characteristics. *Journal of Pain and Symptom Management*, **38** (6), 882–893.

17 Silverberg, M.J. *et al.* (2009) Age and racial/ethnic differences in the prevalence of reported symptoms in human immunodeficiency virus-infected persons on antiretroviral therapy. *Journal of Pain and Symptom Management*, **38** (2), 197–207.

18 Silverberg, M.J. *et al.* (2004) Prevalence of clinical symptoms associated with highly active antiretroviral therapy in the women's interagency HIV study. *Clinical Infectious Diseases*, **39** (5), 717–724.

19 Cervia, L.D., McGowan, J.P. & Weseley, A.J. (2010) Clinical and demographic variables related to pain in HIV-infected individuals treated with effective, combination antiretroviral therapy (cART). *Pain Medicine*, **11** (4), 498–503.

20 Miaskowski, C. *et al.* (2011) Occurrence and characteristics of chronic pain in a community-based cohort of indigent adults living with HIV infection. *The Journal of Pain*, **12** (9), 1004–1016.

21 Karon, J.M. *et al.* (2001) HIV in the United States at the turn of the century: an epidemic in transition. *American Journal of Public Health*, **91** (7), 1060–1068.

22 Centers for Disease Control and Prevention (2011) *Vital Signs: HIV Prevention Through Care and Treatment – United States* MMWR: Morbidity and Mortality Weekly Report. CDC, Atlanta, pp. 1618–1623.

23 Sullivan, L.W. & Eagel, B.A. (2005) Leveling the playing field: recognizing and rectifying disparities in management of pain. *Pain Medicine*, **6** (1), 5–10.

24 Dobalian, A., Tsao, J.C. & Duncan, R.P. (2004) Pain and the use of outpatient services among persons with HIV: results from a nationally representative survey. *Medical Care*, **42** (2), 129–138.

25 Breitbart, W. *et al.* (1996) The undertreatment of pain in ambulatory AIDS patients. *Pain*, **65** (2–3), 243–249.

26 Breitbart, W. *et al.* (1996) Pain in ambulatory AIDS patients. I: Pain characteristics and medical correlates. *Pain*, **68** (2–3), 315–321.

27 Nguyen, M. *et al.* (2005) Access to care for chronic pain: racial and ethnic differences. *The Journal of Pain*, **6** (5), 301–314.

28 Chen, I. *et al.* (2005) Racial differences in opioid use for chronic nonmalignant pain. *Journal of General Internal Medicine*, **20** (7), 593–598.

29 Cleeland, C.S. *et al.* (1997) Pain and treatment of pain in minority patients with cancer. *The Eastern Cooperative Oncology Group Minority Outpatient Pain Study. Annals of Internal Medicine*, **127** (9), 813–816.

30 Tsao, J.C. & Soto, T. ((2009)) Pain in persons living with HIV and comorbid psychologic and substance use disorders. *Clinical Journal of Pain*, **25** (4), 307–312.

31 Bair, M.J. *et al.* (2003) Depression and pain comorbidity: a literature review. *Archives of Internal Medicine*, **163** (20), 2433–2445.

32 Frich, L.M. & Borgbjerg, F.M. (2000) Pain and pain treatment in AIDS patients: a longitudinal study. *Journal of Pain and Symptom Management*, **19** (5), 339–347.

33 Gonzalez-Duarte, A., Robinson-Papp, J. & Simpson, D.M. (2008) Diagnosis and management of HIV-associated neuropathy. *Neurologic Clinics*, **26** (3), 821–832, x.

34 Evans, S.R. *et al.* (2011) Peripheral neuropathy in HIV: prevalence and risk factors. *AIDS*, **25** (7), 919–928.

35 Lichtenstein, K.A. *et al.* (2005) Modification of the incidence of drug-associated symmetrical peripheral neuropathy by host and disease factors in the HIV outpatient study cohort. *Clinical Infectious Diseases*, **40** (1), 148–157.

36 Ellis, R.J. *et al.* (2010) Continued high prevalence and adverse clinical impact of human immunodeficiency virus-associated sensory neuropathy in the era of combination antiretroviral therapy: the CHARTER study. *Archives of Neurology*, **67** (5), 552–558.

37 Kirkland, K.E. *et al.* (2012) Headache among patients with HIV disease: prevalence, characteristics, and associations. *Headache*, **52** (3), 455–466.

38 Merlin, J.S., Childers, J. & Arnold, R.M. (2013) Chronic pain in the outpatient palliative care clinic. *The American Journal of Hospice & Palliative Care*, **30** (2), 197–203.

39 Hemkens, L.G. & Bucher, H.C. (2014) HIV infection and cardiovascular disease. *European Heart Journal*, **35** (21), 1373–1381.

40 Willig, A.L. & Overton, E.T. (2014) Metabolic consequences of HIV: pathogenic insights. *Current HIV/AIDS Reports*, **11** (1), 35–44.

41 Shiels, M.S. *et al.* (2009) A meta-analysis of the incidence of non-AIDS cancers in HIV-infected individuals. *Journal of Acquired Immune Deficiency Syndromes*, **52** (5), 611–622.

42 Petoumenos, K. *et al.* (2011) Rates of cardiovascular disease following smoking cessation in patients with HIV infection: results from the D:A:D study(*). *HIV Medicine*, **12** (7), 412–421.

43 Neuhaus, J. *et al.* (2010) Markers of inflammation, coagulation, and renal function are elevated in adults with HIV infection. *Journal of Infectious Diseases*, **201** (12), 1788–1795.

44 Balderson, B.H. *et al.* (2013) Chronic illness burden and quality of life in an aging HIV population. *AIDS Care*, **25** (4), 451–458.

45 Campsmith, M.L., Nakashima, A.K. & Davidson, A.J. (2003) Self-reported health-related quality of life in persons with HIV infection: results from a multi-site interview project. *Health and Quality of Life Outcomes*, **1**, 12.

46 Oursler, K.K. *et al.* (2011) Association of age and comorbidity with physical function in HIV-infected and uninfected patients: results from the Veterans Aging Cohort Study. *AIDS Patient Care and STDs*, **25** (1), 13–20.

47 Berg, K.M. *et al.* (2009) Self-efficacy and depression as mediators of the relationship between pain and antiretroviral adherence. *AIDS Care*, **21** (2), 244–248.

48 Horberg, M.A. *et al.* (2013) Missed office visits and risk of mortality among HIV-infected subjects in a large healthcare system in the United States. *AIDS Patient Care and STDs*, **27** (8), 442–449.

49 Merlin, J.S. *et al.* (2013) Pain is independently associated with impaired physical function in HIV-infected patients. *Pain Medicine*, **14** (12), 1985–1993.

50 Shen, J.M., Blank, A. & Selwyn, P.A. (2005) Predictors of mortality for patients with advanced disease in an HIV palliative care program. *Journal of Acquired Immune Deficiency Syndromes*, **40** (4), 445–447.

51 Koeppe, J., Lyda, K. & Armon, C. (2013) Association between opioid use and health care utilization as measured by emergency room visits and hospitalizations among persons living with HIV. *Clinical Journal of Pain*, **29** (11), 957–961.

CHAPTER 2

Pathophysiology of chronic pain in individuals with HIV

Michael A. Owens[1] and Burel R. Goodin[2]

[1] *Department of Psychology, University of Alabama at Birmingham, Birmingham, AL, USA*
[2] *Department of Psychology, Department of and Anesthesia and Perioperative Medicine, University of Alabama at Birmingham, Birmingham, AL, USA*

Introduction

Pain is a ubiquitous experience among humans as well as many animal species. It is commonly understood to be a normal sensation triggered in the nervous system as an alert to injury, or the possibility of injury, and the need for rest and recuperation. In this way, the experience of acute pain is adaptive and can be considered an expected consequence of illness, injury, and surgery, which typically resolves with healing.

However, the experience of chronic pain is an entirely different matter. There is pathophysiological activation of the peripheral and central nervous systems (CNSs). Pain signals keep firing in the nervous system for weeks, months, even years beyond the expected period of healing or resolution of the source of pain. Chronic pain does not appear to serve an instrumental role in protecting the sufferer or in otherwise promoting adaptation and adjustment. For those afflicted and their caregivers, chronic pain all too commonly exerts deleterious effects on sense of well-being and quality of life.

The experience of pain is widely conceptualized to represent "an unpleasant sensory and emotional experience associated with actual or potential tissue damage, or described in terms of such damage [1]." Pain is a highly subjective experience that can vary substantially from one individual to the next [2]. How individuals learn the application of the word "pain" can result from social, cultural, and gender-based experiences related to injury in early life [3]. These early life experiences have implications for how future painful information will be appraised and interpreted. Thus, the individual experience of pain is a physiological process, but it is important to bear in mind that it is heavily influenced by a complex interacting system of psychological and social factors.

A basic understanding of the anatomy and physiology underlying acute and chronic pain is essential to increase appreciation of what pain is, what is not, and how both pharmacologic and nonpharmacologic interventions can help to manage it. The purpose of this chapter is threefold and seeks to accomplish the following: (1) provide a general outline of the anatomy and physiology pertaining to the pain sensory system, (2) characterize the contributions of peripheral and central sensitization to the experience of chronic pain, and (3) address pathophysiological mechanisms that may contribute to development and maintenance of chronic pain conditions specifically in individuals infected with HIV.

The pain sensory system

According to the International Association for the Study of Pain (IASP), it is important to

Chronic Pain and HIV: A Practical Approach, First Edition.
Edited by Jessica S. Merlin, Peter A. Selwyn, Glenn J. Treisman and Angela G. Giovanniello.

distinguish between the concepts of nociception and pain [1]. The term "nociception" refers to afferent activity in the peripheral and CNSs produced in response to tissue damage caused by intense chemical (e.g., capsaicin), mechanical (e.g., pinching and crushing), or thermal (e.g., heat and cold) stimulation [4]. This nomenclature was first introduced in the early 1900s when Charles Scott Sherrington proposed the existence of primary sensory neurons that are activated by stimuli capable of causing tissue damage [5]. The term "pain," on the other hand, is the perceptual experience that typically accompanies nociception [6]. The process of nociception describes the normal processing of pain and the responses to noxious stimuli that are damaging or potentially damaging to normal tissue. Basic processes involved in nociception include (1) transduction, (2) transmission, (3) perception, and (4) modulation [7].

Generally, relay of the nociceptive signal and the ultimate percept of pain is a sequential process that, in its simplest form, involves a chain of three anatomically and functionally distinct subpopulations of neurons [8,9]. The first subpopulation of neurons in the chain, the primary afferent neurons, are responsible for the transduction (i.e., conversion) of noxious stimulation into nociceptive signals and the transmission of these signals from the peripheral tissues to second-order neurons in the dorsal horn of the spinal cord. The second-order neurons in the chain, the spinal neurons, receive input from the primary afferent neurons and project to third-order neurons in the brainstem and thalamus. These third-order supraspinal neurons integrate signals from the spinal neurons and project to the subcortical and cortical areas, where pain is finally perceived.

The component parts of the pain sensory system are further described in what follows. We begin by describing how the pain sensory system relates to the experience of acute pain in healthy individuals under normal conditions. We have included this information because one must understand the *normal* pain state of acute pain in order to understand the *abnormal* pain state of chronic pain. We then describe the pathophysiology of chronic pain.

Pathophysiology of the normal acute pain response

Primary afferent neurons

Nociception is initiated by the transduction of a noxious stimulus into an electrical signal. The mechanism responsible for transduction is the nociceptor [10]. Nociceptors are the free nerve endings of neurons that have their cell bodies outside the spinal column in the dorsal root ganglion (DRG). The DRG is a special type of afferent spinal nerve that is located in the peripheral nervous system and transmits nociceptive signals from the nociceptors to the spinal cord [11]. A bifurcated axon emanates from each cell body within the DRG. At its central end, this axon forms a synapse within the spinal cord. At the peripheral end, this axon produces the nociceptor sensory endings that are distributed in cutaneous structures (skin), somatic structures (joints and bones), and visceral structures (body organs). Following a noxious stimulus, if sufficient numbers of nociceptors are activated, the energy at the site of noxious stimulation will be transduced into a nociceptive signal [12].

The primary afferent neurons are classified according to their diameter, degree of myelination, and conduction velocity. There are two classes of primary afferent nociceptors including the small diameter, myelinated A-delta (Aδ) and the unmyelinated C polymodal fibers [8]. Most Aδ and C polymodal fibers respond maximally to only noxious stimuli and represent the first-order neurons of nociceptive transmission. In general, the more rapidly conducting Aδ fibers are responsible for triggering a fast and sharp pain response that is often referred to as "first pain." The more slowly conducting C polymodal fibers are responsible for producing a delayed and aching pain response commonly referred to as "second pain [10]." For example, one may initially experience a feeling of "sharp" pain when hitting their thumb with a hammer, proceeded by a prolonged "aching." The first pain is thought to be mediated by the faster Aδ fibers, whereas the second pain is the result of the slower C polymodal fibers.

In addition to the small diameter Aδ and C polymodal nociceptors, there is also a class of large diameter primary afferent fibers called A-beta (Aβ). These Aβ fibers respond maximally to light touch and/or moving stimuli, and they are primarily present in nerves that innervate the skin [13]. In healthy individuals, the activity of these fibers does not produce pain; therefore, Aβ fibers are not classified as nociceptors. It is important to mention the Aβ class of primary afferents because many of these fibers have collateral branches that terminate within the spinal cord dorsal horn. Through an inhibitory mechanism, these collateral branches can block the activity of the Aδ and C polymodal nociceptors and thereby prevent nociceptive signals from ascending the spinal cord [14]. This mechanism has been termed the gate-control theory of pain modulation and appears to play a significant role in control of the pain sensory system [15].

Primary afferent nociceptors are not simply passive messengers of nociceptive signals but also play an active role in modifying the nociceptive signal via release of polypeptide mediators. Noxious stimuli have been found to initiate the release of pain-promoting (algesiogenic) polypeptides from primary afferent nociceptors including substance P, neurokinin A, glutamate, calcitonin gene-related peptide, prostaglandins, and bradykinin among others [4,8,12]. To illustrate, several lines of evidence have shown that the polypeptide known as substance P is released in response to noxious stimulation and promotes the transmission of nociceptive signals from primary afferent nociceptors to the dorsal horn of the spinal cord [16]. Substance P is also a potent vasodilator, degranulates mast cells, is a chemoattractant for leukocytes, and increases the production and release of inflammatory cytokines. Interestingly, depletion or antagonism of substance P has been shown to decrease the severity of pain generated from a noxious stimulus [17].

Spinal neurons

The first-order primary afferent Aδ and C polymodal fibers, and ultimately the nociceptive signal, enter the spinal cord and terminate in the dorsal horn, where they synapse with the second-order spinal neurons. There are two main types of nociceptive spinal neurons

in the dorsal horn (projection neurons and interneurons), and these neurons are organized into layers or laminae. The dorsal horn of the spinal cord gray matter has been divided into six roughly horizontal bands; the most dorsal is designated as lamina I [18]. Spinal neurons that mediate nociception are located within lamina I (marginal layer), lamina II (substantia gelatinosa), and lamina V. The spinal neurons that are located primarily in laminae I and II receive input directly from primary afferent Aδ and C fibers and are called nociceptive-specific (NS) neurons [19]. Spinal neurons located chiefly in lamina V receive both nociceptive and nonnociceptive inputs and are classified as wide dynamic range (WDR) neurons [19]. The WDR neurons are sometimes referred to as convergent neurons. The interneurons located within the dorsal horn play a key role in gating and modulating nociceptive signals [20].

The second-order spinal neurons (i.e., NS and WDR cells) have axonal projections that immediately cross the spinal cord at the midline and ascend contralaterally to supraspinal areas in the midbrain, where they synapse with third-order supraspinal neurons. Electrical and chemical signals are relayed from the second-order spinal neurons to the third-order supraspinal neurons through one of three major ascending nociceptive pathways. These three pathways are the spinothalamic tract, the spinoreticular tract, and the spinomesencephalic tract [9,21]. The spinothalamic tract is the major pathway for projecting nociceptive signals from the spinal cord to appropriate supraspinal destinations. The spinothalamic tract consists of medial and lateral components that each project to the third-order supraspinal neurons located within the thalamus. The medial component of this tract projects to the medial nuclei of the thalamus. From there, third-order supraspinal neurons transmit nociceptive input to the limbic system (e.g., the anterior cingulate cortex). Alternatively, the lateral component of the spinothalamic tract projects to the lateral thalamic nuclei and from there, to the somatosensory cortex. The spinoreticular tract projects to the reticular formation in the brainstem (e.g., the medulla and pons). Similarly, this tract then travels to thalamic nuclei and then to the somatosensory cortex. The reticular formation is a part of the brainstem, which is involved in stereotypical actions, such as walking, sleeping, and lying down. Projections within the spinoreticular tract terminate in close apposition to regions that are involved in blood pressure and motor control and the descending inhibition of pain. Thus, it appears that this pathway is involved in the basic autonomic, motor, and endogenous analgesic responses to nociceptive input. The spinomesencephalic tract also projects to the reticular formation, in addition to the periaqueductal gray (PAG) matter in the midbrain. The PAG plays an important role in the integration and modulation of nociceptive input at the supraspinal level. The sites of termination for the spinomesencephalic tract suggest that some of its components are involved in more organized and integrated motor, autonomic, and antinociceptive responses to noxious input, such as orienting, quiescence, defense, and confrontation.

Supraspinal neurons

The brain does not have a discrete pain center, so when nociceptive signals arrive at the thalamus and other brainstem structures, the signals are directed to multiple areas of the brain by third-order supraspinal neurons, where they are ultimately processed [22]. Perception of pain is the end result of the neuronal activity involved in nociceptive transmission and where pain becomes a conscious multidimensional experience. The experience of pain has sensory-discriminative, affective-motivational, as well as emotional and behavioral components [23]. Brain imaging studies, incorporating both positron emission tomography (PET) and functional magnetic resonance imaging (fMRI), have confirmed that multiple cortical areas are engaged in the processing of nociceptive signals that ultimately result in the perception of pain [24]. In particular, evidence suggests that three cortical areas are critical in the perception of pain: (1) the reticular system, (2) the somatosensory cortex, and (3) the limbic system [25]. The reticular system is responsible for the autonomic and motor response to pain as well as for motivating the individual to react, for example, automatically removing a hand

when it touches a hot stove. It also plays a role in the affective-motivational response to pain such as looking at and assessing the injury to the hand once it has been removed from the hot stove. The somatosensory cortex is involved with the perception and interpretation of nociceptive signals. It identifies the intensity, type, and location of the nociceptive signal and relates it to memories of past painful experiences. It identifies the nature of the painful stimulus before it elicits an emotional response, which includes where the pain is located, the intensity of the pain, and what the pain feels like. Lastly, the limbic system is responsible for the emotional and behavioral responses to pain. Important structures such as the anterior cingulate cortex, hippocampus, and amygdala are involved in the attentional and emotional components of pain processing.

Modulation

The nociceptive signal is subject to modulation not only during its ascending transmission from the primary afferent nociceptors to supraspinal structures but also during descending transmission from these supraspinal structures back down to the spinal cord [26]. The descending modulation of incoming nociceptive stimuli is manifested via pathways that originate at the level of the cerebral cortex, the thalamus, and the brainstem (i.e., pons and medulla). The multiple, complex pathways involved in the modulation of nociceptive signals are referred to as the descending modulatory pain pathways. It is important to note that these descending modulatory pain pathways can lead to either an increase in the transmission of nociceptive signals (excitation) or a decrease in transmission (inhibition) [27]. Activation of the descending modulatory pain pathways often involves the supraspinal release of inhibitory neurotransmitters that include endogenous opioid agonists such as endorphins and enkephalins. In addition to other inhibitory neurotransmitters, such as serotonin and norepinephrine, endogenous opioids suppress (at least partially) the transmission of nociceptive signals and thereby decrease the perceived severity of pain. Descending modulatory pain pathways help to explain the wide variation in the perception of pain across different people as individuals produce different amounts of inhibitory neurotransmitters.

Pathophysiology of chronic pain

Chronic pain conditions are defined as nociceptive when they are generated by noxious stimuli, inflammatory when produced by tissue injury and/or immune cell activation, or neuropathic when due to a lesion of the nervous system. It is important to attempt to identify which of these discrete categories best describes a given patient's pain. This is because treatments are often tailored to the type (i.e., category) of chronic pain and the unique pathophysiologic mechanisms that generate it. However, it is important to acknowledge that much of the time a patient's chronic pain cannot be neatly placed into one of these categories. Sometimes, more than one category is involved; other times, it may be difficult to determine whether a patient's chronic pain fits into any of the above categories. This lack of clarity regarding the type of chronic pain being experienced by the patient can result in others questioning the validity of the pain and ultimately lead to the patient feeling invalidated.

Current understanding of the mechanisms that drive chronic pain – pain that persists beyond the period of normal tissue healing, or even pain that exists in the absence of local injury – has grown considerably. It is generally understood that development of chronic pain depends in part on sensitization of the pain sensory system [28]. Peripheral sensitization can occur at the level of the primary afferent nociceptors, whereas central sensitization can occur at the level of the dorsal horn of the spinal cord.

Peripheral sensitization

Peripheral sensitization can occur when inflammatory mediators (e.g., bradykinin, prostaglandins, leukotrienes, and nerve growth factor) are released from damaged or inflamed tissue and stimulate primary afferent nociceptors directly [8]. When intense, repeated, or prolonged stimuli are applied to these damaged or inflamed tissues, the threshold for activating

primary afferent nociceptors is lowered, and the frequency of firing is higher for all stimulus intensities [29]. This neuronal plasticity is manifest as peripheral sensitization, and the result is increased pain sensitivity [30]. The process of eliciting peripheral sensitization takes place via receptor-mediated second messenger action. Cyclic AMP, protein kinase A, and protein kinase C are important second messengers involved in peripheral sensitization of primary afferent nociceptors given their role in prompting an increase in the production, transport, and membrane insertion of chemically gated and voltage-gated ion channels [8]. These ion channels include members of multiple gene families, which are responses to various stimuli. Voltage-gated sodium and calcium channels, transient receptor potential (TRP) channels, acid-sensing ion channels (ASIC), ligand-gated ion channels, P2X, NMDA, AMPA, and Kainate receptors all make significant contributions to the pathogenesis of pain and ultimately, peripheral sensitization [31]. A striking example of peripheral sensitization is sunburned skin, in which severe pain can be produced by a light slap on the back (i.e., hyperalgesia) or a warm shower (i.e., allodynia). Hyperalgesia refers to an enhanced perception of pain in response to a noxious stimulus, whereas allodynia refers to the novel perception of a normally innocuous stimulus as being painful [32].

Central sensitization

It has been suggested that peripheral sensitization acts to increase the total nociceptive afferent barrage (i.e., the number and intensity of nociceptive signals) to the spinal cord, which is likely instrumental to the development of central sensitization [33]. Current evidence indicates that increased primary afferent discharges into the spinal cord initiate a state of central sensitization, but neuroplastic changes within the CNS maintain the long-term sensitized status of the spinal dorsal horn [34]. The net effect is that previously subthreshold synaptic inputs come together to generate an increased or augmented action potential output, a state of nociceptive facilitation, potentiation, or amplification. An important implication of this central sensitization phenomenon is the possibility that the experience of chronic pain might not necessarily reflect the presence of an ongoing peripheral noxious stimulus. People learn from everyday experiences interacting with their external environment to interpret pain as the result of a peripheral damaging stimulus, and indeed this is critical to its protective function in the acute context. However, central sensitization introduces another dimension to the understanding of chronic pain, one where the CNS can change, distort, or amplify pain, increasing its degree, duration, and spatial extent in a manner that no longer directly reflects the specific qualities of peripheral noxious stimuli, but rather the particular functional states of circuits in the CNS. The end result is that the phenomenon of central sensitization may act to maintain chronic pain in the absence of any peripheral noxious stimulus, or long after the peripherally damaging noxious stimulus that initially elicited the pain has subsided [28,33,34].

What has become clear is that there is no single defining molecular mechanism of central sensitization. Indeed, central sensitization is a general phenomenon that produces distinct changes in somatosensory processing by eliciting different cascades of molecular activity. In response to primary afferent nociceptor input, these molecular cascades can (1) increase membrane excitability, (2) facilitate synaptic strength, or (3) decrease inhibitory influences in dorsal horn neurons. The first major mechanistic insight was that the induction and maintenance of acute central sensitization was dependent on *N*-methyl-ᴅ-aspartate (NMDA) receptors, revealing a key involvement of glutamate and its receptors [35]. After decades of scientific study across numerous laboratories around the world, it is now generally appreciated that central sensitization comprises two temporal phases, each with specific mechanisms. The early phosphorylation-dependent and transcription-independent phase results mainly from rapid changes in glutamate receptor and ion channel properties. The later, longer-lasting, transcription-dependent phase drives synthesis of the new proteins responsible for the longer-lasting form of central sensitization observed in multiple chronic pain conditions including fibromyalgia, complex

regional pain syndrome, headache, low back pain, and osteoarthritis among others.

Before central sensitization was identified, there were two major models describing the pain sensory system. The first model posited that pain processing was "straight through" system, in which specific pain pathways were activated only by particular peripheral noxious stimuli and that the amplitude and duration of pain was determined solely by the intensity and timing of these noxious inputs [36]. The second model described "gate controls" in the CNS, which could augment or diminish the percept of pain when open or closed, respectively [20,23]. However, neither model accounted for the possibility that pain could arise as a result of changes in the properties of neurons in the CNS, such as those changes described by the phenomenon of central sensitization. It is now widely accepted that there are indeed specific nociceptive pathways and that they are subject to complex modulatory controls that can facilitate and inhibit nociceptive signals, and ultimately the percept of pain. Further, it is also appreciated that changes in the functional properties of the neurons in these nociceptive pathways are sufficient to reduce pain threshold, increase the magnitude and duration of responses to noxious input, and permit normally innocuous inputs to generate pain sensations. Pain is not then simply a reflection of peripheral inputs or pathology but is also a dynamic reflection of central neuronal plasticity. This plasticity profoundly alters pain sensitivity (i.e., more pain sensitivity), thereby making it a major contributor to many chronic pain conditions and representing an important target for therapeutic intervention.

Pathophysiology of chronic pain in patients with HIV

Although HIV-infected individuals appear to be at substantial risk for experiencing chronic pain, the pathophysiological mechanisms underlying chronic pain development and maintenance within this population remain unclear. At present, the majority of what is known regarding the pathophysiological mechanisms of chronic pain development in HIV-infected individuals has come from previous studies examining the classically described syndrome of HIV neuropathy [37]. For a detailed description of the pathophysiology of HIV neuropathy, see Chapter 6. It is important to note, however, that HIV-infected individuals in the current treatment era often experience other chronic pain conditions not related to neuropathy, such as nonspecific chronic low back pain and other regional musculoskeletal pain syndromes [38]. It may be that there is an overlap between neuropathic and nonneuropathic pain conditions in terms of their pathophysiological mechanistic underpinnings; however, this is not clear at this time. In addition, it stands to reason that the pathophysiologic mechanisms described earlier in this chapter apply both to the neuropathic and nonneuropathic pain conditions seen in individuals with HIV; however, this possibility has not yet been specifically investigated. On balance, the unique aspects of chronic pain pathophysiology in individuals with HIV are not yet known.

One additional approach to understanding chronic pain pathophysiology in the general population may be particularly applicable to individuals with HIV: the biopsychosocial model. Pathophysiological changes at the cellular level initiate, maintain, and modulate the experience of chronic pain among HIV-infected individuals. However, the biopsychosocial model maintains that the experience of chronic pain is determined by the interaction among biological (i.e., pathophysiological), psychological, and social factors [3]. In the emerging field of pain psychology, often studied psychological factors include cognition, affect, and behavior, while corresponding social factors include the cultural contexts that influence a person's perception of, and response to, physical signs and symptoms of pain. Compared to previous theories and models conceptualizing chronic pain development, the biopsychosocial model posits a much broader, multidimensional, and complex perspective.

Although advances have been made in specifying the theoretical relationships among biological, psychological, and social process, the actual evidence base addressing which constructs (and their respective interactions) within the biopsychosocial model are most effective for explaining chronic pain outcomes

in HIV-infected individuals remains underdeveloped. One group of authors has postulated that psychological and social factors common in individuals with HIV, such as psychological distress from comorbid mental illness, traumatic life events, stigma, and social isolation, may be particularly relevant [39]. However, the role of these factors has not yet been formally tested. At present, the full potential of the biopsychosocial model for advancing our understanding of chronic pain outcomes remains untapped.

Implications for pain treatment

As evidenced by the above, the mechanisms that underlie chronic pain are complex and varied. They include both peripheral and central processes and have both biological and psychosocial components. Traditionally, chronic pain has been treated within the biomedical model. In the biomedical model, the focus has been on pain as a purely biological process that can be addressed with pharmacologic treatments alone. Not surprisingly, this approach has been met with limited success. Given the information presented in this chapter, it stands to reason that for most individuals with chronic pain, a comprehensive approach that addresses multiple mechanisms is needed [40]. For example, in a patient with knee osteoarthritis, a combination of nonsteroidals to address ongoing peripheral inflammation and cognitive behavioral therapy to address emotional distress and help with coping may be the best approach. In Chapter 10, we will provide a comprehensive overview of both the pharmacologic and nonpharmacologic (including behavioral) treatments for chronic pain.

Conclusion

The processing of nociceptive signals and ultimate perception of pain is a complex process. This process involves excitation of primary afferent nociceptors in the periphery, local interactions within the spinal dorsal horn, and the activation of ascending and descending pathways that comprise a loop from the spinal cord to supraspinal structures, which can both facilitate and inhibit nociceptive inputs at the spinal level. Although the pain pathways described in this chapter appear to be part of normal pain processing, the system demonstrates a remarkable ability to undergo neuroplastic transformations when nociceptive inputs are extended over time. These transformations of the peripheral and CNS pave the way for sensitization of the pain sensory system, which now appears to be an important component of chronic pain development. The extent to which this cascade of pathophysiological processes helps to explain the experience of chronic pain for HIV-infected individuals remains unclear. New translational studies are currently needed to take what has already been learned from animal models addressing HIV and chronic pain development and apply it to humans. Mechanistic studies aimed at better understanding the ascending and descending pain facilitatory pathways as well as related neuroplastic changes may provide for the design of rational therapies that do not interfere with normal sensory processing. Treatments designed to diminish nociceptive inputs from the periphery may effectively disrupt the maintenance of the sensitized pain state and ultimately thwart the development of chronic pain for HIV-infected individuals.

References

1 Merskey, H. & Bogduk, N. (1994) Classification of chronic pain. In: Merskey, H. & Bogduk, N. (eds), *Part III: Pain Terms, A Current List with Definitions and Notes on Usage. IASP Task Force on Taxonomy*. IASP Press, Seattle, pp. 209–214.

2 Koyama, T., McHaffie, J.G., Laurienti, P.J. & Coghill, R.C. (2005) The subjective experience of pain: where expectations become reality. *Proceedings of the National Academy of Sciences of the United States of America*, **102** (36), 12950–12955.

3 Gatchel, R.J., Peng, Y.B., Peters, M.L., Fuchs, P.N. & Turk, D.C. (2007) The biopsychosocial approach to chronic pain: scientific advances and future directions. *Psychological Bulletin*, **133** (4), 581–624.

4 Julius, D. & Basbaum, A.I. (2001) Molecular mechanisms of nociception. *Nature*, **413** (6852), 203–210.

5 Sherrington, C.S. (1906) *The Integrative Action of the Nervous System*. Scribner, New York.

6 Coghill, R.C. (2010) Individual differences in the subjective experience of pain: new insights into mechanisms and models. *Headache*, **50** (9), 1531–1535.

7 Vanderah, T.W. (2007) Pathophysiology of pain. *The Medical Clinics of North America*, **91** (1), 1–12.

8 Basbaum, A.I., Bautista, D.M., Scherrer, G. & Julius, D. (2009) Cellular and molecular mechanisms of pain. *Cell*, **139** (2), 267–284.

9 Brooks, J. & Tracey, I. (2005) From nociception to pain perception: imaging the spinal and supraspinal pathways. *Journal of Anatomy*, **207** (1), 19–33.

10 Basbaum, A.I. & Jessell, T. (2000) The perception of pain. In: Kandel, E.R., Schwartz, J. & Jessell, T. (eds), *Principles of Neuroscience*. Appleton and Lange, New York, pp. 472–491.

11 Wall, P.D. & Devor, M. (1983) Sensory afferent impulses originate from dorsal root ganglia as well as from the periphery in normal and nerve injured rats. *Pain*, **17** (4), 321–339.

12 Petho, G. & Reeh, P.W. (2012) Sensory and signaling mechanisms of bradykinin, eicosanoids, platelet-activating factor, and nitric oxide in peripheral nociceptors. *Physiological Reviews*, **92** (4), 1699–1775.

13 McGlone, F., Olausson, H., Boyle, J.A. *et al.* (2012) Touching and feeling: differences in pleasant touch processing between glabrous and hairy skin in humans. *The European Journal of Neuroscience*, **35** (11), 1782–1788.

14 Braz, J., Solorzano, C., Wang, X. & Basbaum, A.I. (2014) Transmitting pain and itch messages: a contemporary view of the spinal cord circuits that generate gate control. *Neuron*, **82** (3), 522–536.

15 Moayedi, M. & Davis, K.D. (2013) Theories of pain: from specificity to gate control. *Journal of Neurophysiology*, **109** (1), 5–12.

16 O'Connor, T.M., O'Connell, J., O'Brien, D.I., Goode, T., Bredin, C.P. & Shanahan, F. (2004) The role of substance P in inflammatory disease. *Journal of Cellular Physiology*, **201** (2), 167–180.

17 Malmberg, A.B. & Yaksh, T.L. (1992) Hyperalgesia mediated by spinal glutamate or substance

P receptor blocked by spinal cyclooxygenase inhibition. *Science*, **257** (5074), 1276–1279.

18 Kandel, E.R., Schwartz, J. & Jessell, T. (2000) *Principles of Neural Science*. Vol. **4**. McGraw-Hill, New York.

19 D'Mello, R. & Dickenson, A.H. (2008) Spinal cord mechanisms of pain. *British Journal of Anaesthesia*, **101** (1), 8–16.

20 Wall, P.D. (1978) The gate control theory of pain mechanisms. A re-examination and re-statement. *Brain: A Journal of Neurology*, **101** (1), 1–18.

21 Almeida, T.F., Roizenblatt, S. & Tufik, S. (2004) Afferent pain pathways: a neuroanatomical review. *Brain Research*, **1000** (1–2), 40–56.

22 Millan, M.J. (1999) The induction of pain: an integrative review. *Progress in Neurobiology*, **57** (1), 1–164.

23 Melzack, R. (1999) From the gate to the neuromatrix. *Pain*, (Suppl 6), S121–126.

24 Treede, R.D., Kenshalo, D.R., Gracely, R.H. & Jones, A.K. (1999) The cortical representation of pain. *Pain*, **79** (2–3), 105–111.

25 Willis, W.D. & Westlund, K.N. (1997) Neuroanatomy of the pain system and of the pathways that modulate pain. *Journal of Clinical Neurophysiology: Official Publication of the American Electroencephalographic Society*, **14** (1), 2–31.

26 Millan, M.J. (2002) Descending control of pain. *Progress in Neurobiology*, **66** (6), 355–474.

27 Heinricher, M.M., Tavares, I., Leith, J.L. & Lumb, B.M. (2009) Descending control of nociception: specificity, recruitment and plasticity. *Brain Research Reviews*, **60** (1), 214–225.

28 Graven-Nielsen, T. & Arendt-Nielsen, L. (2002) Peripheral and central sensitization in musculoskeletal pain disorders: an experimental approach. *Current Rheumatology Reports*, **4** (4), 313–321.

29 Woolf, C.J. & Ma, Q. (2007) Nociceptors – noxious stimulus detectors. *Neuron*, **55** (3), 353–364.

30 Nielsen, L.A. & Henriksson, K.G. (2007) Pathophysiological mechanisms in chronic musculoskeletal pain (fibromyalgia): the role of central and peripheral sensitization and pain disinhibition. *Best Practice & Research. Clinical Rheumatology*, **21** (3), 465–480.

31 McCleskey, E.W. & Gold, M.S. (1999) Ion channels of nociception. *Annual Review of Physiology*, **61**, 835–856.

32 Sandkuhler, J. (2009) Models and mechanisms of hyperalgesia and allodynia. *Physiological Reviews*, **89** (2), 707–758.

33 Latremoliere, A. & Woolf, C.J. (2010) Synaptic plasticity and central sensitization: author reply. *The Journal of Pain: Official Journal of the American Pain Society*, **11** (8), 801–803.

34 Woolf, C.J. (2011) Central sensitization: implications for the diagnosis and treatment of pain. *Pain*, **152** (3 Suppl), S2–15.

35 Woolf, C.J. & Thompson, S.W. (1991) The induction and maintenance of central sensitization is dependent on N-methyl-D-aspartic acid receptor activation; implications for the treatment of post-injury pain hypersensitivity states. *Pain*, **44** (3), 293–299.

36 Melzack, R. (1993) Pain: past, present and future. *Canadian Journal of Experimental Psychology = Revue canadienne de psychologie experimentale*, **47** (4), 615–629.

37 Cornblath, D.R. & Hoke, A. (2006) Recent advances in HIV neuropathy. *Current Opinion in Neurology*, **19** (5), 446–450.

38 Merlin, J.S., Westfall, A.O., Raper, J.L. *et al.* (2012) Pain, mood, and substance abuse in HIV: implications for clinic visit utilization, antiretroviral therapy adherence, and virologic failure. *Journal of Acquired Immune Deficiency Syndromes*, **61** (2), 164–170.

39 Merlin, J.S., Zinski, A., Norton, W.E. *et al.* (2014) A conceptual framework for understanding chronic pain in patients with HIV. *Pain Practice: The Official Journal of World Institute of Pain*, **14** (3), 207–216.

40 Gordon, D.B., Dahl, J.L., Miaskowski, C. *et al.* (2005) American Pain Society recommendations for improving the quality of acute and cancer pain management: American Pain Society Quality of Care Task Force. *Archives of Internal Medicine*, **165** (14), 1574–1580.

CHAPTER 3

Chronic pain assessment, diagnostic testing, and management, with an emphasis on communication about these topics to individuals with HIV

Christopher A. Hess[1] and Antje M. Barreveld[2]

[1] *Harvard Medical School, Brigham and Women's Hospital, 75 Francis St, Boston, MA, USA*
[2] *Tufts University School of Medicine, Newton-Wellesley Hospital, 2014 Washington St, Newton, MA, USA*

Introduction

Patients with chronic pain present multi-faceted challenges to providers. Successful communication and patient–provider rapport are paramount to helping patients adequately treat their symptoms and cope with living with chronic pain. As stated by AW Frank, "All the interventions that treat the body as an object, and that consequently understand pain as something inside the body, will never be enough for many patients … Sooner or later, what affects pain is the relationship between the patient and the clinician [1–3]."

In this chapter, we begin with an overview of challenges to patient–provider communication about chronic pain; we also discuss special considerations in HIV-infected individuals. We then provide a general overview of strategies to optimize patient–provider communication about assessment, diagnostic testing, and management.

Why communication with patients with chronic pain and HIV can be complex?

Historically, chronic pain has been viewed as a symptom of an underlying disease, such as arthritis or cancer. However, in the past decade, we have come to view chronic pain as its own chronic condition (see Chapter 1, Introduction) [4]. As such, chronic pain has a unique pathophysiology (see Chapter 2, Pathophysiology of Chronic Pain) and is associated with suboptimal health outcomes. For example, chronic pain can affect all aspects of patients' lives, leading to severely impaired physical and emotional function, difficulty with close personal relationships, and financial strain due to loss of employment [5,6]. In addition, in the past 10 years, there have been substantial advances in understanding the risks associated with long-term opioid therapy and the benefits of other nonopioid pharmacologic therapies and

Chronic Pain and HIV: A Practical Approach, First Edition.
Edited by Jessica S. Merlin, Peter A. Selwyn, Glenn J. Treisman and Angela G. Giovanniello.
© 2016 John Wiley & Sons, Ltd. Published 2016 by John Wiley & Sons, Ltd.

nonpharmacologic therapies. In our experience, patient and provider misunderstandings about what chronic pain is, what causes it, and how it should be treated often lead to communication challenges.

There is also evidence to suggest that patients and providers place different priorities on chronic pain. For example, in one study of primary care patient–provider dyads, patients were more likely than providers to rank painful conditions as their top medical priority [6]. In addition, providers and patients may not have the same impressions of key issues that arise during chronic pain management, such as opioid misuse. In a study of patient–provider dyads in an HIV primary care clinic, providers judged there to be misuse of prescribed opioids more often than their patients, especially in younger African–American patients [7].

There are numerous patient and provider-specific barriers to chronic pain communication that merit consideration. The patient experience of living with chronic pain is affected by a myriad of biological, psychological, and social factors [8,9]. The biological factors involved are described in Chapter 2 (Pathophysiology of Chronic Pain); psychological and social factors include psychiatric and substance use comorbidities, perceived stigma associated with chronic pain and other chronic diseases such as HIV, and lack of social support [2,10–13]. All of these added stressors may color how patients communicate with their providers about chronic pain. For example, a patient who is depressed may come across as lacking interest in engaging in chronic pain care. In addition, suboptimal coping strategies such as catastrophizing (e.g., fear that chronic pain will result in dying) and pain behaviors (e.g., pacing or moaning) may be present. Compounding matters, patients may have previous experience with providers who have reacted negatively. Providers may use emotion-laden language to describe these patients as "drug-seeking" or otherwise difficult (see Chapter 13, The Difficult Patient with HIV and Chronic Pain) [14]. In our experience, this may make understanding the basis of such behaviors more difficult and is distressing to the patient. Other patient-specific barriers include cognitive impairment, low health literacy, and pain-related cultural beliefs.

There are also many provider-specific barriers to effective chronic pain communication. Most providers are trained in a biomedical model that relies on abnormal test results to establish a diagnosis. As described in Chapter 2 (Pathophysiology of Chronic Pain), there is no biomarker for chronic pain. Therefore, one of the most challenging aspects of managing chronic pain for providers is that reports of pain may correlate poorly with physical exam findings or other "objective" tests such as MRIs [15,16].

In addition, providers may have explicit or subconscious biases that affect the encounter. Explicit biases may include overt frustration with caring for patients with chronic pain, and especially those with psychiatric or substance use comorbidities [17]. This can be exacerbated by lack of provider experience managing pain and time pressures common in primary care practices. Recognizing these barriers early allows providers to self-reflect and reframe their thinking during the patient encounter. Examples of subconscious biases may include prescribing opioids less often to African–Americans [18] and monitoring them on long-term opioid therapy more closely [19].

Communication with HIV-infected individuals with chronic pain may pose additional challenges. For instance, HIV-infected patients with chronic pain have higher rates of psychiatric illness and substance abuse than individuals with HIV or chronic pain alone, which may affect their ability to effectively communicate with providers (see Chapter 8, Psychiatric Comorbidities). HIV-infected individuals also have a unique biopsychosocial milieu that includes issues such as social isolation and addiction that may prove to be problematic for their healthcare givers [20]. In addition, providers may be uncomfortable with their dual role as an HIV provider and chronic pain provider [21]. They may worry that failure to continue to provide opioids to patients may lead to patients leaving HIV care and be unsure of how to navigate that conversation (Starrels JL PD, Fox AD, Merlin J, Arnsten JH, Cunningham CO. HIV Treatment Providers' Perspectives on Opioid Prescribing for Chronic Pain: The Overriding Concern to Retain Patients in Care [oral abstract presentation]. Paper presented at: Association of Medical

Education and Research in Substance Abuse, November 8, 2013, Bethesda M.).

The following sections describe strategies and examples of effective communication with patients with HIV and chronic pain, keeping in mind the aforementioned patient and provider barriers when formulating a successful dialogue and pain management care plan.

Principles of successful patient–provider communication

Patient–provider communication begins as soon as the patient enters the room through both verbal and nonverbal cues and thus these initial patient–provider interactions ultimately determine the fate of the encounter [22]. The provider must be aware of potential barriers to effective communication as discussed above in order to guarantee the most successful encounter. It is essential for the provider to ensure early on that the patient feels welcome, calm, and free to discuss issues openly [23].

A simple way to frame the interview is by using the *WIPS* mnemonic (Table 3.1).

Makoul suggests starting this endeavor by building rapport, being aware of the patient's true concerns, incorporating active listening, understanding where the patient is coming from, encouraging the patient to understand their condition, collaborating to create an effective treatment plan, and closing the encounter with a summary (Table 3.2) [24]. Shaping a healing relationship requires a substantial effort by both the provider and the patient and, notably, is a process that takes time [24]. As the interview progresses, special attention is made to building rapport and nonverbal cues, such as constant eye contact, frequent head nods

Table 3.1 WIPS mnemonic for framing the patient encounter [23].

W: *Welcome* patients into your practice
I: Make patients feel they are *important*
P: Ensure their *perspective* was understood
S: Ensure that patients feel *secure* that you the provider will meet their needs.

Table 3.2 Essential elements of the patient interview [24].

- *Step 1: build the doctor–patient relationship*
- *Step 2: open the discussion*
- *Step 3: gather information*
- *Step 4: understand the patient's perspective*
- *Step 5: share information*
- *Step 6: reach agreement on problems and plans*
- *Step 7: provide closure.*

---

and expressions of understanding, and facing toward the patient at eye level [22,24].

Another essential principle of effective patient–provider communication is the concept of shared medical decision-making (SMD). In SMD, the patient maintains autonomy during a two-way interview process, where the provider and the patient develop a treatment plan while keeping the preferences of the patient in mind [2,25,26]. There are limits to the use of SMD, based on patient, provider, and situational factors, and it should be tailored to the discretion of the provider. The following scenarios contrast a one-sided, paternalistic communication approach with a modified SMD approach to illustrate some of the above interviewing principles.

Examples of poor and effective communication
Case scenario
Mr Jones is a 55-year-old male patient with HIV and poorly controlled diabetes who has developed painful peripheral neuropathy.

Example of less effective communication
Provider: Mr Jones, your pain is from your HIV and your diabetes. We need to get your sugars under control in addition to starting a new medication for your pain.
Mr Jones: Okay, but I didn't think it's because of my diabetes. I don't understand why I have it. It's really affecting what I am able to do.
Provider: I think it is from your diabetes. I am also going to prescribe gabapentin and you will take one pill three times daily for the next 2 weeks and then we can increase the dose until it works for you.

Mr Jones: Well, okay but I have a few questions. What about side effects?

Provider: I will have my nurse schedule a follow-up appointment for you. Please take the medication as I prescribed it for you. You might feel a little tired, but the side effects are minimal.

Example of more effective communication
Beginning of encounter
Provider: Hello Mr Jones, it is nice to see you again, I'm sorry to hear about your increased pain. Tell me about your pain ... Where do you think your pain is coming from? ... Are you able to do the things you want to on a daily basis? ...

Middle of encounter
Provider: Do you have ideas about how you would like to best treat your pain?

End of the encounter
Provider: Now that we have both come up with a plan, can you tell me in your own words how we are going to treat your nerve pain? ... I will have you schedule an appointment with me in the next couple of weeks to discuss your progress and I would like you to keep a log of your sugar levels, your daily pain and functioning, and any medication side effects. If you experience any problems with this medication, please call my office and we can discuss the next steps. Do you have any other questions?

The above scenarios reinforce the concept that open and bilateral communication is linked to positive patient outcomes in emotional health, pain control, and functional status – the fundamental goals in pain management [27].

The art of assessing pain history

Although history-taking is a fundamental skill learned early in training [10,16,28,29], we present several useful pearls that can assist the provider in developing a diagnostic and therapeutic plan.

The story
Assessing pain is an art form that requires providers to delve into the personal, subjective, and multidimensional life of both the patient and providers while instilling empathy and trust. Often providers struggle with balancing the typical learned assessment skills, scientific method, their personal style, and experiences when assessing pain. One widely cited assessment technique is the concept of the *personal pain narrative* in written as well as spoken form. Rita Charon, MD, PhD, suggests that a key concept of narrative medicine is for the provider to pay attention to the important emotional details, comprehend the meaning of patients' statements, and respond empathically to their personal narratives [30]. Charon writes, "A scientifically competent medicine alone cannot help a patient grapple with the loss of health or find meaning in suffering. Along with scientific ability, physicians need the ability to listen to the narratives of the patient, grasp and honor their meanings, and be moved to act on the patient's behalf [30]." In essence, the provider takes in what a patient has to say, processes it not just scientifically but also emotionally, then reflects on that story in order to comprehend the core issues the patient is emotionally drawn to. Pain narratives therefore permit direct insight into patients' pain experiences [15].

Examples of open-ended questions to guide the patient in their pain narrative
Case scenario: Mrs Farley is a 38-year-old woman with HIV and depression who presents to discuss with you what to do for her multiple joint and muscle complaints especially in her neck and shoulders and arms.

Provider: Hello Mrs Farley. How are you doing?

Mrs Farley: Doctor, I don't know what to do. Sometimes, I can't get out of bed in the morning, I can't sleep, and something has to be done. What is wrong with me? Why is this happening?

Provider: Mrs Farley, it sounds like you have been suffering a lot from your pain and I'm sorry to hear this. Why don't you start by telling me more? What was going on in your life when you first noticed the pain? ... What do you do for yourself when the pain is very bad? ... Is there anyone who is helping support you through this? ... Perhaps so I can better understand what is going on in your life and with your pain you could write down your pain story for me and we can discuss it together. I think this could be very helpful for you and for me.

Table 3.3   Pain assessment mnemonic "OPQRST [31]."

O: Onset of symptoms – when did the pain start? What happened when you first noticed pain? Anything particularly stressful at the time?

P: Palliating and/or provoking factors – What makes the pain better or worse?

Q: Qualitative and quantitative factors – How would you describe your pain? What number from 0 to 10 would you rate your pain on average?

R: Radiating to different areas – Does the pain move to anywhere else?

S: Severity of symptoms – How does the pain affect your daily life? Ability to work? Be with family?

T: Timing of symptoms – Are there certain times of the day or activities that worsen your pain?

The standard pain history

Every pain history should include directed questions. For instance, a frequently used mnemonic in assessing acute pain, "OPQRST," can also be applied to chronic pain and may provide a framework for the patient's assessment (see Table 3.3).

In addition, other key historical data, with an emphasis on the patient's current functional status, should be obtained during any chronic pain assessment. This includes the following:

- A thorough current and past medical history and a detailed history of surgeries, medical treatments, and therapies tried for treating their pain including medications, interventions, physical therapy, and alternative treatments
- A focused psychological and psychiatric history, including hospitalizations, medical and behavioral treatments, history of physical or sexual abuse, in addition to current update their mood and any depression or anxiety
- A social history emphasizing support systems
- A substance use history
- An employment and disability history
- A detailed description of physical and emotional function that may include questions on the patient's ability to perform daily activities, how they spend their time during the day, sleep patterns, exercise, and number of work days missed secondary to pain.

Structured assessment tools

Various assessment tools can serve as a framework to guide the interview and ensure important information is gathered. Notably, one of the most common pain assessment tools is the 0–10 numeric rating scale for pain severity. This tool can be a useful initial question for understanding someone's pain, as it is widely used in primary care practices, most patients and providers are familiar with it, and it may provide a baseline pain level from which response to treatment can be measured. However, the numeric rating scale has limitations. It was initially designed for use in acute pain and has never been validated among individuals with chronic pain. Furthermore, among individuals with chronic pain, scale values are highly variable from person to person and even within one person during the course of the day and may reflect not only the pain itself but also an individual's affective response to pain.

In contrast, one of the best-studied and most useful pain assessment tools among HIV-infected individuals is the Brief Pain Inventory [32]. This tool takes approximately 10 min to administer and assesses not only pain severity but also its impact on seven functional domains (general activity, mood, walking ability, normal work, relations with other people, sleep, and enjoyment of life). One approach is to administer this assessment electronically prior to the encounter and use the results as a starting point for the discussion [3,31]. Similarly, standardized assessment tools that have been well-studied among individuals with HIV include the PHQ-9 for depression, the PHQ anxiety module for anxiety/panic disorders, the AUDIT-C for alcohol use disorders, and the ASSIST for illicit substance use disorders.

Special considerations when discussing psychiatric illness and/or addiction in individuals with chronic pain

Chronic pain, psychiatric illness, and addiction often (but not always) occur together (see Chapter 8). When present, treatment of these comorbidities and treatments that rely heavily on psychological and behavioral approaches (e.g., cognitive behavioral therapy) are an integral part of successfully treating chronic pain.

Helping patients to make these connections can be challenging. Patients may perceive us as telling them that their pain is "all in their head" or that they are just "drug seeking." In addition, we are working with our patients to identify and change behaviors that are detrimental to their recovery from chronic pain (e.g., avoidance of physical and social activity, overreliance on pain medications), or to begin new healthy behaviors (e.g., seeing a psychologist).

Again, for such difficult conversations, the authors have found that Motivational Interviewing can be an invaluable tool. Motivational interviewing is a technique that allows patients and providers to talk about behavior change in a way that diffuses resistance (Miller and Rollnick, Motivational Interviewing). Instead of the typical approach in which the provider tells the patient about all the things the patient must do in order to get well, Motivational Interviewing relies on the provider reflecting on the patient's concerns, asking open-ended questions, and affirming any positive forward progress (however small). It also allows patients to come up with their own goals and ways of achieving them, with help and suggestions from the provider.

The following case scenario illustrates how using Motivational Interviewing can help to reduce resistance during a conversation about the importance of cotreating mood disorders and chronic pain:

Ms Greene: I feel like people think that I'm crazy because I'm anxious, and the pain is in my head.
Provider: Your pain is not all in your head, and it's about more than just your anxiety.

Ms Greene: Right – if my pain was better, I wouldn't be anxious!
Provider: You have anxiety and you have pain, and you are looking for solutions to both.
Ms Greene: So you want me to see a shrink?
Provider Well, would you be open to some ideas about how we could treat both your anxiety and your pain together?
Ms Greene: Sure, I'll try anything to feel better.
Provider: We have someone here who specializes in helping patients with pain and anxiety. If you'd like, I can explain a little more about why some of our other patients have found her to be very helpful.
Ms Greene: Sure.
Provider: For many people, anxiety and pain feed off of each other. What I mean by that is, if you have a day when you're feeling particularly anxious, it might make your pain worse, and if you have a day when you're hurting more, it might make you more anxious. Pretty soon it's hard to figure out which came first, and it can become a viscous cycle. Has that ever happened to you?
Ms Greene: Yes, I know exactly what you mean.
Provider: The person I have in mind for you to see is like a coach – she helps people who are in the same situation you are – with anxiety and pain – come up with strategies of how to manage both together in their daily lives. I imagine you already have strategies to manage your pain and anxiety – you were able to get out of bed to come here today! How did you do that?
Ms Greene: Well, I just push myself. I take my time. And sometimes I take pain medication to help too.
Provider: Great! Well, the person I'd like you to see – she is trained as a psychologist but helps to coach people with HIV and chronic pain – she can help you work on the strategies you are already using, and come up with new ones. It sounds like you are already pretty good at this, but everyone can use a coach to get even better!
Ms Greene: That sounds like something I could try.
Provider: I think that's a great idea. What do you think would be a good next step toward seeing your new coach?
Ms Greene: I will stop by the front desk today to make an appointment, would that be OK? I'd like to see her soon.
Provider: Definitely. You want to see her soon – when do you think you would like to see her?
Ms Greene: I'd like to see her before I come back to see you again, maybe in the next month?

Provider: That sounds like a great goal. The next time we see each other, I look forward to hearing how it went!

This is just one example of the usefulness of Motivational Interviewing techniques in such encounters. Motivational Interviewing is typically taught in 1- to 3-day workshops, and is learnable skill. For more information on training in Motivational Interviewing, we recommend that you visit http://www .motivationalinterviewing.org/.

Communication about diagnostic testing

Evidence-based diagnostic testing for the most common painful conditions among individuals with HIV is covered in their respective chapters. However, choosing and discussing the indication for diagnostic testing can pose significant challenges. Patients may request a variety of tests that are not indicated. In addition, providers may become frustrated when evidence-based diagnostic testing does not reveal an obvious underlying diagnosis and may order unnecessary studies that lead to complex workups. To help navigate these challenges, it is important to keep in mind the idea of shared decision-making. It is also important to recognize that every test has risks and benefits, and as a result, limits must be set based on what is reasonable and safe for the patient to endure.

Diagnostic testing is sometimes used to identify an underlying cause of someone's chronic pain (e.g., rheumatoid arthritis), and other times used to identify whether a procedural intervention may be indicated (e.g., low back imaging in a patient with sciatica, or joint imaging in a patient with knee pain). The purpose of imaging should be discussed with the patient when it is ordered, so that the patient understands the implications of a positive or negative result. For example, a negative spinal MRI in someone with low back pain and sciatica does not mean that their pain is particularly worrisome or cannot be treated, but rather, that physical therapy may be more effective than an injection.

In addition to diagnostic testing to evaluate the etiology of chronic pain, urine drug testing is typically used to monitor an individual with chronic pain who is on long-term opioid therapy (see Chapter 12). When ordering urine drug testing, individuals with chronic pain should be informed that this is done routinely for all patients with chronic pain for the purposes of monitoring adherence to pain medications and the presence of substances that could be dangerous, such as nonprescribed medications and other illicit substances. Discussing routine urine drug testing is often accomplished in the context of an opioid treatment agreement, when other monitoring strategies are also reviewed.

Explaining the diagnosis

Patient education regarding the nature of chronic pain as a chronic illness and the role of both the patient and provider in the patient's recovery is a key element to successful communication. Many patients may feel that providers do not believe that they are in pain or that the "pain is in my head." Establishing rapport is critical to encouraging an open dialogue and recognizing the patient's concerns. Providers need to pay attention to "words that heal, words that harm": avoiding medical jargon and words that invoke fear, but rather focusing on simple terminology, reassurance, and encouragement [33]. Examples of empathic statements are as follows:

- *You have been through so much and I know we can help you. This just might take time.*
- *This must be very hard for you.*
- *It is okay to feel shocked or scared; we can get through this together. You are not alone. You will get through this. You are strong. Think about how far you have come since you first started having pain.*

Closing statements can also leave lasting impressions on the patient and should be chosen thoughtfully, void of medical complexity and potential ambiguity. When providers make statements that suggest recovery is unlikely, such as "you have the worst back I have ever seen" or "I don't know how you are even able to walk," patients are more likely to suffer long-term disability. It is important that providers understand that regardless of the degree of functional disability or the results of an imaging study, patients with chronic pain have the ability to recover through both pharmacologic and nonpharmacologic treatments. Other examples of discouraging statements are as follows:

- *You don't have the right outlook on this diagnosis.*
- *That's the wrong way to think.*
- *You need to pull yourself up by your bootstraps.*
- *People have been through so much more than you have been through.*
- *This is just chronic neuropathic pain, we can treat it.*
- *Your immune system is attacking your nerves.*
- *You spinal canals have become stenosed.*

Framing expectations

Framing expectations is a critical step in communicating the pain treatment plan. In the authors' experience, reiterating the nature of pain as a chronic disease to be managed rather than a symptom to be treated is helpful. Along these lines, we also advise patients that while we wish we had a treatment that would make their pain go away completely, no such treatment exists. We explain that multimodal therapies, including both pharmacologic and nonpharmacologic therapies, are successful in helping patients with chronic pain lead happy, full lives, and achieve their goals.

Management of chronic pain focuses on functional goals. Setting goals, such as increasing one's physical activity, often involves behavior change. The authors have found that motivational interviewing is a technique that can be very helpful in discussing such behavior change and can be a way to open the conversation about goal setting. It is critical that the patient come up with those goals, often with guidance from the provider.

Patients should identify both short- and long-term goals. Learning more about the patient's hobbies, interests, and current or prior occupations can help the provider assist a patient who is struggling in identifying long-term goals. Long-term goals might include returning to work or reinitiating a hobby. In order to build a patient's self-efficacy, it is also important to also set achievable short-term goals, such as leaving the house for a scheduled social activity once a week or walking to the mailbox. Any progress toward these goals, however modest, should be celebrated, and the provider should ask the patient to reflect on strategies used.

The following case scenario of Mrs Smith who has HIV and neuropathy illustrates principles in framing expectations and setting functional goals:

Provider: Mrs Smith, I would like to work with you to come up with a plan. So that I can better understand your thoughts, what are your goals in regard to your pain management?… What are you hoping to have happen with your treatments?… What is something you used to like to do that you feel you cannot do anymore?… Why don't we set a time line for the next few months of goals you would like to work toward. It is also very important that we address your pain from multiple angles as I'm also hearing that your pain is clearly worse when your mood is low.

Discussing treatment components

Every pain management plan can be divided into categories such as medications, interventions, specialists, physical therapy, behavioral therapy, dietary modifications, alternative medicine therapies, and support groups. A multidisciplinary and multimodal approach has been shown to have the greatest impact on reaching functional goals and decreasing pain scores [34]. In addition, a collaborative communication style in initial and follow-up appointments positively affects patient treatment outcomes and medication adherence [35]. Patients may complete a functional pain log daily to help monitor and track their pain, daily activities, and response to treatments.

Scheduling follow-up and discussing possible referrals

Continuity of care

An integral part of treating patients with chronic pain includes maintaining continuity of care and information sharing among different specialties. This can be done by a variety of means in today's digital era; however, what is central to this paradigm is the primary care provider's role as the coordinator of information. Patients with HIV and chronic pain often have many providers and specialists responsible for their care. Coordination among this diverse team is essential to ensuring that a unified diagnosis and treatment plan is communicated to patients. One medical provider, such as the primary care provider, should be responsible for ensuring this successful care coordination and regular follow-up with the patient.

Family and social support

Consider involving family members or other social support when discussing the plan with the patient. These individuals can play a key role in helping the patient emotionally, physically, or even financially. Providers should reach out to the patient and discuss the potential of involving others.

Conclusion

For some providers, assessing and treating patients with chronic pain can be overwhelming, emotionally draining, and time consuming – but it does not have to be this way! Treating patients with chronic pain can be a rewarding and fulfilling experience. Communication is most effective using the following guiding principles: understanding provider and patient biases, focusing on shared decision-making and bidirectional communication, encouraging a patient's pain narrative with open and empathic interviewing techniques, accurately assessing pain using organized and potentially quantitative assessment modalities to track progress, framing expectations with an emphasis on reaching both functional and emotional goals, and skillfully delivering a multimodal and multidisciplinary plan with adequate follow-up and collaboration with the patient, family members, and specialists. Clear, open, and empathic communication will engender patients' respect, trust, satisfaction, and hope, as they cope with a condition that can cause significant stress and disability: chronic pain.

References

1 Frank, A.W. (2003). In: Dostrovsky, J.O., Carr, D.B. & Koltzenburg, M. (eds), *How Stories Remake What Pain Unmakes*. International Association for the Study of Pain (Iasp) Press, Seattle, pp. 619–630.

2 Frantsve, L.M. & Kerns, R.D. (2007) Patient–provider interactions in the management of chronic pain: current findings within the context of shared medical decision making. *Pain Medicine*, **8** (1), 25–35.

3 Perry, B.A., Westfall, A.O., Molony, E. *et al.* (2013) Characteristics of an ambulatory palliative care clinic for HIV-infected patients. *Journal of Palliative Medicine*, **16** (8), 934–937.

4 Institute of Medicine (US) Committee on Advancing Pain Research, Care, and Education (2011) *Relieving Pain in America: A Blueprint for Transforming Prevention, Care, Education, and Research* The National Academies Collection: Reports funded by National Institutes of Health. National Academies Press, Washington (DC).

5 Turk, D.C., Wilson, H.D. & Cahana, A. (2011) Treatment of chronic non-cancer pain. *Lancet*, **377** (9784), 2226–2235.

6 Zulman, D.M., Kerr, E.A., Hofer, T.P., Heisler, M. & Zikmund-Fisher, B.J. (2010) Patient–provider concordance in the prioritization of health conditions among hypertensive diabetes patients. *Journal of General Internal Medicine*, **25** (5), 408–414.

7 Vijayaraghavan, M., Penko, J., Guzman, D., Miaskowski, C. & Kushel, M.B. (2011) Primary care providers' judgments of opioid analgesic misuse in a community-based cohort of HIV-infected indigent adults. *Journal of General Internal Medicine*, **26** (4), 412–418.

8 Engel, G.L. (1977) The need for a new medical model: a challenge for biomedicine. *Science*, **196** (4286), 129–136.

9 Engel, G.L. (1980) The clinical application of the biopsychosocial model. *The American Journal of Psychiatry*, **137** (5), 535–544.

10 Dansie, E.J. & Turk, D.C. (2013) Assessment of patients with chronic pain. *British Journal of Anaesthesia*, **111** (1), 19–25.

11 John, C., Schwenk, T.L., Roi, L.D. & Cohen, M. (1987) Medical care and demographic characteristics of 'difficult' patients. *The Journal of Family Practice*, **24** (6), 607–610.

12 Levenstein, J.H., McCracken, E.C., McWhinney, I.R., Stewart, M.A. & Brown, J.B. (1986) The patient-centred clinical method. 1. A model for the doctor–patient interaction in family medicine. *Family Practice*, **3** (1), 24–30.

13 Jamison, R.N. & Edwards, R.R. (2013) Risk factor assessment for problematic use of opioids for chronic pain. *The Clinical Neuropsychologist*, **27** (1), 60–80.

14 Merlin, J.S., Turan, J.M., Herbey, I. *et al.* (2014) Aberrant drug-related behaviors: a qualitative analysis of medical record documentation in patients referred to an HIV/chronic pain clinic. *Pain Medicine*, **15** (10), 1724–1733.

15 Moore, R.J. (2012) *Handbook of Pain and Palliative Care: Biobehavioral Approaches for the Life Course*. Springer, New York, London xxvi, 865 p.

16 McGuire, D.B. (1992) Comprehensive and multidimensional assessment and measurement of pain. *Journal of Pain and Symptom Management*, **7** (5), 312–319.

17 Dobscha, S.K., Corson, K., Flores, J.A., Tansill, E.C. & Gerrity, M.S. (2008) Veterans affairs primary care clinicians' attitudes toward chronic pain and correlates of opioid prescribing rates. *Pain Medicine*, **9** (5), 564–571.

18 Burgess, D.J., Nelson, D.B., Gravely, A.A. *et al.* (2014) Racial differences in prescription of opioid analgesics for chronic noncancer pain in a national sample of veterans. *The Journal of Pain*, **15** (4), 447–455.

19 Becker, W.C., Starrels, J.L., Heo, M., Li, X., Weiner, M.G. & Turner, B.J. (2011) Racial differences in primary care opioid risk reduction strategies. *Annals of Family Medicine*, **9** (3), 219–225.

20 Merlin, J.S., Zinski, A., Norton, W.E. *et al.* (2014) A conceptual framework for understanding chronic pain in patients with HIV. *Pain Practice: The Official Journal of World Institute of Pain*, **14** (3), 207–216.

21 McCance-Katz, E.F., Lum, P.J., Beatty, G., Gruber, V.A., Peters, M. & Rainey, P.M. (2012) Untreated HIV infection is associated with higher blood alcohol levels. *Journal of Acquired Immune Deficiency Syndromes*, **60** (3), 282–288.

22 Roter, D.L., Frankel, R.M., Hall, J.A. & Sluyter, D. (2006) The expression of emotion through nonverbal behavior in medical visits. Mechanisms and outcomes. *Journal of General Internal Medicine*, **21** (Suppl 1), S28–34.

23 Fishman, S., Ballantyne, J., Rathmell, J.P. & Bonica, J.J. (2010) *Bonica's Management of Pain*, 4th edn. Lippincott, Williams & Wilkins, Baltimore, MDxxxiii, 1661 p..

24 Makoul, G. (2001) Essential elements of communication in medical encounters: the Kalamazoo consensus statement. *Academic Medicine: Journal of the Association of American Medical Colleges*, **76** (4), 390–393.

25 Murray, E., Charles, C. & Gafni, A. (2006) Shared decision-making in primary care: tailoring the Charles et al. model to fit the context of general practice. *Patient Education and Counseling*, **62** (2), 205–211.

26 Moulton, B. & King, J.S. (2010) Aligning ethics with medical decision-making: the quest for informed patient choice. *The Journal of Law, Medicine & Ethics: A Journal of the American Society of Law, Medicine & Ethics.*, **38** (1), 85–97.

27 Stewart, M.A. (1995) Effective physician–patient communication and health outcomes: a review. *CMAJ: Canadian Medical Association Journal = journal de l'Association medicale canadienne*, **152** (9), 1423–1433.

28 Smith, R.C., Lyles, J.S., Mettler, J. *et al.* (1998) The effectiveness of intensive training for residents in interviewing. A randomized, controlled study. *Annals of Internal Medicine*, **128** (2), 118–126.

29 Makoul, G. & Curry, R.H. (2007) The value of assessing and addressing communication skills. *JAMA, the Journal of the American Medical Association*, **298** (9), 1057–1059.

30 Charon, R. (2001) The patient–physician relationship. Narrative medicine: a model for empathy, reflection, profession, and trust. *JAMA, the Journal of the American Medical Association*, **286** (15), 1897–1902.

31 Powell, R.A.D.J., Ddungu, H. & Mwangi-Powell, F.N. (2010) Pain management and assessment. In: Kopf, A. & Patel, N.B. (eds), *Guide to Pain Management in Low-Resource Settings*. IASP: International Association for the Study of Pain, Seattle, pp. 67–79.

32 Merlin, J.S., Cen, L., Praestgaard, A. *et al.* (2012) Pain and physical and psychological

symptoms in ambulatory HIV patients in the current treatment era. *Journal of Pain and Symptom Management*, **43** (3), 638–645.

33 Bedell, S.E., Graboys, T.B., Bedell, E. & Lown, B. (2004) Words that harm, words that heal. *Archives of Internal Medicine*, **164** (13), 1365–8.

34 Guzman, J., Esmail, R., Karjalainen, K., Malmivaara, A., Irvin, E. & Bombardier, C. (2002) Multidisciplinary biopsychosocial rehabilitation for chronic low back pain. *The Cochrane Database of Systematic Reviews*, **1**, CD000963.

35 Bultman, D.C. & Svarstad, B.L. (2000) Effects of physician communication style on client medication beliefs and adherence with antidepressant treatment. *Patient Education and Counseling*, **40** (2), 173–185.

CHAPTER 4

HIV and chronic pain: musculoskeletal pain

Jessica Robinson-Papp

Department of Neurology, Icahn School of Medicine at Mount Sinai, New York, NY, USA

Introduction

Chronic musculoskeletal pain is a common, disabling problem in HIV-infected patients [1]. Musculoskeletal pain includes muscular pain, joint pain, bone pain, and other complex chronic musculoskeletal pain syndromes. In this chapter, we present a practical and clinically oriented approach to chronic musculoskeletal pain in HIV, recognizing that such symptoms may be related to a wide variety of underlying disorders. We review what is known about the epidemiology of musculoskeletal pain in HIV and its potential mechanisms and offer an approach to diagnosis. For a comprehensive discussion of the treatment of chronic pain in HIV-infected patients, see Chapter 10; however, we briefly mention treatment approaches specific to the disorders described herein. We also specifically address three of the most common and challenging chronic musculoskeletal pain syndromes: low back pain, widespread pain including fibromyalgia, and myofascial pain syndrome.

Epidemiology

Chronic musculoskeletal pain is highly prevalent in the general population. Approximately 30% of adults report some form of chronic pain,[2] most of which is musculoskeletal. Estimates of the prevalence of chronic, painful musculoskeletal conditions in HIV were mostly made prior to the current HIV treatment era [3]. Current estimates arise mainly from resource-limited settings, where infectious etiologies such as septic arthritis, osteomyelitis, and pyomyositis predominate [4,5]. However, even in these settings, noninfectious causes of chronic pain such as arthralgias, spondyloarthropathies, osteonecrosis, myopathy, and fibromyalgia have been reported [4,5].

Large epidemiologic studies of chronic musculoskeletal pain in populations with well-controlled HIV are lacking. Therefore, the prevalence of chronic musculoskeletal pain in developed countries in the current HIV treatment era is unknown. However, clinical experience suggests chronic musculoskeletal pain in HIV is common, and some estimates of its prevalence can be made based on available data. The prevalence of chronic pain in HIV-infected patients is estimated to be between 39% and 85% [see Chapter 1] [6,7]. In three series of patients with HIV and chronic pain, more than half of patients reported musculoskeletal pain, predominantly low back pain, but also leg, hip, shoulder, neck, and joint pain [1,6,8].

Underlying mechanisms

The underlying mechanisms of most of the conditions that cause chronic musculoskeletal pain in HIV have not been definitively established. Hypothesized mechanisms include direct effects of HIV itself, direct and indirect

Chronic Pain and HIV: A Practical Approach, First Edition.
Edited by Jessica S. Merlin, Peter A. Selwyn, Glenn J. Treisman and Angela G. Giovanniello.
© 2016 John Wiley & Sons, Ltd. Published 2016 by John Wiley & Sons, Ltd.

effects of antiretroviral therapy (ART), chronic inflammation, neurologic mechanisms, psychosocial influences, and the presence of painful comorbidities.

HIV and ART may have direct effects on the musculoskeletal system. HIV has been detected within muscle in both endomysial macrophages and myocytes [9]. HIV has also been associated with decreased bone mineral density [10]. ART, particularly high-dose AZT, can be directly toxic to muscle [11]. ART may also alter muscle metabolism via adverse effects on glucose transport [12]. In bone, initiation of ART causes an initial loss in bone mineral density with subsequent stabilization, independent of regimen [13,14]. Less directly, the metabolic effects of ART could contribute to musculoskeletal pain via changes in body composition. For example, loss of muscle mass and increased central obesity may alter body mechanics and lead to pain [15,16].

Even when treated with ART, HIV is associated with chronic low-level inflammation and immune activation [17,18]. Circulating proinflammatory cytokines can lead to a clinical syndrome of exaggerated pain and physiological and behavioral changes, which constitute the "sickness response [19]." This chronic inflammation may also contribute to the development of certain painful musculoskeletal conditions such as avascular necrosis (AVN)[20] and is a proposed mechanism of accelerated aging and frailty,[18] which exacerbate most musculoskeletal disorders.

There are multiple neurologic mechanisms that may contribute to chronic pain including peripheral and central sensitization. These mechanisms are addressed in Chapter 2. The recent finding of an association between small fiber neuropathy and fibromyalgia suggests a novel neurologic mechanism for some forms of chronic musculoskeletal pain [21,22]. Small nerve fibers are responsible for pain and temperature sensation and also for sensing internal milieu and conveying this information to the central nervous system. This "sixth sense" has been termed interoception and is believed to be important in establishing a sense of physical well-being [23]. Thus, it is postulated that its malfunction could cause feelings of illness, including diffuse musculoskeletal pain and

other somatic symptoms. This may be particularly relevant in HIV-infected patients, in whom neuropathy is a common and clinically important condition (Chapter 6).

Musculoskeletal pain is also strongly influenced by psychosocial factors (for a discussion of psychosocial factors in chronic pain in general, see Chapters 2, 8, and 9). In the fear-avoidance model of chronic musculoskeletal pain, an initial minor musculoskeletal injury can lead to chronic pain when excessive fear and/or anxiety causes avoidance and disuse, which in turn exacerbates disability and perpetuates pain [24]. Risk factors for transition from minor acute musculoskeletal pain into a chronic pain syndrome are highly prevalent in HIV-infected individuals and include psychiatric disorders, greater burden of medical illness, and social isolation [25,26].

HIV-infected patients are at a higher risk for the development of certain comorbidities than the general population [see epidemiology (Chapter 1) and multimorbidity (Chapter 7)]. These comorbidities may have painful musculoskeletal sequelae. For example, hepatitis C infection is associated with multiple rheumatologic manifestations including arthritis, arthralgias, and myalgias,[27] and osteoporosis may lead to pain due to fractures.

Clinical manifestations

Clinical manifestations of musculoskeletal pain are diverse but can be grouped into two general forms: myalgia and arthralgia. Myalgia refers to pain in muscle and arthralgia to pain in joints. Myalgia and arthralgia can be diffuse, regional, or focal and may be described as deep, aching, or throbbing. Myalgia may also be described as cramping, and arthralgia as stiffness.

While myalgia and arthralgia may indicate an underlying disorder of the muscle or joint, respectively, they may also be nonspecific "constitutional" symptoms of illness or be reflective of a chronic widespread pain syndrome such as fibromyalgia. It is also important to recognize that patients may have difficulty describing their pain precisely and may not ascribe it to the correct anatomic structure. Thus, when applying the diagnostic approaches outlined below, it may sometimes be necessary to pursue more than one potential etiology of the pain.

Diagnostic and treatment approaches

The evaluation of chronic musculoskeletal pain begins with a detailed history as described in Chapter 3. The physical examination begins with the general appearance of the patient including body habitus, posture, and general level of fitness. Based on the nature of the specific pain symptoms, examination of joints may be important including visual inspection for physical deformities or erythema, palpation for temperature and focal tenderness, and assessment of active and passive range of motion. Palpation of tendons may be performed to assess for focal tenderness or signs of inflammation. Neuromuscular examination includes palpation of muscles, functional and manual muscle strength testing, and assessment of deep tendon reflexes and sensation. These findings are particularly relevant for patients with muscular pain in whom myopathy is suspected and patients with back pain in whom radiculopathy is suspected (e.g., those with pain radiating into a limb). In patients with diffuse or regional pain syndromes, taut bands of muscle and trigger points may also be sought. Points of increased tenderness, particularly at the base of the skull, in the shoulder area, in the buttocks, elbows, or knees are potentially consistent with fibromyalgia,[28] and trigger points within taut bands are seen in myofascial pain syndrome [29].

The diagnostic testing required, if any, will vary greatly depending on the nature of the pain complaint and so must be planned on an individualized basis. Tests that may be appropriate include blood tests, imaging, and nerve conduction studies and electromyography (EMG). Appropriate diagnostic testing is addressed in greater detail in the following sections. However, in planning a diagnostic evaluation, the clinician and patient should both be aware that a definitive cause of musculoskeletal pain may be elusive and that the goal of diagnostic testing should be to reasonably

exclude serious treatable conditions rather than to exhaustively pursue a precise etiology of the pain.

Painful disorders of muscle

Muscular disorders are typically characterized by muscular pain, or myalgia. Myalgia is often diffuse and can be described as deep, aching, cramping, or throbbing. Myalgia may indicate an underlying primary muscle disorder, such as HIV-associated myopathy, or be reflective of a muscular pain not due to underlying muscle damage such as fibromyalgia. The majority of HIV-infected individuals with myalgia do not have objective evidence of a primary muscle disorder. If there is no objective proximal muscle weakness and creatine phosphokinase (CPK) levels are normal, further diagnostic testing for myopathy (e.g., EMG and muscle biopsy) is not necessary. Such patients will often have symptoms in addition to myalgias, including other types of pain, other somatic symptoms, and cognitive and mood symptoms. This is discussed in more detail in the following section on complex chronic pain syndromes.

Several primary muscle disorders occur in patients with HIV, ranging in severity from asymptomatically elevated CPK to rhabdomyolysis. Elevated CPK in otherwise asymptomatic HIV-infected individuals is relatively common with about 15% of patients experiencing transient elevations and about 4% experiencing sustained elevations [30]. These patients likely have a mild form of HIV-associated myopathy and do not require specific treatment.

More severe muscle disorders are very rare. The best characterized is HIV-associated myopathy, also known as HIV-associated polymyositis. HIV-associated myopathy is clinically and pathologically similar to autoimmune polymyositis in HIV-negative patients. It may occur at any stage of HIV disease and is characterized by diffuse myalgias, and slowly progressive, proximal, symmetric muscle weakness [31]. Proximal muscle weakness may manifest as difficulty performing tasks such as holding the arms up over the head, or difficulty climbing stairs or arising from a chair unassisted. The presence of such symptoms combined with objective evidence of proximal weakness on examination is suggestive of the diagnosis, which is confirmed by elevated serum CPK, myopathic findings on EMG, and a myopathic muscle biopsy. Due to the rarity of HIV-associated myopathy, the prognosis and best course of treatment are not well established and rely on data from small case series. It is prudent to begin treatment by eliminating myotoxic medications, such as statins. In one case series ($n = 13$), over half of those treated with corticosteroids attained complete remission and were able to discontinue therapy after a mean of 9 months [32]. The remainder of the patients improved over months to years. A case series from Africa ($n = 14$) showed similar steroid responsiveness [33]. Based on the treatment of polymyositis in HIV-uninfected individuals, other immunomodulatory treatments such as IVIG can also be considered. Steroid-sparing agents, such as methotrexate and azathioprine, have also been used. However, there is concern over their immunosuppressant toxicity and little evidence of efficacy [32].

Other even less common primary muscle disorders in HIV have been reported in the literature. For example, HIV-associated myopathy has been described as a manifestation of IRIS [34]. Zidovudine (AZT) has been associated with a toxic myopathy,[35] which can manifest as either fixed weakness or exercise intolerance. This disorder, which resolves upon cessation of the drug, was mainly associated with high-dose AZT and is rare today. Inclusion body myositis and polymyalgia rheumatica have also been reported in HIV-infected individuals, but it is unclear if there is any association [36,37].

Painful disorders of joint and bone

A common cause of joint pain in HIV is AVN [20]. AVN, also known as osteonecrosis, is more common among HIV-infected individuals. It occurs most commonly in the portion of bones adjacent to joints, likely due to a predilection for vascular insufficiency in such areas. AVN is most common in the hip but may also arise in other locations and may involve multiple joints in some cases. AVN commonly presents with pain, particularly with weight bearing on the affected joint. Pain at rest may be a feature of more advanced disease. Although

there were reports of AVN prior to the current ART treatment era, the prevalence now appears to be higher [38]. Thus, both ART and HIV itself likely contribute to the development of AVN. Proposed mechanisms include metabolic effects of ART on bone, and an HIV-induced proinflammatory state that may promote bone resorption or vascular insufficiency to bone via atherosclerosis or thromboemboli. Diagnosis of AVN is made with MRI. Medical treatments have limited utility, and in cases where AVN is severe and causing significant functional impairment, surgery is often necessary.

Mild, intermittent, polyarticular arthralgias involving the knees, shoulders, and metacarpophalangeal joints have been described as a common symptom in HIV, although it is unclear whether this is a specific syndrome [3]. An association between certain forms of inflammatory arthritis and HIV has been reported. Reiter's syndrome is a triad of arthritis, uveitis, and urethritis that occurs as a reaction to infection, most often a gastrointestinal or sexually transmitted infection. A high prevalence of Reiter's syndrome in HIV has been reported in some studies, mainly prior to the current treatment era, although the association may be spurious due to high rates of sexually transmitted infections in these populations [39]. The prevalence of psoriatic arthritis in HIV may also be increased [40]. Psoriatic arthritis presents with pain and stiffness in joints, particularly in the morning, and psoriatic skin lesions. Inflammatory arthritis may be accompanied by tendonitis [41]. Treatment of inflammatory arthritis may require disease-modifying antirheumatic drugs, typically in consultation with a rheumatologist.

In addition to the disorders described above, joint pains in an HIV-infected individual may be due to disorders unrelated to HIV such as autoimmune disease (e.g., lupus) or other infections (e.g., disseminated gonococcus). Osteoarthritis is common among older people in the general population and will likely become increasingly common among HIV-infected individuals as the population ages (see Chapter 1, epidemiology). Osteoarthritis is characterized by pain with movement of the affected joint and commonly involves fingers, knees, hips, and the spine. Radiographic evidence of degenerative changes in symptomatic joints supports the diagnosis. Pain from osteoarthritis is typically managed with a combination of exercise therapy and NSAIDS. Persistent pain may require referral to a specialist, such as a rheumatologist, and in cases of severe disease, a surgeon for consideration of joint replacement.

Isolated or generalized aches and pains in bones are most often nonspecific symptoms, but less commonly may be due to osteomalacia. Osteomalacia results from severe vitamin D deficiency[42] and has also been reported as a side effect of tenofovir accompanied by hypophosphatemia and renal toxicity [43]. Vitamin D deficiency and insufficiency are very common among HIV-infected individuals although typically not of the severity required to cause osteomalacia. This high prevalence is in part attributable to demographics and lifestyle factors although vitamin D deficiency has also been linked to nonnucleoside reverse transcriptase inhibitor use, particularly efavirenz [44]. The importance of vitamin D in bone metabolism is undisputed. Links between vitamin D and several other musculoskeletal conditions have been postulated including muscle weakness and osteoarthritis [42]. This has not been studied specifically in HIV. Vitamin D deficiency is detected with measurement of serum 25-hydroxy vitamin D. Osteomalacia is diagnosed with plain radiographs. Vitamin D deficiency and osteomalacia are treated with oral vitamin D supplementation, usually with calcium.

Other chronic musculoskeletal pain syndromes

Several musculoskeletal pain syndromes that do not fit cleanly into the aforementioned categories have been described. We present three of the most common of these syndromes: chronic low back pain, chronic widespread pain including fibromyalgia, and myofascial pain syndrome.

Chronic low back pain

Chronic low back pain may be caused by a number of different etiologies. When a structural cause is apparent, it is usually a combination of degenerative disc disease, bony changes such as osteophytes, and ligamentous hypertrophy, which combine to cause narrowing of the spinal canal. When such narrowing involves the neural foramina, nerve root irritation and/or compression may occur, resulting in radiculopathy. Radiculopathy classically presents with asymmetric neuropathic pain radiating in the distribution of a nerve root. For example, S1 radiculopathy causes pain radiating into the buttock, posterior thigh, calf and into the foot and is often referred to as "sciatica." As radiculopathy progresses, focal neurologic deficits may occur including numbness and weakness in the nerve root distribution. Patients with clear radicular signs and symptoms require neuroimaging, preferably with MRI [45]. Those with an abnormal neurologic examination are usually referred for surgical evaluation. This evaluation is done emergently if there are acute neurologic deficits.

The patient with chronic axial low back pain without radiation or focal neurologic signs or symptoms is quite different. This syndrome, which is also referred to as chronic nonspecific low back pain, is a complex biopsychosocial disorder, which may overlap with or evolve into other chronic widespread pain syndromes, such as fibromyalgia [46]. Chronic nonspecific low back pain is exceedingly common in the general population and is very costly due to treatment, lost productivity, and disability [26].

In a patient presenting with chronic low back pain without neurologic signs or symptoms, neuroimaging such as MRI is of questionable benefit. Quite often no clear etiology is found. Even when abnormalities are discovered, they must be interpreted with caution since many asymptomatic patients also have MRI abnormalities in the lumbar spine [47]. Lumbar MRI in general should be reserved for those patients in whom a potentially serious pathology such as infection, cancer, or vertebral fracture is suspected. History of cancer, unexpected weight loss, fevers, recent bacterial infection, intravenous drug use, significant trauma, osteoporosis, and immunocompromised state are considered "red flags" that might increase the utility of spinal imaging [26].

There is a very large evidence base for the treatment of chronic low back pain in the general population. A useful synthesis of this literature is provided by numerous recent meta-analyses, systematic reviews, and guidelines, including several Cochrane reviews (available at www.back.cochrane.org). Regardless of the etiology, initial treatment involves promoting self-care, including advising the patient to remain active, and providing evidence-based, patient-oriented reading material on back care [48]. Pharmacologic therapy may be added when pain is more severe. The risks and benefits of specific medications must be weighed for each patient on an individual basis, and all therapies should be monitored for efficacy and discontinued if they do not provide benefit. First-line pharmacologic treatments are usually acetaminophen and nonsteroidal anti-inflammatory drugs (NSAIDS), in conjunction with physical therapy [48]. In patients who do not respond to these agents, a number of other classes of medications may be tried. Among antidepressants, duloxetine, a serotonin–norepinephrine reuptake inhibitor (SNRI) is FDA approved for chronic musculoskeletal pain including chronic low back pain [49]. The tricyclic antidepressants and muscle relaxants also have limited evidence for efficacy,[50,51] but must be used with caution and in carefully selected patients due to their sedating side effects. Similarly, there is little evidence as to the efficacy of benzodiazepines and opioids[52] and significant known risks; opioids are discussed in detail in Chapters 10 and 11.

Nonpharmacologic options should be offered to all HIV-infected patients with chronic low back pain and are often more effective than pharmacologic therapies. Evidence-based treatments for chronic low back pain include spinal manipulation, various exercise and rehabilitative therapies, massage, yoga, acupuncture, cognitive behavioral therapy, and relaxation techniques [48]. For a more detailed description of the rationale for and role of nonpharmacologic therapies in chronic pain, see Chapter 10. A theme common to many of the effective treatments is that they contain some combination of psychological and physical intervention. For example, "low back pain schools" are evidence based and combine coping techniques with stretching and strengthening exercises. In practice, most traditional healthcare settings will not have all of these treatment modalities

available, particularly for patients without the means to pay for them independently. Thus, the particular modality chosen will depend on local resources. While often performed in clinical practice, the evidence base for interventional and surgical treatment for chronic nonspecific low back pain is very limited, and these therapies are not generally recommended [53]. This is particularly relevant in HIV patients, in whom systemic Cushingoid features have developed in patients on protease inhibitors following local steroid injections [54].

Chronic widespread pain and fibromyalgia

Chronic widespread pain is defined as pain on both sides of the body and pain in the axial skeleton for more than 3 months [55]. One of the most common types of chronic widespread pain is fibromyalgia. Fibromyalgia is distinguished from other widespread pain by its associated symptoms, which include fatigue, waking unrefreshed, and cognitive difficulty [28,56]. Pain may be migratory and multifocal, and physical examination is usually normal except for muscle tenderness, which may be more noticeable at certain tender points in the torso and limbs. The prevalence of fibromyalgia in HIV is unknown, but one study demonstrated a median of five pain locations in an HIV-infected population, suggesting that it may be common [6]. Guidelines recommend that fibromyalgia be diagnosed promptly in the primary care setting based on the classic clinical presentation. A simple diagnostic evaluation to exclude other causes should include a thorough physical examination, serologies (complete blood count, erythrocyte sedimentation rate, C reactive protein, and thyroid stimulating hormone), with further diagnostic testing only if this evaluation suggests some underlying condition (e.g., rheumatoid factor if joint inflammation is present on exam). Prompt diagnosis of fibromyalgia is important as it allows patients to avoid unnecessary diagnostic testing and specialist referrals and receive prompt initiation of treatment.

In most cases, the pain of fibromyalgia cannot be attributed to local tissue damage or inflammation. However, recent studies have found a higher prevalence of small fiber neuropathy in fibromyalgia patients compared to controls [21,22]. Small fiber neuropathy is defined as a neuropathy that exclusively involves small nerve fibers, which are responsible for pain and temperature sensation. The classic symptoms of small fiber neuropathy are hyperalgesia and dysesthesia in a stocking and glove distribution. The clinical implications of the association between fibromyalgia and small fiber neuropathy is not yet clear, but it may be that small fiber neuropathy is the underlying cause of fibromyalgia-like symptoms in some patients. This is particularly interesting in the context of HIV, where peripheral neuropathy, including small fiber neuropathy, is very common [57]. Thus, HIV-infected patients with fibromyalgia should have a careful clinical assessment for signs of small fiber neuropathy including decreased distal pinprick and temperature sensation. Neurologic referral can be considered for confirmation of the diagnosis. However, treatments for pain associated with small fiber neuropathy are very similar to those used for fibromyalgia, and so definitive diagnosis may not significantly change management.

The treatment of fibromyalgia is similar to that of chronic low back pain in that it requires recognition of the biopsychosocial aspects of the disorder. Patients with HIV have by definition experienced a chronic, serious illness, and the subsequent development of fibromyalgia can easily be interpreted catastrophically as an ill omen for their overall health status. Effort must be made to replace this perception with an active patient-driven management plan including goals for treatment outcomes. This should include simple measures such as encouragement of a health-promoting lifestyle, maintenance of as normal a level of function as possible, and a plan for a graduated exercise program [58]. In the authors' clinical practice, many patients view their pain as inseparable from HIV and are helped by the social support of regular interaction with peers who are experiencing similar symptoms.

Pharmacologic therapy for fibromyalgia should also be considered in conjunction with psychologically focused treatments, due to the high prevalence of psychiatric comorbidity in fibromyalgia [59]. As discussed in Chapter 10 on treatment, comorbid psychiatric illnesses such as mood disorders should be aggressively treated.

In addition, there are three FDA-approved pharmacologic treatments for fibromyalgia: duloxetine and milnacipran, which are SNRIs, and pregabalin, which is an antiepileptic [60]. Comorbidities should be carefully considered while choosing an agent. SNRIs are relatively contraindicated in liver disease, and pregabalin is renally excreted and must be dose-adjusted in patients with renal insufficiency.

Myofascial pain syndrome

Myofascial pain syndrome is a common muscular pain syndrome characterized by the presence of taut bands and painful trigger points within the muscle [29]. The pain of myofascial pain syndrome is typically focal or regional, as opposed to the more generalized pain of fibromyalgia, although there is overlap between these syndromes. The patient may report a history of trauma or repetitive use of the affected muscles. Physical examination should include palpation of the affected muscles to identify taut bands and painful trigger points within these bands. Range of motion should also be assessed, as pain with stretching of affected muscles is characteristic. Evidence guiding the best treatment of myofascial pain syndrome is scant although most authors advocate similar treatment modalities. Physical therapy is recommended and involves targeted stretching often preceded by the application of a topical cooling agent (e.g., ethyl chloride). Trigger point injections with saline, local anesthetic, and botulinum toxin have been reported to have similar efficacy to needle insertion without injection, leading to the hypothesis that the disruption of the trigger point with the needle is the therapeutic part of the procedure. The prevalence of myofascial pain syndrome in HIV is unknown.

Conclusion

Chronic musculoskeletal pain is common among HIV-infected patients and is a challenging problem for clinicians involved in the long-term care of this population. Such pain may be caused by a specific HIV-associated condition such as myopathy or AVN, or it may be due to a condition that is not clearly related to HIV, such as osteoarthritis. In addition, many HIV patients experience other less well-defined chronic musculoskeletal pain syndromes such as low back pain, widespread pain including fibromyalgia, and regional myofascial pain syndromes. Diagnostic evaluation varies based on the particular syndrome and the suspected etiology, but a general guiding principle is to perform the simplest diagnostic workup that will reasonably exclude serious causative disorders requiring specific treatment. This approach will minimize excessive testing and medicalization of the patient, which can be counterproductive to the goal of maintaining as normal functioning as possible. Although management of chronic musculoskeletal pain in HIV will be tailored to the individual, general principles include combination of pharmacological interventions such as NSAIDS or SNRIs, with physical modalities designed to prevent or reverse deconditioning, and psychological modalities designed to enhance coping.

References

1 Perry, B.A., Westfall, A.O., Molony, E. *et al.* (2013) Characteristics of an ambulatory palliative care clinic for HIV-infected patients. *Journal of Palliative Medicine*, **16** (8), 934–937.

2 Institute of Medicine Committee on Advancing Pain Research, Care, and Education (2011) *Relieving Pain in America: A Blueprint for Transforming Prevention, Care, Education, and Research*. The National Academies Press, Washington, DC.

3 Lawson, E. & Walker-Bone, K. (2012) The changing spectrum of rheumatic disease in HIV infection. *British Medical Bulletin*, **103** (1), 203–221.

4 Zhang, X., Li, H., Li, T., Zhang, F. & Han, Y. (2007) Distinctive rheumatic manifestations in 98 patients with human immunodeficiency virus infection in China. *Journal of Rheumatology*, **34** (8), 1760–1764.

5 Kole, A.K., Roy, R. & Kole, D.C. (2013) Musculoskeletal and rheumatological disorders in HIV infection: experience in a tertiary referral center. *Indian Journal of Sexually Transmitted Diseases*, **34** (2), 107–112.

6 Miaskowski, C., Penko, J.M., Guzman, D., Mattson, J.E., Bangsberg, D.R. & Kushel, M.B. (2011) Occurrence and characteristics of chronic pain in a community-based cohort of indigent adults living with HIV infection. *The Journal of Pain*, **12** (9), 1004–1016.

7 Lee, K.A., Gay, C., Portillo, C.J. *et al.* (2009) Symptom experience in HIV-infected adults: a function of demographic and clinical characteristics. *Journal of Pain and Symptom Management*, **38** (6), 882–893.

8 Johnson, A., Condon, K.D., Mapas-Dimaya, A.C. *et al.* (2012) Report of an HIV clinic-based pain management program and utilization of health status and health service by HIV patients. *Journal of Opioid Management*, **8** (1), 17–27.

9 Seidman, R., Peress, N.S. & Nuovo, G.J. (1994) In situ detection of polymerase chain reaction-amplified HIV-1 nucleic acids in skeletal muscle in patients with myopathy. *Modern Pathology*, **7** (3), 369–375.

10 Bruera, D., Luna, N., David, D.O., Bergoglio, L.M. & Zamudio, J. (2003) Decreased bone mineral density in HIV-infected patients is independent of antiretroviral therapy. *AIDS*, **17** (13), 1917–1923.

11 Dalakas, M.C., Illa, I., Pezeshkpour, G.H., Laukaitis, J.P., Cohen, B. & Griffin, J.L. (1990) Mitochondrial myopathy caused by long-term zidovudine therapy. *New England Journal of Medicine*, **322** (16), 1098–1105.

12 Sathekge, M., Maes, A., Kgomo, M., Stolz, A., Ankrah, A. & Van de Wiele, C. (2010) Evaluation of glucose uptake by skeletal muscle tissue and subcutaneous fat in HIV-infected patients with and without lipodystrophy using FDG-PET. *Nuclear Medicine Communications*, **31** (4), 311–314.

13 Brown, T.T., McComsey, G.A., King, M.S., Qaqish, R.B., Bernstein, B.M. & da Silva, B.A. (2009) Loss of bone mineral density after antiretroviral therapy initiation, independent of antiretroviral regimen. *Journal of Acquired Immune Deficiency Syndromes*, **51** (5), 554–561.

14 Duvivier, C., Kolta, S., Assoumou, L. *et al.* (2009) Greater decrease in bone mineral density with protease inhibitor regimens compared with nonnucleoside reverse transcriptase inhibitor regimens in HIV-1 infected naive patients. *AIDS*, **23** (7), 817–824.

15 Wearing, S.C., Hennig, E.M., Byrne, N.M., Steele, J.R. & Hills, A.P. (2006) Musculoskeletal disorders associated with obesity: a biomechanical perspective. *Obesity Reviews*, **7** (3), 239–250.

16 Toda, Y., Segal, N., Toda, T., Morimoto, T. & Ogawa, R. (2000) Lean body mass and body fat distribution in participants with chronic low back pain. *Archives of Internal Medicine*, **160** (21), 3265–3269.

17 Brenchley, J.M., Price, D.A. & Douek, D.C. (2006) HIV disease: Fallout from a mucosal catastrophe? *Nature Immunology*, **7** (3), 235–239.

18 Deeks, S.G. (2011) HIV infection, inflammation, immunosenescence, and aging. *Annual Review of Medicine*, **62**, 141–155.

19 Watkins, L.R. & Maier, S.F. (2000) The pain of being sick: Implications of immune-to-brain communication for understanding pain. *Annual Review of Psychology*, **51**, 29–57.

20 Mehta, P., Nelson, M., Brand, A. & Boag, F. (2013) Avascular necrosis in HIV. *Rheumatology International*, **33** (1), 235–238.

21 Oaklander, A.L., Herzog, Z.D., Downs, H.M. & Klein, M.M. (2013) Objective evidence that small-fiber polyneuropathy underlies some illnesses currently labeled as fibromyalgia. *Pain*, **154** (11), 2310–2316.

22 Uceyler, N., Zeller, D., Kahn, A.K. *et al.* (2013) Small fibre pathology in patients with fibromyalgia syndrome. *Brain*, **136** (Pt 6), 1857–1867.

23 Craig, A.D. (2002) How do you feel? Interoception: the sense of the physiological condition of the body. *Nature Reviews Neuroscience*, **3** (8), 655–666.

24 Leeuw, M., Goossens, M.E., Linton, S.J., Crombez, G., Boersma, K. & Vlaeyen, J.W. (2007) The fear-avoidance model of musculoskeletal pain: current state of scientific evidence. *Journal of Behavioral Medicine*, **30** (1), 77–94.

25 Chou, R. & Shekelle, P. (2010) Will this patient develop persistent disabling low back pain? *JAMA*, **303** (13), 1295–1302.

26 Morlion, B. (2013) Chronic low back pain: pharmacological, interventional and surgical strategies. *Nature Reviews Neurology*, **9** (8), 462–473.

27 Lormeau, C., Falgarone, G., Roulot, D. & Boissier, M.C. (2006) Rheumatologic manifestations of chronic hepatitis C infection. *Joint, Bone, Spine*, **73** (6), 633–638.

28 Wolfe, F., Smythe, H.A., Yunus, M.B. *et al.* (1990) The American College of Rheumatology 1990 criteria for the classification of fibromyalgia. Report of the multicenter criteria committee. *Arthritis and Rheumatism*, **33** (2), 160–172.

29 Giamberardino, M.A., Affaitati, G., Fabrizio, A. & Costantini, R. (2011) Myofascial pain syndromes and their evaluation. *Best Practice & Research. Clinical Rheumatology*, **25** (2), 185–198.

30 Manfredi, R., Motta, R., Patrono, D., Calza, L., Chiodo, F. & Boni, P. (2002) A prospective case–control survey of laboratory markers of skeletal muscle damage during HIV disease and antiretroviral therapy. *AIDS*, **16** (14), 1969–1971.

31 Simpson, D.M. & Bender, A.N. (1988) Human immunodeficiency virus-associated myopathy: analysis of 11 patients. *Annals of Neurology*, **24** (1), 79–84.

32 Johnson, R.W., Williams, F.M., Kazi, S., Dimachkie, M.M. & Reveille, J.D. (2003) Human immunodeficiency virus-associated polymyositis: a longitudinal study of outcome. *Arthritis and Rheumatism*, **49** (2), 172–178.

33 Heckmann, J.M., Pillay, K., Hearn, A.P. & Kenyon, C. (2010) Polymyositis in African HIV-infected subjects. *Neuromuscular Disorders*, **20** (11), 735–739.

34 Sellier, P., Monsuez, J.J., Evans, J. *et al.* (2000) Human immunodeficiency virus-associated polymyositis during immune restoration with combination antiretroviral therapy. *American Journal of Medicine*, **109** (6), 510–512.

35 Cupler, E.J., Danon, M.J., Jay, C., Hench, K., Ropka, M. & Dalakas, M.C. (1995) Early features of zidovudine-associated myopathy: histopathological findings and clinical correlations. *Acta Neuropathologica*, **90** (1), 1–6.

36 Cupler, E.J., Leon-Monzon, M., Miller, J., Semino-Mora, C., Anderson, T.L. & Dalakas, M.C. (1996) Inclusion body myositis in HIV-1 and HTLV-1 infected patients. *Brain*, **119** (Pt 6), 1887–1893.

37 Solinger, A.M. & Hess, E.V. (1993) Rheumatic diseases and AIDS – is the association real? *Journal of Rheumatology*, **20** (4), 678–683.

38 Calza, L., Manfredi, R., Mastroianni, A. & Chiodo, F. (2001) Osteonecrosis and highly active antiretroviral therapy during HIV infection: report of a series and literature review. *AIDS Patient Care and STDs*, **15** (7), 385–389.

39 Hochberg, M.C., Fox, R., Nelson, K.E. & Saah, A. (1990) HIV infection is not associated with Reiter's syndrome: data from the Johns Hopkins Multicenter AIDS Cohort Study. *AIDS*, **4** (11), 1149–1151.

40 Buskila, D., Gladman, D.D., Langevitz, P., Bookman, A.A., Fanning, M. & Salit, I.E. (1990) Rheumatologic manifestations of infection with the human immunodeficiency virus (HIV). *Clinical and Experimental Rheumatology*, **8** (6), 567–573.

41 Tehranzadeh, J., Ter-Oganesyan, R.R. & Steinbach, L.S. (2004) Musculoskeletal disorders associated with HIV infection and AIDS. part II: non-infectious musculoskeletal conditions. *Skeletal Radiology*, **33** (6), 311–320.

42 Holick, M.F. (2007) Vitamin D deficiency. *New England Journal of Medicine*, **357** (3), 266–281.

43 Woodward, C.L., Hall, A.M., Williams, I.G. *et al.* (2009) Tenofovir-associated renal and bone toxicity. *HIV Medicine*, **10** (8), 482–487.

44 Kwan, C.K., Eckhardt, B., Baghdadi, J. & Aberg, J.A. (2012) Hyperparathyroidism and complications associated with vitamin D deficiency in HIV-infected adults in New York City, New York. *AIDS Research and Human Retroviruses*, **28** (9), 1025–1032.

45 Chou, R., Qaseem, A., Owens, D.K., Shekelle, P. & Clinical Guidelines Committee of the American College of Physicians (2011) Diagnostic imaging for low back pain: advice for high-value health care from the American College of Physicians. *Annals of Internal Medicine*, **154** (3), 181–189.

46 Kindler, L.L., Jones, K.D., Perrin, N. & Bennett, R.M. (2010) Risk factors predicting the development of widespread pain from chronic back or neck pain. *The Journal of Pain*, **11** (12), 1320–1328.

47 Jensen, M.C., Brant-Zawadzki, M.N., Obuchowski, N., Modic, M.T., Malkasian, D. & Ross, J.S. (1994) Magnetic resonance imaging of the lumbar spine in people without back pain. *New England Journal of Medicine*, **331** (2), 69–73.

48 Chou, R., Qaseem, A., Snow, V. *et al.* (2007) Diagnosis and treatment of low back pain: a joint clinical practice guideline from the American College of Physicians and the American Pain Society. *Annals of Internal Medicine*, **147** (7), 478–491.

49 Skljarevski, V., Desaiah, D., Liu-Seifert, H. *et al.* (2010) Efficacy and safety of duloxetine in patients with chronic low back pain. *Spine (Phila Pa 1976)*, **35** (13), E578–E585.

50 Staiger, T.O., Gaster, B., Sullivan, M.D. & Deyo, R.A. (2003) Systematic review of antidepressants in the treatment of chronic low back pain. *Spine (Phila Pa 1976)*, **28** (22), 2540–2545.

51 van Tulder, M.W., Touray, T., Furlan, A.D., Solway, S., Bouter, L.M. & Cochrane Back Review Group (2003) Muscle relaxants for nonspecific low back pain: a systematic review within the framework of the cochrane collaboration. *Spine (Phila Pa 1976)*, **28** (17), 1978–1992.

52 Chou, R., Huffman, L.H., American Pain Society & American College of Physicians (2007) Medications for acute and chronic low back pain: a review of the evidence for an American Pain Society/American College of Physicians clinical practice guideline. *Annals of Internal Medicine*, **147** (7), 505–514.

53 Chou, R., Loeser, J.D., Owens, D.K. *et al.* (2009) Interventional therapies, surgery, and interdisciplinary rehabilitation for low back pain: an evidence-based clinical practice guideline from the American Pain Society. *Spine (Phila Pa 1976)*, **34** (10), 1066–1077.

54 Hyle, E.P., Wood, B.R., Backman, E.S. *et al.* (2013) High frequency of hypothalamic-pituitary-adrenal axis dysfunction after local corticosteroid injection in HIV-infected patients on protease inhibitor therapy. *Journal of Acquired Immune Deficiency Syndromes*, **63** (5), 602–608.

55 Hunt, I.M., Silman, A.J., Benjamin, S., McBeth, J. & Macfarlane, G.J. (1999) The prevalence and associated features of chronic widespread pain in the community using the 'Manchester' definition of chronic widespread pain. *Rheumatology (Oxford)*, **38** (3), 275–279.

56 Wolfe, F., Clauw, D.J., Fitzcharles, M.A. *et al.* (2010) The American College of Rheumatology

preliminary diagnostic criteria for fibromyalgia and measurement of symptom severity. *Arthritis Care & Research (Hoboken)*, **62** (5), 600–610.

57 Morgello, S., Estanislao, L., Simpson, D. *et al.* (2004) HIV-associated distal sensory polyneuropathy in the era of highly active antiretroviral therapy: the Manhattan HIV Brain Bank. *Archives of Neurology*, **61** (4), 546–551.

58 Fitzcharles, M.A., Ste-Marie, P.A., Goldenberg, D.L. *et al.* (2013) 2012 Canadian guidelines for the diagnosis and management of fibromyalgia syndrome: executive summary. *Pain Research & Management*, **18** (3), 119–126.

59 Arnold, L.M., Hudson, J.I., Keck, P.E., Auchenbach, M.B., Javaras, K.N. & Hess, E.V. (2006) Comorbidity of fibromyalgia and psychiatric disorders. *Journal of Clinical Psychiatry*, **67** (8), 1219–1225.

60 Hauser, W., Petzke, F. & Sommer, C. (2010) Comparative efficacy and harms of duloxetine, milnacipran, and pregabalin in fibromyalgia syndrome. *The Journal of Pain*, **11** (6), 505–521.

CHAPTER 5

Headache in HIV

Olga Fermo and Jason D. Rosenberg

Department of Neurology, Johns Hopkins University, Baltimore, MD, USA

Headache is the most commonly reported pain condition among patients with HIV [1]. Headaches are classified as either *secondary*, with pain *symptoms* arising from underlying diseases or *primary syndromes* such as tension type, migraine, and cluster that are otherwise idiopathic and fortunately far more common than their more sinister cousins [2]. Migraines, by virtue of being both highly prevalent, affecting approximately 12% of the US adult population, and severe enough to cause cessation of normal activities – even to the point of bed rest – make up the bulk of headache-related disability,[3] even among patients with HIV, and thus will be the focus of this chapter.

Those living with stable HIV infection appear to suffer from primary headaches at a similar rate to the general population, again with migraines making up the bulk of the disability burden [1,4–6]. Infection with HIV could potentially interact with headache disorders in a variety of ways. HIV itself could affect the prevalence or severity of any given primary headache syndrome, whether preexisting prior to infection or *de novo* – theoretically, by inducing changes in glutamate expression, lipid distribution, or cytokine profiles [7]. There could be links through shared comorbidities, an example being psychiatric disorders, known to be more prevalent in the HIV population as well as risk factors for migraine expression [8]. Further, the medications used for treatment might well affect headaches themselves and certainly impact treatment choices due to potential drug interactions with ARVs (antiretrovirals).

In terms of specific HIV-related secondary headaches, HIV itself can cause headaches, and so can the opportunistic diseases as well as the treatment of infections [4–6]. Only in the immunocompromised, with CD4 counts less than 200 cells/µL, do secondary headaches assume a disproportionate burden compared with the non-HIV-infected population, opportunistic diseases such as toxoplasmosis, cryptococcal meningitis, lymphoma, and encephalitis become more of a concern [1].

Workup of a headache complaint

Primary headaches should not – and in fact *cannot* – be diagnosed by international criteria unless secondary causes have been considered and effectively ruled out [2]. Diagnosis involves "ruling in" for clinical criteria, with the caveat that the disease is "not attributable to another disorder." The warning signs ("red flags") of dangerous secondary headaches can be remembered by the mnemonic HPAIN, as per Table 5.1 [9]. In particular, a change of pattern – anything new, sudden ("thunderclap"), or unusually severe should prompt a workup.

In a well-looking patient with a new headache presentation but no focal complaints, the eye exam assumes great importance – acuity, pupillary response, visual field screening (to clinically evaluate the occipital lobes), and especially the fundoscopic exam. All patients with headache should be evaluated for optic disc swelling and for the presence of normal spontaneous central retinal venous pulsations to screen for high intracranial pressure.

Chronic Pain and HIV: A Practical Approach, First Edition.
Edited by Jessica S. Merlin, Peter A. Selwyn, Glenn J. Treisman and Angela G. Giovanniello.
© 2016 John Wiley & Sons, Ltd. Published 2016 by John Wiley & Sons, Ltd.

Table 5.1   HPAIN – headache "red flags [9]."

Host factors:	Age >50
(Conferring increased risk for an	Pregnancy
underlying disease)	Cancer
	Immunosuppression (e.g., CD4 < 200 cells/µL)
	Serious medical comorbidities
Pattern:	Constant
	Worsening or progressing
	Thunderclap (maximum intensity reached in seconds)
	New quality (compared to previous headache)
	New level of pain ("worst of life")
Associated symptoms:	Fever
	Neck stiffness
	Weight loss
	Malaise
	Rash
	Temporal artery tenderness, jaw claudication
Increased/provoked by:	Head trauma/cervical trauma or manipulation
	Valsalva or cough
	Exertion
	Standing
	Sleep
	Intercourse
Neurological symptoms or signs:	Seizure
	Weakness
	Rapid numbness
	Atypical visual symptoms
	Papilledema

If there are no HPAIN red flags, and the neurologic and eye exam is normal (or explainable if abnormal), *and* the patient meets the definition for migraine or tension-type headache (TTH, defined below), further diagnostic workup is typically not indicated and empiric treatment begun; as a rule, imaging is not warranted for uncomplicated headache presentations [10,11]. If these conditions cannot be met, there is heightened worry for an underlying condition causing secondary headache and a workup should proceed, tailored to the nature of the red flags.

Secondary headaches

A review of the hundreds of secondary headaches is beyond the scope of this chapter, but they are detailed in the International Classification of Headache Disorders (ICHD) [2]. Having seen that the diagnosis of primary headache starts with eliminating secondary causes, the next section addresses some key conditions pertinent to the HIV population.

Headaches related to infections

Headache is usually the first symptom of an intracranial infection, but it is the accompanying fever, focal neurologic sign, altered mental status, or seizure (i.e., HPAIN warning signs) that raises concern [2], the difference in the HIV population being a lower threshold of suspicion, and a wider array of infectious possibilities. Again, the majority of HIV positive patients with headaches have primary headache [4,6,8], and those with isolated headaches are no more likely to have opportunistic infection (OI) or CSF pleocytosis than those without headaches [8].

A lymphocyte-predominant meningoencephalitis (sometimes fulminant) is a rare but possible presentation of primary HIV infection, or of antiretroviral treatment interruption [12]. A relentless, dull, bilateral headache is sometimes attributed to ongoing HIV infection itself, provided OIs have been ruled out, but it is very difficult to distinguish this entity from primary TTH. To be "definitely" attributed to HIV infection, the headache must develop at the onset of HIV infection, and worsen with disease severity or improve with disease treatment [2].

Unknown to most patients (and many healthcare providers) sinusitis almost never causes *recurring* headaches, especially without other symptoms of infection; "sinus headache" is a misnomer, being nearly always a migraine [13].

Complications of infections
Persistent postinfectious headache
For reasons poorly understood, persistent headaches can develop at the time of an intracranial infection (meningitis, encephalitis, and ventriculitis) and continue despite resolution of the inciting illness. Workup with imaging (including nuclear medication studies) and lumbar punctures (LPs) will be unrevealing [2]. Treatment is symptom management.

Septic thrombosis
This is a very rare complication of bacterial infection, but given the high mortality rate it is a "do-not-miss" diagnosis. Infections of the face, paranasal sinuses, middle ear, mastoid, and meninges can cause subsequent septic thrombosis, most commonly in the cavernous sinus, but also lateral sinus and superior sagittal sinus. Most patients are terribly ill, with other signs or symptoms, but in all comers, headache is found to be the initial symptom [14].

Immune reconstitution inflammatory syndrome (IRIS)
The immune reconstitution inflammatory syndrome (IRIS) is defined by clinical symptoms consistent with an inflammatory process in a patient with recent initiation of antiretroviral therapy, who has a recovering CD4 count and decreasing viral load. Several infections that present with CNS manifestations are associated with IRIS. Any combination of headache, meningismus, seizure, and neurologic focality can be caused by cryptococcal or mycobacterial IRIS, or less commonly by IRIS due to progressive multifocal leukoencephalopathy (PML), toxoplasmosis, HSV, VZV, or parvovirus 19. There are several ways to distinguish IRIS from active infection. With cryptococcal IRIS, opening pressure and CSF WBC will be higher (>20) than with infection, and CSF cultures will be negative. The white matter lesions of PML IRIS will enhance with contrast compared to active PML [15].

Headaches related to the cerebral vasculature

Reversible cerebral vasoconstriction syndrome (RCVS)
Reversible cerebral vasoconstriction syndrome (RCVS), a disorder of diffuse, multifocal narrowing of the cerebral arteries is an important "do-not-miss" cause of secondary headache. This self-limited syndrome classically presents with recurrent thunderclap headaches mimicking subarachnoid hemorrhage (seldom ignored by patients or clinicians) and sometimes with features of migraine. Mild cases may go unrecognized, but at its worst strokes, brain edema or even death can result. Over half of cases are linked to identifiable risk factors, including the use of marijuana or recreational drugs but also pregnancy, use of SSRIs, triptans, cyclophosphamide, and decongestants [16].

Ischemic and hemorrhagic stroke
Evidence suggests that HIV patients treated with highly active antiretroviral therapy (HAART) are at a higher risk for ischemic and hemorrhagic stroke, both of which can be associated with acute headache, particularly the latter, but nearly always with focal neurological symptoms. Several mechanisms have been

proposed for this increased risk of cerebrovascular disease, including accelerated atherosclerosis due to HAART, vasculitis caused by secondary infections, and endothelial dysfunction caused by HIV itself [17].

Posterior reversible encephalopathy syndrome (PRES)

Posterior reversible encephalopathy syndrome (PRES) may be encountered in an ill HIV-infected patient with headaches; typically, there will be other signs including altered mental status, abnormal neurologic exam, and/or seizure. While classically a clinical and radiographic diagnosis in patients with severe hypertension, case reports have described advanced HIV patients with triggers of end-stage renal disease, hypercalcemia, disseminated infections of blastomycosis, tuberculosis, and varicella zoster virus (VZV), and one case where no specific cause was found [18]. There may be pathophysiological overlap with RCVS.

Iatrogenic headaches related to treatment and procedures

Medication side effects

Virtually all members of every class of antiretroviral agents can cause headache as an adverse effect. In fact, the few *exceptions* are worth noting: etravirine (NNRTI), enfuvirtide (entry inhibitor), saquinavir, and nelfinavir (protease inhibitors) [19]. Whether to alter or abandon an otherwise successful HAART regimen for a *possible* headache side effect, negatively impacting quality of life is no easy decision; even diagnostic "drug holidays" are not without risk.

Postdural puncture headache

It is not uncommon for patients with HIV to undergo diagnostic LP, often as part of a headache workup. LP itself can result in a postdural puncture headache. Nearly always a positional headache developing within a few days of an LP, it is expected to improve or even resolve with recumbency and to worsen with upright posture and Valsalva. The headache typically resolves spontaneously within 2 weeks, or more rapidly to epidural lumbar blood patch, but may persist [2]. To evaluate for this, question if the headache changed after the LP.

Medication overuse headache (MOH)

Medication overuse headache (MOH, sometimes called "rebound") is a secondary chronic daily headache (CDH, defined as having headaches 15+ days per month) that results from transformation of an episodic primary headache (typically migraine) *because of* excessive (more than 2–3 days/week) use of analgesics. The history is one of escalating headache frequency in the setting of mounting pill usage, occurring over weeks to months; the longer time course distinguishes "rebound" from "recurrence" of a partially treated single headache attack. The drugs most implicated in MOH are the butalbital compounds and opiates, but combination analgesics (e.g., with caffeine), triptans, and even NSAIDs may be causative as well. Headache features are variable, but there is a characteristic reduced responsiveness to acute treatments. Critically, this relentless CDH can occur even when pain-relieving drugs are used for nonheadache pain, placing chronic pain patients at high risk.

Treatment of MOH involves discontinuation of the offending agent, typically with the initiation of rational headache prevention therapy. Most weans can be safely accomplished in the outpatient setting over several weeks. In a rapid wean, the offending agent is stopped abruptly, with simultaneous "bridge" treatment (discussed below) and rapid up-titration of a preventive agent. Butalbital compounds or opiates should *not* be abruptly discontinued without additional therapy to prevent withdrawal. Attempts to stop any analgesic the patient perceives as necessary is likely to produce misgivings, and many patients will initially worsen before improving; nonadherence and resumption of the offending pattern of drug use is common. Patients with a long history of overuse or psychiatric comorbidities may be best served by a hospital or inpatient interdisciplinary program [20].

MOH is far easier to prevent than to treat. Use of acute headache treatments should be limited to 2 days/week on average. The most specific medications for headache type should be chosen so that treatment is as effective as possible, reducing the need for multiple doses. Acute treatment should also be taken as early as possible in the individual headache attack to maximize responsiveness ("treat early but not often"). There should be a preventive regimen in place (discussed below) if headaches are frequent. As a rule, butalbital compounds and opiates should be avoided in headache patients, *even for the treatment of nonheadache pain* [11,20,21].

Primary headaches

Tension type

TTH is the most common headache *outside* of the medical setting; it is seldom severe enough to become a chief complaint. Pain is bilateral, nonpulsatile, mild or moderate, not aggravated by routine activity, and is not associated with nausea, vomiting or both photophobia and phonophobia [2]. Patients may describe it as a "tight band" around the head. Despite the name, there is no actual overactivity of muscles in TTH, although there may be tenderness. As the headache is "just pain," the diagnosis is made clinically by ruling out HPAIN red flags and migraines. TTH is reportedly precipitated most commonly by stress but may also be brought on by hunger, dehydration, or change in sleep patterns. NSAIDs are treatments of choice for infrequent episodic TTH; combinations of aspirin, acetaminophen, and caffeine can also be used. Triptans are ineffective, except perhaps in migraineurs. For frequent TTH, effort should be made to reduce potential triggers – regulate sleep, meals, and exercise. Physical therapy, massage, and stress reduction techniques may be useful. If warranted due to frequency, daily pharmacological preventive therapy typically employs agents used for migraines, particularly tricyclic antidepressants (TCAs) and serotonin–norepinephrine reuptake inhibitors (SNRIs) [22].

Migraine

Migraine is a neurobiological primary headache disorder characterized by at least five attacks of headache lasting 4–72 h, accompanied by various other nonheadache features. To meet the formal definition, two of the following four major criteria are required: moderate-to-severe pain, unilateral, pulsating, and aggravation by routine activity (it is the latter feature that makes them so disabling). It must also be accompanied by either nausea/vomiting or both photophobia and phonophobia [2].

Explain to patients that they have inherited a "hypersensitive brain," one susceptible if provoked to produce hangover-like headaches. In this way, a migraineur is like an asthmatic; both have chronic diseases with episodic manifestations when triggered; both are managed symptomatically and, if warranted, preventively.

Treatment of migraine attacks

The goal of acute treatment is to resolve the headache phase of the migraine attack as quickly as possible (not just the pain but also any nausea and heightened stimulus sensitivity), without headache recurrence, and with minimal side effects. Acute agents include triptans, ergot alkaloids, dopaminergic antiemetics, NSAIDs, non-opiate analgesics, and – ideally only in exceptional cases – barbiturate compounds and opiates.

NSAIDs (aspirin, ibuprofen, and naproxen sodium) or combination analgesics (acetaminophen, aspirin, and caffeine) are reasonable first-line choices for mild-to-moderate migraines. For moderate-to-severe migraine, there is uniform agreement backed by multiple double-blind, placebo-controlled trials that triptans are appropriate *first-line* agents; they are also appropriate when nonspecific agents are ineffective. Intranasal (sumatriptan and zolmitriptan), subcutaneous (sumatriptan), and newer transdermal (sumatriptan) triptan preparations are available if significant nausea precludes the oral route. While all triptans are $5HT_{1B/D/F}$ agonists, patients may find that one is preferred. Triptans can and often should be *combined* with NSAIDs (sumatriptan–naproxen is available as a single tablet) to increase effectiveness. Triptans should not be used in patients with known or suspected heart disease, stroke, *uncontrolled* hypertension, or the exceedingly uncommon hemiplegic migraine. Dihydroergotamine (DHE) in the form of nasal spray, SC, or IM (and possibly soon as an oral inhalation) is a reasonable choice for moderate-to-severe migraine if triptans have failed and there are no contraindications [23], although potential serious drug interactions with ARVs especially protease inhibitors are of concern.

Relief of nausea is an important part of migraine treatment. Fortuitously, dopaminergic antiemetics such as metoclopramide, prochlorperazine, and chlorpromazine also have pharmacological antimigraine properties [23,24]. While these are often combined with other agents to maximize relief, they can be quite effective as monotherapy, especially useful when there are contraindications to NSAIDs, triptans, or DHE (e.g., gastric ulcer, cardiac disease, and pregnancy). The class is quite useful with intravenous DHE regimen because significant nausea can otherwise limit its benefit. $5HT_3$ receptor antagonists (e.g., ondansetron, which is available as an oral dissolving generic tablet) are not useful for pain relief but may be used to control nausea with few side effects when dosed orally [23].

Nonspecific analgesics with strong potential for overuse and dependency are not recommended as part of an acute treatment regimen. The point bears repeating again here: avoid butalbital-containing analgesics (Fioricet®), butorphanol nasal spray, and parenteral or oral opiates [11,21,23].

Whatever acute treatment method is chosen, it is commonly accepted that *combined total use of all analgesics* should be kept to a maximum of 2–3 days/week (on average) as more liberal use substantially increases the risk of MOH. For headaches occurring in frequencies approaching or above this limit, preventive treatment should be revised.

Migraine rescue and bridge therapy

Rescue therapy is employed when first-line acute attack agents have failed to provide relief, or when the maximum weekly allotment of acute treatments has been used. Butalbital combinations and opiates are sometimes used for rescue once NSAIDs or migraine-specific agents have failed, but as a rule they are best avoided [25]. Opiates in particular are overutilized, despite evidence that they have no beneficial effect on migraine pathophysiology;

further, they increase sensitization to pain in migraineurs and may even reduce triptan effectiveness [26]. We recommend use of a rescue regimen containing a dopamine antagonist and antihistamine and, depending on the clinical setting, adjunctive steroids.

At times "bridge" treatment is utilized for patients where rapid treatment or treatment changes are being made, for example, when detoxifying from medication overuse in the case of rebound headaches. In these cases, we employ either round-the-clock NSAIDs (naproxen, typically) or corticosteroids (i.e., a methylprednisolone dose pack, dexamethasone, or high-dose prednisone for 7–10 days) to "hold the patient over" until a preventive effect is seen or the offending agent has been weaned [20]. Inpatient admission for repetitive parenteral DHE is another option along the same line, as discussed below under status migrainosus. Peripheral nerve branch blocks (supraorbital, greater and lesser occipital) are sometimes utilized by headache specialists for this purpose as well.

Migraine preventive therapy

In a patient with mild or infrequent attacks, acute treatment alone may suffice, but for many, daily preventive medication is required, along with lifestyle modification and nonpharmacological approaches. A successful migraine preventive regimen will reduce migraine frequency, severity, or duration, and will reduce dependence on acute therapies. Daily medication is employed when migraines are frequent, or when infrequent migraines are debilitating, significantly reducing quality of life. In clinical practice, *preventive medications are underutilized*. A good rule of thumb is to ask the patient, "Would it be worth your while to take a proven effective medication every single day – headache or not – to cut your headaches in half?" When the answer is affirmative, or "it depends," proceed. Unfortunately, no currently available migraine preventive was developed specifically for this purpose; all have been ported over to migraine management from other classes, particularly from the antihypertensives, antidepressants, and antiepileptics. A few moments of patient education regarding treatment rationale may reduce the chance for confusion and nonadherence to the offered treatment.

Antihypertensives may prove to be excellent choices in selected populations due to limited cognitive side effects and generally weight-neutral profiles. The nonsympathomimetic beta-blockers (propranolol, timolol, atenolol, metoprolol, and nadolol) have well-established efficacy, with propranolol and timolol FDA-approved for migraine prevention. Use may be limited by side effects of fatigue, weight gain, slight increased risk for diabetes, reduced exercise tolerance, and sexual side effects. Calcium channel blockers (verapamil and diltiazem), the ACE inhibitor lisinopril, and angiotensin receptor blocker candesartan may be better tolerated, the latter having few drug interactions (avoid with lithium) and strong evidence supporting its use [27].

Drugs marked for mood disorders are especially useful for prevention of migraine in HIV given higher prevalence of depression, anxiety, and neuropathic and other pain disorders. The widely used (off-label) TCAs can be a good starting point due to well-established efficacy [25]. Side effects such as fatigue, weight gain, and dry mouth can limit compliance; start low and titrate over weeks to a minimum effective dose. Nighttime amitriptyline or nortriptyline is a good starting choice when depression or insomnia is present. Morning protriptyline may be useful when stimulation is the desired side effect, or when weight gain becomes a burden.

When TCAs are not tolerated, ineffective, or there is a strong need to use a weight-neutral agent, we employ the off-label use of SNRIs; venlafaxine is "probably effective [27]." Duloxetine is not included in current guidelines, but it is well established for the treatment of neuropathic pain and fibromyalgia and we often use it when these are comorbid conditions [28].

Several antiepileptic drugs are used for migraine prevention; out of all, only valproate and topiramate are actually FDA indicated for this purpose. Valproate's potential side effects may limit the use of this otherwise efficacious drug. These commonly include weight gain, nausea, tremor, and hair loss; encephalopathy, hepatitis, pancreatitis, and agranulocytosis are rare but serious occurrences [25]. The drug is contraindicated in pregnancy and generally avoided in women of childbearing age [19]. Valproate may be a good prophylactic option for men with HIV or nonchildbearing women, as HAART interactions are few. It is also a good choice when a mood-stabilizing agent is needed, or when the patient has a concomitant seizure disorder.

Topiramate has an excellent HAART interaction profile, making it a good first-line agent [19]. The drug is especially useful when weight *loss* is a desired side effect. Some patients will report cognitive slowing and word finding difficulty, others perioral or distal tingling. These effects can be mitigated by titrating slowly to minimally effective doses (starting at 25 mg QHS, working up by 25 mg/week to 50 mg BID divided, or higher if needed and tolerated). We would not recommend using the drug in poorly controlled HIV, however, as symptoms of cognitive dulling and weight loss could be the result of either disease progression or the drug, resulting in diagnostic confusion.

Gabapentin and pregabalin are sometimes used off-label, and with little supporting data for migraine prevention [27]. Neither has significant interactions with any class of HAART medications and therefore may be useful adjunctive therapy especially when there is co-occurring neuropathic pain [19]. Both have mild pro-appetite effects.

Some general rules to preventive pharmacology apply. Specific choice of a preventive agent is often dependent on the patient's other health problems – depression, mood disorder, insomnia, epilepsy, pain, obesity, hypertension, and so on. Performing a drug–drug interaction check is crucial when starting headache medication in a patient on HAART not only to prevent loss of HAART effectiveness but also to avoid supratherapeutic levels. When a preventive agent is chosen, it should be started at the lowest dose and titrated slowly (usually weekly) until clinical benefit is seen or maximum dose is reached. An agent should not be considered "failed" until the therapeutic dose (or maximally tolerated dose) has been trialed for 2–3 months. Treatment response should be tracked with a headache diary or validated scales. When therapy is limited by side effects, nonmedical adjunctive approaches should be employed.

In practical terms, a clinician should have at the ready one familiar drug from each of the three main preventive categories – antihypertensives, antidepressants, and antiepileptics. In so doing, the vast majority of outpatient migraineurs can be managed successfully by their primary medical provider.

Nonpharmacological and complementary therapy

Comprehensive migraine treatment should also include nonmedication approaches to prevention. Lifestyle modification, behavioral therapies, and complementary/alternative medicine are meant to increase the efficacy of pharmacologic approaches – allowing for better headache control, headache prevention, and minimization of pharmacotherapies with dose-limiting side effects. At the very least, they can produce a sense of internal control and through this reduce symptoms of anxiety and depression [29].

Despite lack of rigorous evidence, it makes sense to identify potential migraine "triggers" and strive to remove them. Some, like weather and stressful events (or "let down" after a stressful period), are generally unavoidable, but many others can be managed. These include excessive or irregular consumption of caffeine, insomnia, or otherwise poor sleep hygiene, irregular meals, alcohol, and perhaps foods containing MSG, aspartame, nitrites, or tyramine (chocolate and cheese) [29,30]. A headache diary can help identify migraine-provoking factors.

Behavioral interventions aim to teach the patient about the connection between stress and headache, and to mitigate adverse responses to stress as well as pain itself. The techniques with the best evidence in migraine are relaxation training, biofeedback, and cognitive behavioral therapy, with some studies showing 50% improvement in up to half of patients through these methods [30]; further, the beneficial effects seem to be at least additive with pharmacotherapy.

Several nutritional supplements/vitamins/ "nutraceuticals" may reduce migraine attacks. These include – in order of ranked evidence – butterbur, riboflavin (B2), magnesium, and coenzyme Q10 [31]. Based on other small studies, nightly melatonin has been used for migraine prevention, especially in patients suffering from insomnia related to sleep phase delay (i.e., "night owls"); 3 mg 1 h or so prior to regular bedtime may suffice [32].

Cefaly®, an external supraorbital nerve stimulator available by prescription, has recently won FDA-approval as a migraine preventive device, when worn for 20 min each day [33]. Operating expenses are low – it uses AAA batteries and proprietary reusable electrode pads – but the initial ~$350 cost is generally not reimbursed by insurance.

Aerobic exercise may reduce migraine frequency when performed for 40 min, three times per week [34].

Chronic migraine

Migraine is no longer conceptualized as a purely episodic disorder, but rather a chronic condition with episodic exacerbation, with the potential for progression [35]. When attacks occur on more than 15 days/month, the patient is said to be suffering from chronic migraine (CM) [2]. Epidemiological studies have reported that between 3% and 14% of patients with episodic migraine (EM) progress to CM over a 1-year period [36]. Several modifiable risk factors for this progression have been identified (Table 5.2).

Early acute treatment and aggressive prevention alone address three risk factors – attack frequency, medication overuse, and allodynia (routine stimulation such as brushing the hair becomes painful, thought to be a central sensitization of neurons). Early and effective treatment of acute migraines may also reduce

Table 5.2   Risk factors for progression to chronic migraine.[a]

Nonmodifiable	Modifiable
Female gender	Attack frequency
Young age	Obesity
Caucasian	Medication overuse
Family history of chronic migraine	Excessive caffeine
Unmarried	Snoring
Lower socioeconomic status	Psychiatric comorbidities
Stressful life event(s)	Cutaneous allodynia during attack

[a]Adapted from Refs. 35 and 36.

attack frequency, by reducing "recurrent" headache and forestalling development of allodynia [35,36].

In terms of other modifiable risks, obesity is clearly related to chronic migraine, perhaps through shared inflammatory pathways. Patients with a BMI ≥30 have fivefold increased odds of developing CM. Comorbid mood disorders should be treated, ideally using a migraine preventive from the TCA or SNRI family, but if needed with a specific additional agent. Excessive (or irregular) caffeine intake is common and remediable. We suggest a *regular* intake of no more than 150 mg/day, about 8 oz. of brewed regular coffee, four cans of cola, or two Excedrin® tablets. *Any* sleep disturbance, from insomnia to sleep apnea, can worsen migraines [36]. Simple sleep hygiene measures can make an enormous difference in migraine expression and patient quality of life. In all high-frequency migraine/CM patients, we recommend screening for sleep apnea, education on sleep hygiene, and maintaining a low threshold for diagnostic sleep studies.

Migraine-related complications

Serious complications of migraine are fortunately rare. Migraines, particularly with aura, confer an increased risk of stroke; some of these occur between headache attacks (migraine-related stroke) and others at the time of an aura (migraine-induced stroke) [37]. We recommend that a patient with a prolonged aura (> 1 h) or lingering neurological symptoms undergo urgent stroke workup including brain MRI with diffusion imaging (part of an "acute stroke protocol").

A more commonly encountered complication of a migraine is that of status migrainosus, present when a severe, debilitating migraine lasts more than 72 h [2]. The efficacy for repetitive intravenous DHE in treating intractable migraine has been well established since Raskin's original study in 1986 [38–42]. Patients commonly are coadministered antiemetics and sometimes diphenhydramine before each dose of IV DHE, and often an NSAID (ketorolac) and steroids. When this type of "Modified Raskin Protocol" is employed, many patients become headache free within the first 48 h and continue to experience benefit on long-term

follow-up. We typically admit these patients to the neurology service, where the physicians and nurses are familiar with a standardized protocol as well as the caveats and side effects of the medications used. The patients must not be pregnant, have no cardiovascular or pharmacological contraindications, and maintain hemodynamic stability after each medication administration.

Ergotism is a condition characterized by diffuse vasospasm (along with hallucinations and other symptoms), by an ergotamine, when combined with potent cytochrome P450 inhibitors. It has been described following coadministration with macrolide antibiotics, cyclosporine, tacrolimus, heparin, and possibly ampicillin [43]. Several case reports have also described ergotism in HIV patients on protease inhibitors, known potent inhibitors of CYP 3A4 [43–46]. Interactions must be checked prior to using DHE in a patient on HAART.

Other primary headaches and neuralgias

Trigeminal autonomic cephalalgias (TAC)

The TACs – the cluster headache "family" – are a group of primary headache disorders characterized by lateralized headache with accompanying ipsilateral autonomic symptoms. These include conjunctival injection, lacrimation, nasal congestion, rhinorrhea, facial sweating, miosis, ptosis, and eyelid edema and are due to activation of a normal trigeminal–parasympathetic reflex arc. Pain is typically, sharp, severe, and maximal in the V1 distribution (often periorbital) [2,47]. These disorders are rare and often disabling – indeed cluster may lead to thoughts of suicide. All should be worked up with imaging, ideally contrast brain MRI, looking especially for pituitary or posterior fossa pathologies. Other than potential medication interactions, we are not aware of other unique HIV-related issues in this patient population. The role of the primary provider is to *recognize* the disease family, obtain initial imaging, and refer promptly for specialty management; diagnostic delay can be devastating for quality of life. Hemicrania continua (with constant symptoms) and paroxysmal hemicrania (recurring brief attacks of <40 min) both respond spectacularly and uniquely to indomethacin, dosed as high as 225 mg/day, in divided doses (being mindful of GI and renal issues) [2].

Trigeminal neuralgia

Trigeminal neuralgia is a syndrome of recurrent, brief, unilateral shock-like pain in the distribution of the trigeminal nerve, usually second or third division. The pain is often triggered by normally innocuous sensory stimuli (shaving, washing, cold wind, and chewing). Patients are asymptomatic between attacks, but over time the attacks can become longer and remissions shorter [2]. Most "idiopathic" cases are in fact due to microvascular compression of the trigeminal nerve, but intracranial diseases causing brainstem lesions or neuropathies, including OIs, can mimic the disorder. Diagnostically, it is important to obtain brain imaging (MRI with thin slices through the brain stem) to rule out brainstem lesions or compression of the trigeminal nerve by tumor. We treat patients with antiepileptic neuropathic pain drugs as maintenance therapy, typically oxcarbazepine (carbamazepine has far more drug interactions). Lamotrigine is useful adjunctively but requires slow titration. Pregabalin and gabapentin may be useful, as they have few drug-drug interactions. Definitive procedures under the care of a neurosurgeon (microvascular decompression, percutaneous rhizotomy, or stereotactic radiosurgery) are indicated in most cases where medications are not tolerated or effective [48]. Initial workup and treatment should be promptly undertaken by the primary practitioner, but, again, a neurology referral is warranted for a more thorough assessment and ongoing management.

Pseudotumor cerebri/idiopathic intracranial hypertension (IIH)

The headache of pseudotumor cerebri/IIH is one of daily, diffuse, nonpulsatile pain, associated with papilledema, enlarging blind spot, decreased visual field, and more rarely cranial nerve 6 palsy, caused by elevated intracranial pressure (ICP). On directed questioning, patients may report a pulsatile tinnitus (whooshing in the ears with heartbeat), particularly at night. IIH is typically seen in obese young women, but is substantially rarer than chronic migraine in this population. It is a "do-not-miss" diagnosis as permanent vision loss can result with treatment delay. Workup should include LP in the lateral decubitus position and legs extended, which will reveal elevated opening pressure (>200 mm CSF if normal weight, >250 mm CSF if obese) and an otherwise normal CSF profile [2]. Because *secondary* causes of intracranial hypertension present in the same way, patients need to be screened for use of substances capable of increasing ICP (vitamin A, tetracyclines, lithium, and corticosteroids) and cerebral venous sinus thrombosis needs to be ruled out through imaging (i.e., MR or CT venography) [49]. These patients should be followed closely by both neurology and ophthalmology.

Approach to a patient with daily headache

The patient presenting to a primary practitioner complaining of a CDH (defined as 15+ days/month) bears special consideration. CDH is descriptive of chronic pain, not a specific diagnosis; the clinician's role is to determine the etiology of the underlying condition or primary headache syndrome as well as any treatable contributors to disease expression or severity. Be certain to review medications including OTCs for possible overuse, as well as those with headaches as a common side effect; we have had several "cures" by something as benign as switching from a proton pump inhibitors to an H_2 blocker. Do not neglect possible derangement of ICP.

Triage should be based on HPAIN. Focus on the temporal pattern and any progression. Remember – the more stable the pattern, the more reassuring. If the pain is of prolonged duration or essentially continuous, try to identify the underlying primary headache disorder by phenotype, either from current symptoms "at its worst" or historically, prior to becoming continuous. In all comers, chronic migraine (with or without medication overuse) will be the most common diagnosis underlying a near constant headache. If featureless, chronic TTH is more likely, or new daily persistent headache (NDPH) if sudden onset is "out of the blue" in a patient with little in the way of prior headache history. NDPH is treated empirically according to headache phenotype, with typically poor outcomes. Consider hemicrania continua if the pain is relentless and side-locked. With frequent unilateral *short*-duration headaches (<4 h), TAC should be considered.

Tracking response to treatment

Whatever treatment approach is chosen for CDH or one of the recurring episodic headaches, accurate assessment of ongoing symptoms is needed. Headaches, like other pain disorders, are subjective and assessed based on reporting, without obvious biomarkers (except for the papilledema and elevated opening pressure of IIH). To minimize recall bias, validated self-assessment scales are available online that can be filled out at the appointment, the most widely used being the Migraine Disability Assessment Test (MIDAS) – assessing "days lost" to headaches over the prior 3 months – and the Headache Impact Test (HIT-6). Because headaches are notoriously variable ("noisy"), fluctuating in severity as well as frequency, a prospective diary of symptoms, treatments, and potential "triggers" is a useful tool to track response to any management program over the long haul, looking for a "signal" in review of month-long blocks. At minimum, a diary can involve simply writing an "H" on a day with a significant headache, or logging pills used for acute attacks. For those so inclined, there are numerous headache tracking smartphone apps available. Remember regression to the mean – if a patient's headaches are "the best ever," at the next visit they will almost certainly be worse, even if treatment is left unchanged (the opposite is true as well).

Encourage patients to be meaningful participants in their own self-care. A diary is an excellent first step in getting "buy in," and compliance and motivation are easily assessed from visit to visit by review. *Cures* of primary

headache disorders are rare. Realistic goal setting is critical. Adequate *management* with improved quality of life is the aim – "good enough" rather than "perfect."

Resources for patients

American Council for Headache Education: http://www.achenet.org
American Headache and Migraine Association: https://ahma.memberclicks.net
Cluster Busters (cluster headache support): https://clusterbusters.org
Facial Pain Association/Trigeminal Neuralgia Association: http://fpa-support.org
National Headache Foundation: http://www.headaches.org

Resources for clinicians

American Headache Society: http://www.americanheadachesociety.org
Headache Classification Website of the International Headache Society: http://ihs-classification.org/en/
MIDAS: Migraine Disability Assessment: http://www.achenet.org/midas/
HIT-6: Headache Impact Test, 6 Question: http://www.headaches.org/sites/default/files/uploaded_files/pdf/HIT-6.pdf
Drug Interactions Database: http://www.hiv-druginteractions.org/

References

1 Sheikh, H.U. & Cho, T.A. (2014) Clinical aspects of headache in HIV. *Headache*, **54** (5), 939–945.
2 Headache Classification Committee of the International Headache Society (IHS) (2013) The international classification of headache disorders, 3rd edition (beta version). *Cephalalgia*, **33** (9), 629–808.
3 Lipton, R.B., Bigal, M.E., Diamond, M. *et al.* (2007) Migraine prevalence, disease burden, and the need for preventive therapy. *Neurology*, **68** (5), 343–349.

4 Mirsattari, S.M., Power, C. & Nath, A. (1999) Primary headaches in HIV-infected patients. *Headache*, **39** (1), 3–10.

5 Evers, S., Wibbeke, B., Reichelt, D., Suhr, B., Brilla, R. & Husstedt, I. (2000) The impact of HIV infection on primary headache. Unexpected findings from retrospective, cross-sectional, and prospective analyses. *Pain*, **85** (1–2), 191–200.

6 Kirkland, K.E., Kirkland, K., Many, W.J. Jr., & Smitherman, T.A. (2012) Headache among patients with HIV disease: prevalence, characteristics, and associations. *Headache*, **52** (3), 455–466.

7 Joshi, S.G. & Cho, T.A. (2014) Pathophysiological mechanisms of headache in patients with HIV. *Headache*, **54** (5), 946–950.

8 Singer, E.J., Kim, J., Fahy-Chandon, B., Datt, A. & Tourtellotte, W.W. (1996) Headache in ambulatory HIV-1-infected men enrolled in a longitudinal study. *Neurology*, **47** (2), 487–494.

9 De Luca, G.C. & Bartleson, J.D. (2010) When and how to investigate the patient with headache. *Seminars in Neurology*, **30** (2), 131–144.

10 American College of Radiology. (2012) *Choosing wisely: five things physicians and patients should question*. URL http://www.choosingwisely.org/ doctor-patient-lists/american-college-of-radiology/ [accessed on 12 January 2014].

11 American Headache Society. (2013) *Choosing wisely: five things physicians and patients should question*. URL http://www.choosingwisely .org/doctor-patient-lists/american-headache-society/ [accessed on 12 January 2014].

12 del Saz, S.V., Sued, O., Falco, V. *et al.* (2008) Acute meningoencephalitis due to human immunodeficiency virus type 1 infection in 13 patients: clinical description and follow-up. *Journal of Neurovirology*, **14** (6), 474–479.

13 Cady, R.K., Dodick, D.W., Levine, H.L. *et al.* (2005) Sinus headache: a neurology, otolaryngology, allergy, and primary care consensus on diagnosis and treatment. *Mayo Clinic Proceedings*, **80** (7), 908–916.

14 Southwick, F.S., Richardson, E.P. Jr., & Swartz, M.N. (1986) Septic thrombosis of the dural venous sinuses. *Medicine (Baltimore)*, **65** (2), 82–106.

15 Beatty, G.W. (2010) Immune reconstitution inflammatory syndrome. *Emergency Medicine Clinics of North America*, **28** (2), 393–407.

16 Yancy, H., Lee-Iannotti, J.K., Schwedt, T.J. & Dodick, D.W. (2013) Reversible cerebral vasoconstriction syndrome. *Headache*, **53** (3), 570–576.

17 Dobbs, M.R. & Berger, J.R. (2009) Stroke in HIV infection and AIDS. *Expert Review of Cardiovascular Therapy*, **7** (10), 1263–1271.

18 Sasson, S.C., Oon, A., Chagantri, J., Brew, B.J., Carr, A. (2013) Posterior reversible encephalopathy syndrome (PRES) in an HIV-1 infected patient with disseminated varicella zoster virus: a case report. *BMC Infectious Diseases*, **13**, 396-2334-13-396.

19 Athenahealth. *Epocrates online* (2013). https:// online.epocrates.com

20 Tepper, S.J. (2012) Medication-overuse headache. *Continuum (Minneap Minn)*, **18** (4), 807–822.

21 American Academy of Neurology. (2013) *Choosing wisely: five things physicians and patients should question*. URL http://www .choosingwisely.org/doctor-patient-lists/ american-academy-of-neurology/ [accessed on 12 January 2014].

22 Kaniecki, R.G. (2012) Tension-type headache. *Continuum (Minneap Minn)*, **18** (4), 823–834.

23 Silberstein, S.D. (2000) Practice parameter: evidence-based guidelines for migraine headache (an evidence-based review): report of the quality standards subcommittee of the American Academy of Neurology. *Neurology*, **55** (6), 754–762.

24 Kelley, N.E. & Tepper, D.E. (2012) Rescue therapy for acute migraine, part 2: neuroleptics, antihistamines, and others. *Headache*, **52** (2), 292–306.

25 Rizzoli, P.B. (2012) Acute and preventive treatment of migraine. *Continuum (Minneap Minn)*, **18** (4), 764–782.

26 Kelley, N.E. & Tepper, D.E. (2012) Rescue therapy for acute migraine, part 3: opioids, NSAIDs, steroids, and post-discharge medications. *Headache*, **52** (3), 467–482.

27 Silberstein, S.D., Holland, S., Freitag, F. *et al.* (2012) Evidence-based guideline update: pharmacologic treatment for episodic migraine prevention in adults: report of the quality standards subcommittee of the American

Academy of Neurology and the American Headache Society. *Neurology*, **78** (17), 1337–1345.

28 Ney, J.P., Devine, E.B., Watanabe, J.H. & Sullivan, S.D. (2013) Comparative efficacy of oral pharmaceuticals for the treatment of chronic peripheral neuropathic pain: meta-analysis and indirect treatment comparisons. *Pain Medicine*, **14** (5), 706–719.

29 Mauskop, A. (2012) Nonmedication, alternative, and complementary treatments for migraine. *Continuum (Minneap Minn)*, **18** (4), 796–806.

30 Nicholson, R.A., Buse, D.C., Andrasik, F. & Lipton, R.B. (2011) Nonpharmacologic treatments for migraine and tension-type headache: how to choose and when to use. *Current Treatment Options in Neurology*, **13** (1), 28–40.

31 Holland, S., Silberstein, S.D., Freitag, F. *et al.* (2012) Evidence-based guideline update: NSAIDs and other complementary treatments for episodic migraine prevention in adults: report of the quality standards subcommittee of the American Academy of Neurology and the American Headache Society. *Neurology*, **78** (17), 1346–1353.

32 Peres, M.F., Zukerman, E., da Cunha, T.F., Moreira, F.R. & Cipolla-Neto, J. (2004) Melatonin, 3 mg, is effective for migraine prevention. *Neurology*, **63** (4), 757.

33 Schoenen, J., Vandersmissen, B., Jeangette, S. *et al.* (2013) Migraine prevention with a supraorbital transcutaneous stimulator: a randomized controlled trial. *Neurology*, **80** (8), 697–704.

34 Varkey, E., Cider, A., Carlsson, J. & Linde, M. (2011) Exercise as migraine prophylaxis: a randomized study using relaxation and topiramate as controls. *Cephalalgia*, **31** (14), 1428–1438.

35 Bigal, M.E. & Lipton, R.B. (2011) Migraine chronification. *Current Neurology and Neuroscience Reports*, **11** (2), 139–148.

36 Bigal, M.E. & Lipton, R.B. (2006) Modifiable risk factors for migraine progression. *Headache*, **46** (9), 1334–1343.

37 Alhazzani, A. & Goddeau, R.P. (2013) Migraine and stroke: a continuum of association in adults. *Headache*, **53** (6), 1023–1027.

38 Raskin, N.H. (1986) Repetitive intravenous dihydroergotamine as therapy for intractable migraine. *Neurology*, **36** (7), 995–997.

39 Silberstein, S.D. & Silberstein, J.R. (1992) Chronic daily headache: long-term prognosis following inpatient treatment with repetitive IV DHE. *Headache*, **32** (9), 439–445.

40 Silberstein, S.D. & Young, W.B. (1995) Safety and efficacy of ergotamine tartrate and dihydroergotamine in the treatment of migraine and status migrainosus. Working panel of the headache and facial pain section of the American Academy of Neurology. *Neurology*, **45** (3 Pt 1), 577–584.

41 Silberstein, S.D. & McCrory, D.C. (2003) Ergotamine and dihydroergotamine: history, pharmacology, and efficacy. *Headache*, **43** (2), 144–166.

42 Saper, J.R. & Silberstein, S. (2006) Pharmacology of dihydroergotamine and evidence for efficacy and safety in migraine. *Headache*, **46** (Suppl 4), S171–81.

43 Eadie, M.J. (2001) Clinically significant drug interactions with agents specific for migraine attacks. *CNS Drugs*, **15** (2), 105–118.

44 Baldwin, Z.K. & Ceraldi, C.C. (2003) Ergotism associated with HIV antiviral protease inhibitor therapy. *Journal of Vascular Surgery*, **37** (3), 676–678.

45 Tribble, M.A., Gregg, C.R., Margolis, D.M., Amirkhan, R. & Smith, J.W. (2002) Fatal ergotism induced by an HIV protease inhibitor. *Headache*, **42** (7), 694–695.

46 Marine, L., Castro, P., Enriquez, A. *et al.* (2011) Four-limb acute ischemia induced by ergotamine in an AIDS patient treated with protease inhibitors. *Circulation*, **124** (12), 1395–1397.

47 Goadsby, P.J. (2012) Trigeminal autonomic cephalalgias. *Continuum (Minneap Minn)*, **18** (4), 883–895.

48 Reddy, G.D. & Viswanathan, A. (2014) Trigeminal and glossopharyngeal neuralgia. *Neurologic Clinics*, **32** (2), 539–552.

49 Chen, J. & Wall, M. (2014) Epidemiology and risk factors for idiopathic intracranial hypertension. *International Ophthalmology Clinics*, **54** (1), 1–11.

CHAPTER 6

HIV and peripheral neuropathy

Nu C. Chai[1] and Justin C. McArthur[2]

[1] Department of Neurology, Johns Hopkins University, Baltimore, MD, USA

[2] Department of Neurology, Johns Hopkins University School of Medicine, Baltimore, MD, USA

Introduction

Peripheral neuropathy (PN) is a common and clinically significant comorbidity in HIV-infected individuals. It was originally described in the setting of HIV and severe immune deficiency. However, peripheral neuropathy in HIV-infected patients has persisted in the current treatment era, despite the substantive reduction in the use of older neurotoxic antiretrovirals and the use of effective antiretroviral (Table 6.1) therapy (ART) [1,2].

Distal sensory polyneuropathy (DSP) is the most common form of HIV-associated neuropathy. DSP is characterized by burning pain in the distal extremities that can be severe and lead to impaired physical function and increased psychological burden. It can be caused by either HIV itself (HIV-associated sensory neuropathy [HIV-SN]) or by neurotoxic antiretrovirals (antiretroviral toxic neuropathy [ATN]). The features of HIV-SN and ATN are identical phenotypically. These two etiologies used to frequently coexist in HIV-infected patients. However, in the current HIV treatment era where neurotoxic ART is less frequently prescribed, HIV-SN is now more common. In this chapter, we consider both entities together under the broader umbrella of DSP. We first briefly discuss the epidemiology and pathophysiology of DSP. This will be followed by an overview of the risk factors for developing this condition and its comorbidities. Then we discuss the clinical features of DSP and outline the various diagnostic tools currently available to clinicians, and close with a discussion on its management.

Epidemiology

The prevalence of DSP (both symptomatic and asymptomatic) is estimated to be as high as 60% worldwide in patients with HIV infection [3]. The rate of DSP among HIV-infected individuals may be higher in Africa compared to Asia [4]. In the United States, the prevalence of neuropathy in HIV-infected individuals has been reported to be as low as 1.5% and as high as 62% depending on the study criteria and social–geographic areas involved [4]. In a recent US-based large longitudinal study of more than 2000 ART-naïve participants who initiated ART, rates of peripheral neuropathy ([PN], defined as having at least mild loss of vibration sensation in both great toes or absent/hypoactive ankle reflexes bilaterally) was 32% at 3 years after initiation of ART. Symptomatic PN ([SPN], defined as peripheral neuropathy and bilateral symptoms) was 8.6% at 3 years after initiation of ART [5]. This is despite 87% of the participants achieving CD4 greater than 350 cells/µL [5]. Further, after about 6 years of ART exposure, the rate of PN and SPN continued to increase to 52.8% and 24% [6].

The 1-year incidence of symptomatic DSP (defined as having decreased or absent ankle jerks, decreased or absent vibratory perception at the toes, or decreased pinprick or temperature in stocking distribution *as well as* paresthesias or

Chronic Pain and HIV: A Practical Approach, First Edition.
Edited by Jessica S. Merlin, Peter A. Selwyn, Glenn J. Treisman and Angela G. Giovanniello.
© 2016 John Wiley & Sons, Ltd. Published 2016 by John Wiley & Sons, Ltd.

Table 6.1 Abbreviations.

ART: antiretroviral therapy
ATN: antiretroviral toxic neuropathy
DSP: distal sensory polyneuropathy
HIV-SN: HIV-sensory neuropathy
PN: peripheral neuropathy
SPN: symptomatic peripheral neuropathy

Table 6.2 Antiretroviral medications associated with peripheral neuropathy.

Category	Name
NRTI	Didanosine (ddI)
	Stavudine (d4T)
	Zidovudine (AZT)
	Zalcitabine (ddC; no longer available)
PI	Amprenavir
	Saquinavir
	Indinavir
	Ritonavir
	Lopinavir

NRTI, nucleoside-analog reverse transcriptase inhibitor; PI, protease inhibitor.

pain) was reported to be approximately 36% in the early HIV treatment era, and is now estimated at 21% in the current treatment era [7,8].

In resource-limited settings where the use of lower cost, earlier generation ART such as stavudine is still common, up to 30% patients develop neuropathy within the first year of treatment. The incidence of ATN will hopefully decline, as the 2013 World Health Organization guidelines for the use of antiretroviral drugs strongly recommended the avoidance of stavudine as a first-line regimen because of its well-known toxicity [9].

Pathogenesis

The nerves primarily affected by DSP are the unmyelinated fibers (C fibers) and small myelinated fibers (Aδ fibers). The characteristic pathological feature of DSP is a length-dependent axonal degeneration [10], though some differences exist between the pathogenesis of HIV-SN and ATN.

HIV-SN is caused not by direct infection of neurons by HIV, but rather, by an inflammatory cascade caused by HIV-infected macrophages within the dorsal root ganglia and along the course of the sensory axon. Specifically, glycoprotein 120 on the surface of the HIV envelope activates macrophages, and prominent macrophage activation can lead to subsequent release of proinflammatory cytokines such as TNF-alpha, interferon gamma, and interleukin-1beta. In addition, in HIV-infected patients with DSP, there is an increased level of mitochondrial DNA (mtDNA) common deletion mutations compared to HIV

patients without DSP [11]. This mtDNA damage is more prevalent in the mitochondria of distal long axons, which may explain the length-dependent feature of DSP [11]. Finally, a common European mitochondrial haplogroup has been identified to be linked with an increased risk of HIV-associated DSP [12], again attesting to the importance of mtDNA in the pathogenesis of HIV-SN.

ATN is caused by direct nerve damage by early-generation nucleoside analog reverse transcriptase inhibitors (NRTIs) and possibly, and to a much lesser extent, by exposure to certain protease inhibitors (PIs) (Table 6.2) [13,14]. NRTIs not only have high affinity for viral DNA polymerase, but can also inhibit human mtDNA polymerase in a dose-dependent manner [14]. With the inhibition of mtDNA polymerase-gamma and subsequent depletion of mtDNA content, metabolic functions become disrupted, leading to increased oxidative damage. The sensitivity to damage by toxic antiretrovirals, specifically by stavudine-based therapy, may be associated with certain genetic polymorphisms [15,16]. Further, mtDNA polymerase gamma inhibition is probably not the sole etiology of DSP associated with toxic antivirals. Didanosine treatment has been associated with reduced brain-derived neurotrophic factor production by Schwann cells in dorsal root ganglia in animal models of ATN [17]. In contrast, zidovudine, a potent inhibitor of mtDNA polymerase gamma, only occasionally causes neuropathy, but may cause toxic myopathy.

While PIs have been associated with an increased risk of DSP in several studies (Table 6.2) [13,14,18], the mechanism of neurotoxicity by PIs is yet to be fully elucidated. One study found that HIV-infected dorsal root ganglion cells exposed to indinavir showed significant reductions in the mean neurite length, the mean number of neurons with processes, and the mean neuronal soma diameter [19].

Risk factors

Several risk factors for DSP have been identified in HIV-infected patients. Some of these risk factors are HIV specific and include low CD4 count, high plasma HIV RNA, and increased duration of HIV infection [20]. Others relate to medical comorbidities such as diabetes, elevated triglycerides, and vitamin B12 deficiency [2,5]. Substance use (especially IV drug use and alcohol abuse) and the number of substance used are both associated with increased incident DSP as well [6,21,22]. Physician-prescribed medications for the treatment of common HIV coinfections (i.e., isoniazid, a key component of tuberculosis treatment) can also be neurotoxic and compound the impact of HIV-related DSP [23].

Further, as HIV becomes a chronic disease and the population with HIV ages, aging nervous systems become increasingly vulnerable to cumulative insults. Age, independent of duration of HIV seropositivity, is strongly associated with the risk of DSP [5]. Older age is also associated with lower odds of recovering from ATN after discontinuation of neurotoxic ART [5]. Other nonmodifiable risk factors for developing HIV-related DSP include taller statue and white or Hispanic race [2,5,22].

Although Hepatitis C has been hypothesized to accentuate the neurotoxic effect of the HIV virus within the peripheral nervous system, clinical data does not support this [24]. Finally, while some of its components (i.e., elevated triglycerides) are associated with increased risk for DSP, metabolic syndrome itself has not been found to correlate with the development of DSP [25].

Clinical features

Patients with DSP from either ATN or HIV-SN usually describe the gradual onset of change in sensation in the bilateral feet – often a sensation of having "sand" or "small rocks" in their shoes, or a "sunburned" sensation on the soles or forefoot. They may also report tingling or stabbing sensations in the feet. The distribution of the dysesthesias will gradually ascend from the feet up to the knees. When lower extremity symptoms reach the knees, patients may also begin to complain of symptoms in the fingertips. With progressive damage to the peripheral nerves, DSP can progress to spontaneous sharp, burning or stabbing pain and numbness in a "stocking and glove" distribution very similar to that observed in other small fiber neuropathies (e.g., secondary to diabetes). The sensation of paresthesias can be constant or vary in intensity throughout the day. It may be worsened when the feet of the patients are rubbed against socks, shoes, or bedsheets. As is typical of many painful neuropathies, patients typically report worse pain at night.

The rate of progression from asymptomatic DSP to symptomatic DSP is variable. While age, CD4 count, and exposure to neurotoxic antiretrovirals are all associated with an increased risk of symptomatic DSP, none of these factors have been shown to be associated with the *time* to symptomatic DSP [3]. While DSP tends to occur in those with low CD4 counts and with more advanced disease, it can exist even in those without a history of persistently low CD4 count and can often persist even with improvement of immunologic function and CD4 counts [5]. Once established, there is no convincing evidence that regeneration of epidermal nerve fibers occurs in DSP, regardless of etiology (HIV or ART). However, those with symptomatic DSP can see improvement of their symptoms spontaneously, occasionally even to a pain-free state, with the prolonged duration of symptoms (presumptively due to "burned out" nerve fibers).

Resource-limited settings

Decreased immunity in those not on ART not only leads to HIV-mediated neuropathy but can also expose patients to infectious diseases that can lead to parainfectious or postinfectious neuropathies. *Mycobacterium tuberculosis* and the use of isoniazid (for the treatment of tuberculosis) in the HIV population can further exacerbate their neuropathy [23]. Opportunistic infections (e.g., CMV, HSV) can lead to progressive polyradiculopathy as well as mononeuritis multiplex, both painful neuropathies with a distribution in the pattern of individual peripheral nerves or nerve roots. Nutritional deficiencies may be particularly salient in this population as well.

Children

DSP is a relatively rare HIV-related symptom in children [26]. Stavudine was a commonly used medication in pediatric ART regimens, principally because of the ease of manufacture and its low cost. While in adults, stavudine is strongly associated with the development of DSP, peripheral neuropathy is rare in children on stavudine based on a South African retrospective study [27]. Over a 4-year period, only two cases of peripheral neuropathy were identified in a cohort of more than 2000 children [27]. While stavudine confers a relatively low risk of peripheral neuropathy in children, zidovudine in comparison has an even lower risk (both for peripheral neuropathy and other toxicities) and is now one of the first-line medications recommended by the WHO for children less than 3 years [9,28].

Impact and comorbidities

The presence and severity of neuropathic pain is associated with decreased quality of life in all domains of health-related quality of life (HRQoL) [29]. Depressive symptoms are worse in those with neuropathic pain compared to those without [2]. Depression is also strongly correlated with a worse quality of life in the HIV population [30]. Further, neuropathic pain in the HIV population is associated with higher levels of unemployment [2]. Specifically, even after adjusting for CD4 count, plasma viral load, neuropsychological impairment, current major depression, and other demographic factors such as age and education, HIV patients

with neuropathic pain of any severity was 1.5 times more likely to be unemployed [2]. This illustrates the vicious cycle leading to significant disability caused by neuropathic pain and comorbid depression in the HIV population.

Diagnosis

Many patients with early-stage, mild DSP have a normal neurologic examination, with intact strength and normal reflexes. Despite complaints of abnormal sensation in the feet, specific sensory modalities such as touch, vibration, and proprioception are often intact with testing. In more advanced disease, vibratory thresholds, sensation to pinprick or temperature and ankle jerk reflexes may be reduced.

A variety of rating scales have been developed for more reliable measurement of peripheral neuropathy and can be of utility for the screening and tracking of DSP and its progression in patients. For example, the brief peripheral neuropathy scale (BPNS) includes both subjective symptoms (e.g., pain, numbness in feet or legs) and examination findings (e.g., perception of vibration, ankle reflexes) and can be easily administered by nonneurologist in 10 min to screen for HIV-DSP [31]. The BPNS has a high positive predictive value (85%) but low negative predictive value (45%) [32]. Another scoring system is the total neuropathy score (TNS). Initially developed for the study of diabetic peripheral neuropathy, it involves five components: sensory symptoms, sensory function, tendon reflexes, quantitative sensory testing (QST), and sural nerve amplitude by nerve conduction study (NCS) [32]. The modified TNS excludes the sensory symptom component and is found to correlate pain levels with the remainder of the components of TNS [3], making it a useful tool for those with neuropathic pain.

All patients with suspected HIV DSP should be tested for other common causes of peripheral neuropathy, including diabetes and B12/folate deficiency, and asked about alcohol use and IV drug use. Comorbid conditions should be addressed if present. Patients with clinical manifestations and physical examinations typical of DSP (including a normal examination) do not need additional diagnostic testing to confirm the diagnosis. In patients in whom the diagnosis of HIV DSP is unclear and who may need additional diagnostic testing, punch skin biopsy, electromyogram(EMG)/nerve conduction study, or lumbar puncture should be considered.

The currently accepted gold standard for evaluating small fiber neuropathies such as DSP is punch skin biopsy. Skin biopsies are performed to evaluate the density and integrity of axons of small nerve fibers. They are usually performed via a 3-mm-punch biopsy taken from a symptomatic location (i.e., distal leg). In patients with HIV DSP, skin biopsies will show reduced nerve fiber densities as well as large nerve fiber swellings indicative of axonal degeneration. The sensitivity (78–92%) and specificity (65–90%) of skin biopsies for diagnosis of small fiber neuropathies including DSP are relatively high. Further, even in asymptomatic individuals, the presence of low epidermal nerve fiber density (< 11 fibers/mm) is associated with an increased risk of developing symptomatic DSP in the next 6 months to 1 year. In HIV-infected patients with advanced disease, epidermal nerve fiber density has been correlated with both the clinical and electrophysiological severity of DSP [33].

We recommend performing punch skin biopsies to confirm DSP in individuals in whom multiple neuropathic disease processes are suspected (e.g., with symptoms of DSP and radiculopathy, in whom the examination can be confusing and not classic for DSP). Punch skin biopsy is also recommended if the patient's examination and/or history is internally inconsistent (i.e., changing patterns of numbness during the examination) to differentiate DSP from conversion disorder, or malingering. In cases where the neuropathy is in an asymmetric or nonlength-dependent pattern, punch skin biopsy will be of low yield (most likely normal, since punch skin biopsies are typically normal in radiculopathy and nerve entrapment syndromes). In these cases, EMG/NCS may be the more appropriate diagnostic test.

EMG/NCS cannot assess the integrity of those small unmyelinated fibers affected in HIV DSP; therefore, they cannot be used to make a diagnosis of DSP, especially early DSP. EMG/NCS are generally only performed when the clinical examination suggests other causes of neuropathy or a mixed picture. For example,

unilateral symptoms or very asymmetric symptoms may suggest polyradiculopathy or mononeuritis multiplex. Sensory complaints in the bilateral fingertips instead of bilateral feet along with areflexia may be early signs of acute inflammatory demyelinating polyneuropathy (AIDP). Sensory symptoms in bilateral lower extremities but with an acute onset may suggest conus medullaris syndrome. Deep limb pain or dysesthesia instead of distal symmetric burning pain may be suggestive of chronic inflammatory demyelinating polyneuropathy (CIDP).

Lumbar puncture, like EMG/NCS, cannot be used to make a diagnosis of DSP. It can be helpful for diagnosing other causes of numbness/neuropathic pain if EMG/NCS is suggestive of etiologies where changes in CSF profile are expected (e.g., infectious or inflammatory). For example, in CMV radiculopathy, neutrophilic pleocytosis is expected. In AIDP or CIDP, elevated CSF protein can be seen with normal cell counts.

When to do which test?

In general, if both examination and history are consistent with DSP, no additional diagnostic testing is needed. If the examination and history show components that could be consistent with DSP (e.g., bilateral lower extremity numbness) but additional components that are not typical of DSP, both punch skin biopsy and EMG/NCS may be needed, as it is possible for one patient to have both DSP and another neuropathy processes. In cases where the neuropathy is in a purely asymmetric or nonlength-dependent pattern, punch skin biopsy will be of low yield (most likely normal, as this is most likely not DSP), and EMG/NCS is most appropriate for making a diagnosis. If the patient's examination and history are not internally consistent (e.g., changing patterns of numbness during examination), punch skin biopsies can be used to differentiate DSP from conversion or malingering.

Resource-limited settings
In resource-limited settings where testing equipment may be limited, the sensitivity of single

question neuropathy screen ("Tingling, burning, or numbness in feet or hands?") has been found to be more than 80% sensitive and specific for identification of those with moderate-to-severe neuropathy [34–36].

Management

Management of symptomatic HIV DSP can be challenging. Once modifiable risk factors have been addressed, HIV DSP should be treated symptomatically. A variety of pharmacologic therapies used for posthepatic neuralgia and diabetic neuropathy have also been tested in HIV-infected patients with variable success [37]. With advanced disease and severe pain, opioids may be considered (see Chapter 11). Evidence-based nonpharmacologic modalities are also an important part of an individualized, multidisciplinary approach to HIV DSP.

Modifiable risk factors

While some risk factors for developing neuropathy such as tall statue and older age are not modifiable, other risk factors can be avoided. Initiation of ART in those not already taking it is recommended [38]. Care should be taken to avoid neurotoxic ART, especially didanosine (ddI) or stavudine (d4T), which are fortunately already rarely used in developed countries [39,40]. Other neurotoxic medications such as metronidazole, nitrofurantoin, and isoniazid should also be assessed. If the patient is already on a neurotoxic ART regimen, the decision to discontinue these medications must be made after careful risk–benefit analysis [38]. Treatment of comorbidities known to increase the risk of DSP, such as diabetes, elevated triglyceride levels, and B12/folate deficiency, should be optimized [25].

Symptomatic treatment

For symptomatic treatment of the painful paresthesias, a variety of antidepressant and antiepileptic medications have been used for their efficacy in general neuropathic pain, such as gabapentin, pregabalin, lamotrigine, and amitriptyline [41]. Of these, only gabapentin and lamotrigine have some evidence for efficacy in HIV-specific neuropathic pain, whereas others have either not shown superiority over placebo in the HIV population or have very limited evidence for use in neuropathic pain in the HIV population, but continue to be used by some clinicians based on their efficacy in management of diabetic neuropathy or mixed neuropathic pain [42,43]. There continues to be a lack of definitive information regarding the relative efficacy of these medications or any synergistic efficacy of specific drug combinations [44,45]; so it is reasonable to select these medications based on their side effect profile, taking into consideration each individual patient's comorbidities such as anxiety, depression, metabolic syndrome, and other drug–drug interactions (Table 6.3) [46].

Antiepileptic medications

Gabapentin is used frequently in those with neuropathic pain. It was found to provide significant pain relief in about one third of patients taking it for general neuropathic pain conditions [47]. There has been only one study on the efficacy of gabapentin with a focus on HIV-specific painful sensory neuropathy [47]. This small study of 26 participants compared gabapentin (titrated up to 2400 mg daily) to placebo over 4 weeks and found improvement in both pain and sleep in the gabapentin group [48].

Lamotrigine also has shown efficacy specifically in the HIV-infected population for neuropathic pain. A 2013 Cochrane review evaluated the evidence for lamotrigine in acute and chronic neuropathic pain and determined that while it was no better than placebo in general neuropathic pain, there may be some efficacy for patients with HIV-DSP based on two placebo-controlled studies [49]. One study (42 participants) used lamotrigine 300 mg/day (titrating by 25 mg doses for 7 weeks) and showed larger declines in pain scores in the lamotrigine group compared to placebo, though almost 50% participants in the lamotrigine arm were lost to follow-up [50]. The other study (227 participants) used lamotrigine 400 mg/day and showed that in those participants also receiving ART, there was improvement of pain in the lamotrigine-treated group compared to

Table 6.3   Medications for neuropathic pain.

Category	Name	Dose/titration	Main side effects	Notes
Antiepileptic	Lamotrigine	Start at 25 mg/day, use up to 400 mg/day, and titrate by 25–50 mg/week	Skin rash, dizziness, somnolence, headache, and nausea	Avoid coadministration with valproate; avoid rapid dose escalation to decrease risk of life-threatening rash; also used in bipolar disorder
	Gabapentin	Start at 300 mg/day, use up to 2400 mg/day (divided BID or TID), and titrate by 300 mg/day	Dizziness, somnolence, peripheral edema, and gait disturbance	Dose adjustment needed for decreased renal function; also used as an adjunct for epilepsy
	Pregabalin	Start at 100 mg/day, use up to 600 mg/day (divided BID or TID), and titrate by 100 mg/day	Somnolence and dizziness	Dose adjustment needed for decreased renal function; also used as an adjunct for epilepsy
Antidepressant	Duloxetine	Start at 30 mg/day, use up to 120 mg/day, and titrate by 30 mg/week	Nausea, dizziness, and somnolence	Avoid coadministration with MAOIs; avoid usage in those with uncontrolled narrow-angle glaucoma; also used in depression
	Amitriptyline	Start at 25 mg/day, use up to 125 mg/day (bedtime only or divided up to TID), and titrate by 50 mg/day	Somnolence, confusion, rash, paralytic ileus, and orthostatic hypotension	Avoid coadministration with MAOIs; avoid during the acute recovery phase of MI; also used in depression
Topical	Capsaicin	8% patch (14 cm × 20 cm = 280 cm^2 = 179 mg capsaicin); maximum 4 patches used for 1120 cm^2; leaving patch for 30–60 min, then remove; can repeat every 3 months	Early treatment associated local pain; patch-related edema, erythema, and pruritus	Must use nitrile gloves when applying Can use local anesthesia (lidocaine) prior to application; can use dry cold compress concurrently with application

BID, twice a day; TID, three times a day; MAOI, monoamine oxidase inhibitors; MI, myocardial infarction.

the placebo group (57% improved compared to 23%) [51].

There are no randomized controlled studies in the HIV-DSP-specific population for carbamazepine, lacosamide, phenytoin, pregabalin, topiramate, or valproic acid. Of these, only pregabalin has reasonably good evidence for efficacy in treating diabetic neuropathic pain, whereas others have either minimal evidence of efficacy or have insufficient evidence in analgesia for any neuropathic pain condition [52,53].

Antidepressant medications

Both tricyclic antidepressants and serotonin–noradrenaline reuptake inhibitors (SNRIs) have been tried in diabetic neuropathic pain. Amitriptyline, a tricyclic antidepressant widely used for treatment of neuropathic pain, showed no evidence of efficacy in treating HIV-related neuropathic pain compared to placebo over 14 weeks at doses of 25–75 mg daily in a small trial [54,55]. However, anecdotally, experts agree that amitriptyline has been used successfully for peripheral neuropathy for at least some patients [55]. Therefore, while no large randomized trials are available to support its efficacy, it may still be beneficial for a small subset of patients with neuropathic pain and can be tried if other medications fail or are contraindicated. No randomized controlled studies exist for any SNRI in the HIV population. However, duloxetine (both at doses of 60 and 120 mg daily) is efficacious for treating pain in diabetic neuropathy[56] and may be tried in those with HIV-DSP.

Topical treatment options

Topical agents such as capsaicin patch and lidocaine patch have also been used for the treatment of neuropathic pain [57,58], though lidocaine 5% gel was not found to be effective in the treatment of HIV-associated painful DSP. Capsaicin, a derivative of hot chili pepper plant, has been used medicinally in either low concentrations (i.e., 0.025% cream) or high concentration (i.e., 8% patch). In Europe, high-concentration capsaicin patch is licensed for HIV-DSP, whereas in the United States, it is only FDA approved for posthepatic neuralgia at the moment [59]. While the most recent Cochrane review found insufficient evidence of efficacy for low-concentration capsaicin in treatment of neuropathic pain [57], high-concentration capsaicin patch has been demonstrated to be efficacious in at least two phase III trials [60,61]. The pooled analysis of these two trials showed that patients using capsaicin 8% were more likely than controls (39% compared to 23%; $p = 0.005$) to achieve greater than 30% reduction in pain. The main drawback for using capsaicin is its associated burning pain and dermal reaction with application, as it works via the transient receptor potential vanilloid (TRPV1) receptor channel leading to calcium and sodium influx, resulting in the unpleasant burning sensation in the area of application and possibly erythema, edema, and pruritus. However, the increased pain usually starts to trend downward after day 2 of application [59,61] and can be ameliorated with pretreatment of the area with low-dose topical anesthetic (i.e., lidocaine) or concurrent use of oral analgesic or topical dry cold compress [59].

Other pharmacologic options

NSAIDs and acetaminophen can also be used concurrently with the aforementioned neuropathic pain medications, though no randomized controlled trials exist for the HIV neuropathy subpopulation. Finally, a small clinical trial of cannabis has shown improvement of pain in HIV patients using smoked cannabis compared to controls [62]. The potential medical value of cannabis will likely be further evaluated with its legalization in certain states.

Nonpharmacologic therapy

Leg splinting, acupuncture, and hypnosis have all seen positive results in small clinical trials and may be worth incorporating in the management of HIV neuropathic pain [63–66]. Cognitive behavioral therapy (CBT) may be beneficial for some HIV-infected patients with neuropathic pain. In one randomized trial involving 61 subjects with HIV-DSP, both the CBT group and the group receiving supportive psychotherapy achieved significant improvement of pain compared to baseline. While the CBT group showed greater improvement in most domains of pain-related functional compared to the supportive psychotherapy group, this was not statistically significant. Moreover, the dropout rate was high in this study in both groups [67]. HIV-infected patients with DSP and coexisting mood disorders may benefit the most from psychotherapy and CBT (see Chapter 10 for nonpharmacologic management of pain).

Conclusion

DSP is a painful neuropathy common in the HIV population and can be caused by HIV or by toxic antiretroviral therapies. The diagnosis of DSP is primarily a clinical one – with patients reporting burning pain in both feet. As DSP primarily damages small nerve fibers, EMG and NCS are often normal, whereas punch skin biopsy can show decreased nerve fiber density and abnormal morphology. If the pattern of distribution for the painful neuropathy is atypical (i.e., unilateral, in the hand and/or arm instead of bilateral feet), EMG and NCS can provide valuable diagnostic information.

Treatment for HIV-related DSP must first focus on removing modifiable risk factors such as (1) careful evaluation of all medications to remove neurotoxic medications if possible, (2) improving overall nutritional status to avoid vitamin deficiencies as well as avoiding uncontrolled hyperglycemia and hypertriglyceridemia, and (3) avoiding alcohol and IV drug use. Neuropathic pain medications such as certain antiepileptics and antipsychotic medications may be used concurrently with NSAIDs and/or acetaminophen. Of the many medications for neuropathic pain, only gabapentin and lamotrigine have evidence for efficacy in the HIV population. Although pregabalin and duloxetine have not been studied specifically in the HIV population, they have shown evidence for efficacy in mixed neuropathic pain or for diabetic neuropathic pain and, therefore, may also be tried. Amitriptyline did not show evidence for HIV-related neuropathic pain in a small study, but has some evidence for painful diabetic neuropathy and mixed neuropathic pain and, therefore, may also be tried if other treatment regimens have failed, with the understanding that satisfactory pain relief may only be achieved by a minority of patients

[55]. Generally, medication selection can be based on side effect profile and tolerability, as no specific study has identified superiority in efficacy for any of the neuropathic pain medications against another for HIV-related DSP. Finally, some studies have shown efficacy with certain nonpharmacologic therapies, including psychotherapy, though definitive evidence is still lacking and compliance can be an issue, limiting firm recommendations for any specific therapy. Those with comorbid mood disorders may benefit most strongly from concurrent psychotherapy in addition to neuropathic pain medications to manage their symptoms.

Overall, clinicians taking care of HIV patients should be able to identify neuropathic pain symptoms and take a multidisciplinary approach to its management. Research in the pathogenesis and treatment for HIV-related DSP pain is ongoing, and our understanding in this topic continues to unfold.

References

1 Cornblath, D.R. & McArthur, J.C. (1988) Predominantly sensory neuropathy in patients with AIDS and AIDS-related complex. *Neurology*, **38** (5), 794–796.

2 Ellis, R.J., Rosario, D., Clifford, D.B. *et al.* (2010) Continued high prevalence and adverse clinical impact of human immunodeficiency virus-associated sensory neuropathy in the era of combination antiretroviral therapy: the CHARTER study. *Archives of Neurology*, **67** (5), 552–558.

3 Simpson, D.M., Kitch, D., Evans, S.R. *et al.* (2006) HIV neuropathy natural history cohort study: assessment measures and risk factors. *Neurology*, **66** (11), 1679–1687.

4 Ghosh, S., Chandran, A. & Jansen, J.P. (2012) Epidemiology of HIV-related neuropathy: a systematic literature review. *AIDS Research and Human Retroviruses*, **28** (1), 36–48.

5 Evans, S.R., Ellis, R.J., Chen, H. *et al.* (2011) Peripheral neuropathy in HIV: prevalence and risk factors. *AIDS*, **25** (7), 919–928.

6 Chen, H., Clifford, D.B., Deng, L. *et al.* (2013) Peripheral neuropathy in ART-experienced patients: prevalence and risk factors. *Journal of Neurovirology*, **19** (6), 557–564.

7 Schifitto, G., McDermott, M.P., McArthur, J.C. *et al.* (2005) Markers of immune activation and viral load in HIV-associated sensory neuropathy. *Neurology*, **64** (5), 842–848.

8 Schifitto, G., McDermott, M.P., McArthur, J.C. *et al.* (2002) Dana consortium on the therapy of HIV Dementia and related cognitive disorders. Incidence of and risk factors for HIV-associated distal sensory polyneuropathy. *Neurology*, **58** (12), 1764–1768.

9 World Health Organization (2013) *Consolidated guidelines on the use of antiretroviral drugs for treating and preventing the infection.* World Health Organization, Geneva.

10 Pardo, C.A., McArthur, J.C. & Griffin, J.W. (2001) HIV neuropathy: insights in the pathology of HIV peripheral nerve disease. *Journal of the Peripheral Nervous System*, **6** (1), 21–27.

11 Lehmann, H.C., Chen, W., Borzan, J., Mankowski, J.L. & Hoke, A. (2011) Mitochondrial dysfunction in distal axons contributes to human immunodeficiency virus sensory neuropathy. *Annals of Neurology*, **69** (1), 100–110.

12 Hulgan, T., Haas, D.W., Haines, J.L. *et al.* (2005) Mitochondrial haplogroups and peripheral neuropathy during antiretroviral therapy: an adult AIDS clinical trials group study. *AIDS*, **19** (13), 1341–1349.

13 Ellis, R.J., Marquie-Beck, J., Delaney, P. *et al.* (2008) Human immunodeficiency virus protease inhibitors and risk for peripheral neuropathy. *Annals of Neurology*, **64** (5), 566–572.

14 Gardner, K., Hall, P.A., Chinnery, P.F. & Payne, B.A. (2014) HIV treatment and associated mitochondrial pathology: review of 25 years of in vitro, animal, and human studies. *Toxicologic Pathology*, **42** (5), 811–822.

15 Domingo, P., Cabeza Mdel, C., Torres, F. *et al.* (2013) Association of thymidylate synthase polymorphisms with acute pancreatitis and/or peripheral neuropathy in HIV-infected patients on stavudine-based therapy. *PLoS One*, **8** (2), e57347.

16 Holzinger, E.R., Hulgan, T., Ellis, R.J. *et al.* (2012) Mitochondrial DNA variation and HIV-associated sensory neuropathy in CHARTER. *Journal of Neurovirology*, **18** (6), 511–520.

17 Zhu, Y., Antony, J.M., Martinez, J.A. *et al.* (2007) Didanosine causes sensory neuropathy in an HIV/AIDS animal model: Impaired mitochondrial and neurotrophic factor gene expression. *Brain*, **130** (Pt 8), 2011–2023.

18 Lorber, M. (2013) A case of possible darunavir/ritonavir-induced peripheral neuropathy: case description and review of the literature. *Journal of the International Association of Providers of AIDS Care*, **12** (3), 162–165.

19 Pettersen, J.A., Jones, G., Worthington, C. *et al.* (2006) Sensory neuropathy in human immunodeficiency virus/acquired immunodeficiency syndrome patients: protease inhibitor-mediated neurotoxicity. *Annals of Neurology*, **59** (5), 816–824.

20 Childs, E.A., Lyles, R.H., Selnes, O.A. *et al.* (1999) Plasma viral load and CD4 lymphocytes predict HIV-associated dementia and sensory neuropathy. *Neurology*, **52** (3), 607–613.

21 Robinson-Papp, J., Gelman, B.B., Grant, I. *et al.* (2012) Substance abuse increases the risk of neuropathy in an HIV-infected cohort. *Muscle & Nerve*, **45** (4), 471–476.

22 Robinson-Papp, J., Gonzalez-Duarte, A., Simpson, D.M. *et al.* (2009) The roles of ethnicity and antiretrovirals in HIV-associated polyneuropathy: a pilot study. *Journal of Acquired Immune Deficiency Syndromes*, **51** (5), 569–573.

23 Breen, R.A., Lipman, M.C. & Johnson, M.A. (2000) Increased incidence of peripheral neuropathy with co-administration of stavudine and isoniazid in HIV-infected individuals. *AIDS*, **14** (5), 615.

24 Cherry, C.L., Affandi, J.S., Brew, B.J. *et al.* (2010) Hepatitis C seropositivity is not a risk factor for sensory neuropathy among patients with HIV. *Neurology*, **74** (19), 1538–1542.

25 Ances, B.M., Vaida, F., Rosario, D. *et al.* (2009) Role of metabolic syndrome components in HIV-associated sensory neuropathy. *AIDS*, **23** (17), 2317–2322.

26 Govender, R., Eley, B., Walker, K., Petersen, R. & Wilmshurst, J.M. (2011) Neurologic and neurobehavioral sequelae in children with human immunodeficiency virus (HIV-1) infection. *Journal of Child Neurology*, **26** (11), 1355–1364.

27 Palmer, M., Chersich, M., Moultrie, H., Kuhn, L., Fairlie, L. & Meyers, T. (2013) Frequency of stavudine substitution due to toxicity in

children receiving antiretroviral treatment in sub-Saharan Africa. *AIDS*, **27** (5), 781–785.

28 Van Dyke, R.B., Wang, L., Williams, P.L. & Pediatric AIDS Clinical Trials Group 219C Team (2008) Toxicities associated with dual nucleoside reverse-transcriptase inhibitor regimens in HIV-infected children. *Journal of Infectious Diseases*, **198** (11), 1599–1608.

29 Jensen, M.P., Chodroff, M.J. & Dworkin, R.H. (2007) The impact of neuropathic pain on health-related quality of life: review and implications. *Neurology*, **68** (15), 1178–1182.

30 Keltner, J.R., Vaida, F., Ellis, R.J. *et al.* (2012) Health-related quality of life 'well-being' in HIV distal neuropathic pain is more strongly associated with depression severity than with pain intensity. *Psychosomatics*, **53** (4), 380–386.

31 Cherry, C.L., Wesselingh, S.L., Lal, L. & McArthur, J.C. (2005) Evaluation of a clinical screening tool for HIV-associated sensory neuropathies. *Neurology*, **65** (11), 1778–1781.

32 Cornblath, D.R., Chaudhry, V., Carter, K. *et al.* (1999) Total neuropathy score: validation and reliability study. *Neurology*, **53** (8), 1660–1664.

33 Zhou, L., Kitch, D.W., Evans, S.R. *et al.* (2007) Correlates of epidermal nerve fiber densities in HIV-associated distal sensory polyneuropathy. *Neurology*, **68** (24), 2113–2119.

34 Cettomai, D., Kwasa, J., Kendi, C. *et al.* (2010) Utility of quantitative sensory testing and screening tools in identifying HIV-associated peripheral neuropathy in western Kenya: pilot testing. *PLoS One*, **5** (12), e14256.

35 Cettomai, D., Kwasa, J.K., Birbeck, G.L. *et al.* (2013) Screening for HIV-associated peripheral neuropathy in resource-limited settings. *Muscle & Nerve*, **48** (4), 516–524.

36 Kandiah, P.A., Atadzhanov, M., Kvalsund, M.P. & Birbeck, G.L. (2010) Evaluating the diagnostic capacity of a single-question neuropathy screen (SQNS) in HIV positive Zambian adults. *Journal of Neurology, Neurosurgery & Psychiatry*, **81** (12), 1380–1381.

37 Cornblath, D.R. & Hoke, A. (2006) Recent advances in HIV neuropathy. *Current Opinion in Neurology*, **19** (5), 446–450.

38 Maritz, J., Benatar, M., Dave, J.A. *et al.* (2010) HIV neuropathy in South Africans: frequency, characteristics, and risk factors. *Muscle & Nerve*, **41** (5), 599–606.

39 Cherry, C.L., Skolasky, R.L., Lal, L. *et al.* (2006) Antiretroviral use and other risks for HIV-associated neuropathies in an international cohort. *Neurology*, **66** (6), 867–873.

40 Dragovic, G. & Jevtovic, D. (2003) Nucleoside reverse transcriptase inhibitor usage and the incidence of peripheral neuropathy in HIV/AIDS patients. *Antiviral Chemistry & Chemotherapy*, **14** (5), 281–284.

41 Gonzalez-Duarte, A., Cikurel, K. & Simpson, D.M. (2007) Managing HIV peripheral neuropathy. *Current HIV/AIDS Reports*, **4** (3), 114–118.

42 Simpson, D.M., Schifitto, G., Clifford, D.B. *et al.* (2010) Pregabalin for painful HIV neuropathy: a randomized, double-blind, placebo-controlled trial. *Neurology*, **74** (5), 413–420.

43 Phillips, T.J., Cherry, C.L., Cox, S., Marshall, S.J. & Rice, A.S. (2010) Pharmacological treatment of painful HIV-associated sensory neuropathy: a systematic review and meta-analysis of randomised controlled trials. *PLoS One*, **5** (12), e14433.

44 Harrison, T., Miyahara, S., Lee, A. *et al.* (2013) Experience and challenges presented by a multicenter crossover study of combination analgesic therapy for the treatment of painful HIV-associated polyneuropathies. *Pain Medicine*, **14** (7), 1039–1047.

45 Chaparro, L.E., Wiffen, P.J., Moore, R.A. & Gilron, I. (2012) Combination pharmacotherapy for the treatment of neuropathic pain in adults. *Cochrane Database of Systematic Reviews*, **7**, CD008943.

46 Brix Finnerup, N., Hein Sindrup, S. & Staehelin, J.T. (2013) Management of painful neuropathies. *Handbook of Clinical Neurology*, **115**, 279–290.

47 Moore, R.A., Wiffen, P.J., Derry, S. & McQuay, H.J. (2011) Gabapentin for chronic neuropathic pain and fibromyalgia in adults. *Cochrane Database of Systematic Reviews*, **3**, CD010567.

48 Hahn, K., Arendt, G., Braun, J.S. *et al.* (2004) A placebo-controlled trial of gabapentin for painful HIV-associated sensory neuropathies. *Journal of Neurology*, **251** (10), 1260–1266.

49 Wiffen, P.J., Derry, S. & Moore, R.A. (2013) Lamotrigine for chronic neuropathic pain and fibromyalgia in adults. *Cochrane Database of Systematic Reviews*, **12**, CD006044.

50 Simpson, D.M., Olney, R., McArthur, J.C., Khan, A., Godbold, J. & Ebel-Frommer, K. (2000) A placebo-controlled trial of lamotrigine for painful HIV-associated neuropathy. *Neurology*, **54** (11), 2115–2119.

51 Simpson, D.M., McArthur, J.C., Olney, R. *et al.* (2003) Lamotrigine for HIV-associated painful sensory neuropathies: a placebo-controlled trial. *Neurology*, **60** (9), 1508–1514.

52 Wiffen, P.J., Derry, S., Moore, R.A. *et al.* (2013) Antiepileptic drugs for neuropathic pain and fibromyalgia - an overview of Cochrane reviews. *Cochrane Database of Systematic Reviews*, **11**, CD010567.

53 Moore, R.A., Straube, S., Wiffen, P.J., Derry, S. & McQuay, H.J. (2009) Pregabalin for acute and chronic pain in adults. *Cochrane Database of Systematic Reviews*, **3**, CD007076.

54 Shlay, J.C., Chaloner, K., Max, M.B. *et al.* (1998) Acupuncture and amitriptyline for pain due to HIV-related peripheral neuropathy: a randomized controlled trial. Terry Beirn community programs for clinical research on AIDS. *JAMA*, **280** (18), 1590–1595.

55 Moore, R.A., Derry, S., Aldington, D., Cole, P. & Wiffen, P.J. (2012) Amitriptyline for neuropathic pain and fibromyalgia in adults. *Cochrane Database of Systematic Reviews*, **12**, CD008242.

56 Lunn, M.P., Hughes, R.A. & Wiffen, P.J. (2014) Duloxetine for treating painful neuropathy, chronic pain or fibromyalgia. *Cochrane Database of Systematic Reviews*, **1**, CD007115.

57 Derry, S., Sven-Rice, A., Cole, P., Tan, T. & Moore, R.A. (2013) Topical capsaicin (high concentration) for chronic neuropathic pain in adults. *Cochrane Database of Systematic Reviews*, **2**, CD007393.

58 Mou, J., Paillard, F., Turnbull, B., Trudeau, J., Stoker, M. & Katz, N.P. (2013) Qutenza (capsaicin) 8% patch onset and duration of response and effects of multiple treatments in neuropathic pain patients. *Clinical Journal of Pain*, **30** (4), 286–294.

59 Baranidharan, G., Das, S. & Bhaskar, A. (2013) A review of the high-concentration capsaicin patch and experience in its use in the management of neuropathic pain. *Therapeutic Advances in Neurological Disorders*, **6** (5), 287–297.

60 Simpson, D.M., Brown, S., Tobias, J. & NGX-4010 C107 Study Group (2008) Controlled trial of high-concentration capsaicin patch for treatment of painful HIV neuropathy. *Neurology*, **70** (24), 2305–2313.

61 Simpson, D.M., Gazda, S., Brown, S. *et al.* (2010) Long-term safety of NGX-4010, a high-concentration capsaicin patch, in patients with peripheral neuropathic pain. *Journal of Pain and Symptom Management*, **39** (6), 1053–1064.

62 Ellis, R.J., Toperoff, W., Vaida, F. *et al.* (2009) Smoked medicinal cannabis for neuropathic pain in HIV: a randomized, crossover clinical trial. *Neuropsychopharmacology*, **34** (3), 672–680.

63 Shiflett, S.C. & Schwartz, G.E. (2011) Effects of acupuncture in reducing attrition and mortality in HIV-infected men with peripheral neuropathy. *Explore (NY)*, **7** (3), 148–154.

64 Sandoval, R., Runft, B. & Roddey, T. (2010) Pilot study: does lower extremity night splinting assist in the management of painful peripheral neuropathy in the HIV/AIDS population? *Journal of the International Association of Physicians in AIDS Care (Chicago, Ill.)*, **9** (6), 368–381.

65 Anastasi, J.K., Capili, B., McMahon, D.J. & Scully, C. (2013) Acu/Moxa for distal sensory peripheral neuropathy in HIV: a randomized control pilot study. *Journal of the Association of Nurses in AIDS Care*, **24** (3), 268–275.

66 Dorfman, D., George, M.C., Schnur, J., Simpson, D.M., Davidson, G. & Montgomery, G. (2013) Hypnosis for treatment of HIV neuropathic pain: a preliminary report. *Pain Medicine*, **14** (7), 1048–1056.

67 Evans, S., Fishman, B., Spielman, L. & Haley, A. (2003) Randomized trial of cognitive behavior therapy versus supportive psychotherapy for HIV-related peripheral neuropathic pain. *Psychosomatics*, **44** (1), 44–50.

CHAPTER 7

Common medical comorbid conditions and chronic pain in HIV

David J. Kim[1] and Christine Ritchie[2]

[1] *University of Alabama at Birmingham, Birmingham, AL, 35233 USA*

[2] *Division of Geriatrics, Department of Medicine, University of California, San Francisco, CA, USA*

Background – the growing prevalence of multimorbidity in the HIV population

Over the past 30 years, AIDS has evolved from a fatal disease of wasting to a chronic condition in most developed countries. The transformation began with the implementation of early prophylaxis against common opportunistic infections in the early 1990s and accelerated shortly thereafter with the introduction of highly active antiretroviral therapy (ART) [1]. Within a matter of a few years, AIDS-related morbidity and mortality declined by 60% in the United States [2]. The success of antiretroviral therapies has led to a demographic shift among persons infected by HIV. Estimates indicate that by 2015, more than 50% of HIV-infected patients will be older than the age of 50. Sixty-five percent of those aged 50–59 years and 70% of those aged 60 years and older have multiple non-AIDS-defining medical comorbidities [3–5]. The transformation of HIV infection from a fatal disease to a chronic condition often accompanied by many other conditions presents a challenge for HIV care providers.

Multimorbidity, commonly defined as the cooccurrence of two or more chronic conditions, is increasingly common in the aging HIV-infected population. Among HIV-infected persons in the United States, the prevalence of multimorbidity is estimated to be around 60–70% and is expected to rise as the population continues to age [5]. In one institution, HIV care providers were asked to report the most commonly seen conditions from their clinical practice. For the 1844 patients receiving care at the institution's HIV clinic, the most prevalent comorbidities were mood disorders, tobacco use, and hypertension. In the general population, multimorbidity has been associated with decreased functional status, quality of life, increased adverse drug events, medical cost, and mortality [4–6]. These burdens are amplified in the aging HIV-infected population. Chronic pain is also one of the most common medical comorbidities in the current HIV treatment era, affecting 39–55% of patients [7]. Management of chronic pain is often complicated by the presence of other comorbidities. **This chapter (1) provides an overview of factors contributing to multimorbidity and pain management complexity in HIV, (2) discusses general principles for chronic pain management in HIV patients with multimorbidity, and (3) presents several case studies to illustrate an approach to evaluating chronic pain management in the context of multimorbidity.**

Chronic Pain and HIV: A Practical Approach, First Edition.
Edited by Jessica S. Merlin, Peter A. Selwyn, Glenn J. Treisman and Angela G. Giovanniello.
© 2016 John Wiley & Sons, Ltd. Published 2016 by John Wiley & Sons, Ltd.

Factors contributing to multimorbidity and pain management complexity in HIV-infected individuals

A number of factors contribute to the development of multimorbidity in HIV-infected patients and add to chronic pain management complexity: chronic inflammation, obesity, aging, cognitive impairment, and polypharmacy.

HIV infection and chronic inflammation

Chronic inflammation and immune dysfunction are common in HIV infection and contribute to higher rates of chronic medical comorbidities in HIV-infected patients [4]. Studies have shown increased development of multiorgan disease (cardiac, hepatic, and renal) among patients on ART with treatment interruptions, supporting the notion that immune dysfunction and chronic virally mediated inflammatory states contribute to the development of other chronic conditions [4]. Even those with long-standing virologic suppression have higher rates of cardiovascular disease, cancer, kidney disease, and neurocognitive disease [8], all of which may directly or indirectly lead to painful complications (e.g., cancer pain, chronic claudication, and falls). Direct virally mediated toxicities contribute to common painful medical comorbidities in HIV-infected patients such as peripheral neuropathy.

Obesity

A growing phenomenon in contemporary HIV care is obesity. The prevalence of obesity among HIV-infected patients now mirrors general population averages. Nearly half of all treatment-naïve HIV patients are either overweight or obese in the current treatment era. Once considered side effects of antiretroviral therapy, conditions such as obesity and dyslipidemia are now observed as baseline conditions for treatment-naïve patients. Recently, investigators have shown that ART side effects account for a modest contribution to weight gain. In one analysis of over 600 patients, nearly half of patients are either overweight or obese prior to ART initiation and 1 in 5 patients move

to a deleterious BMI category within 2 years of ART [9].

While obesity contributes to increased chronic disease morbidity and mortality in the general population, in the setting of a proinflammatory state and immune dysfunction, obesity plays an even larger role in shaping the complexity of patients infected with HIV. With every increase in BMI category, HIV-infected patients are noted to have a greater number of chronic medical comorbidities and more complex disease burdens [5]. Obesity in the context of HIV infection confers increased risks for hypertension, cardiovascular disease, metabolic abnormalities, and multimorbidity [5]. As explained above, these comorbidities can directly and indirectly lead to chronic pain. In addition, obesity itself can lead to avoidance of physical activity, which can lead to the development of joint damage and the perpetuation of chronic pain [10].

Aging

Effective ART has significantly prolonged the life expectancy of people living with HIV/AIDS [11]. Further contributing to an aging HIV-infected population is a greater incidence of HIV infection among older individuals. Nearly a quarter of new AIDS cases in the United States occur in people older than 50 years, which represents a fourfold increase in the cumulative incidence over the last two decades [11,12]

Increased age is one of the strongest risk factors of multimorbidity [13]. Older HIV-infected patients are more likely to suffer from medical comorbidities 10–15 years earlier and have more prescribed medications compared to non-HIV-infected patients with similar baseline characteristics [5,13,14]. The earlier presence of multimorbidity in aging adults with HIV contributes to a greater complexity in pain treatment given the known gastrointestinal and renal toxicity of NSAIDs and the hepatic toxicity of higher doses of acetaminophen.

Cognitive impairment

The older HIV-infected population is more likely to experience cognitive impairment. In a large, single center study, providers reported that 11% of their patient population of over 800 patients with HIV was cognitively impaired [15]. Older adults with HIV and cognitive decline experience poorer adherence to their HIV medications and worse outcomes both related to and independent of HIV infection [16]. Of particular relevance is the issue of pain management in the cognitively impaired patient. Cognitive impairment represents a significant barrier to the treatment of pain in HIV-infected patients. Because pain is inherently subjective, management is largely tailored around one's ability to express symptoms. Pain management becomes increasingly challenging in patients who have difficulty communicating their medical history, as is often the case in those who are cognitively impaired. Declines in cognition may be exacerbated by certain medications, delirium, depression, inadequate social support/neglect, or substance abuse[17,18]. In the context of multimorbidity, care providers must assess for these conditions or circumstances that surround each patient to identify any potential barriers to treatment in this special population. For more information on strategies for communicating with patients with chronic pain, see Chapter 3.

Polypharmacy

Because multimorbidity usually results in the use of multiple medications, the issue of polypharmacy is important to consider in the aging HIV population. Polypharmacy leads to increased risk of drug–drug and drug–food interactions, adverse drug reactions, poor medication adherence, greater healthcare cost, and higher treatment burden. The issue of drug–drug interactions (DDIs) becomes more pressing with older patients as studies have reported the number of prescribed medications nearly doubles in patients older than 50 [14]. Furthermore, current clinical practice guidelines are based on trials that often select for relatively healthy patients with isolated disease. One of the challenges of managing multimorbidity and HIV is whether or not a particular treatment regimen is appropriate given a patient's unique set of comorbid conditions [19]. Two patients with the same chronic pain condition may require different classes of analgesics depending on their ART therapy and comorbid medical conditions. In order to avoid complications related to polypharmacy, care providers must look beyond managing the isolated disease

process with analgesics and consider how introducing a medication will affect downstream processes on a systemic scale. For additional guidance on pharmacologic management of chronic pain, see Chapter 10.

Chronic pain management in the setting of multimorbidity

Challenges arise in the setting of chronic pain and HIV multimorbidity due to lack of evidence-based literature guiding clinical practice. In addition, there are inherent trade-offs when clinicians, in partnership with their patients, must prioritize management of certain conditions over others. While a patient may be concerned about their chronic pain condition, the clinician in a busy primary care practice may feel compelled to focus on the patient's recent hospitalization for diabetic ketoacidosis, elevated blood pressure at triage of 200/100 mm Hg, or may feel that a pharmacologic therapy for chronic pain could exacerbate the patient's other chronic conditions [20].

A model for patient-centered care of older adults with multimorbidity adapted from an American Geriatrics Society expert panel can be applied to the aging HIV-infected population experiencing chronic pain: seek to understand patient preferences, weigh available evidence and the burdens and benefits of interventions, and communicate effectively and decide with the patient on a course of action [20].

One of the first steps in evaluating an HIV-infected patient with chronic pain and multimorbidity is to inquire about the patient's primary goals, treatment preferences, and outcome priorities, that is, whether the patient prefers intensive medical management regardless of side effects, or treatment strategies that take quality of life more into account. While these outcomes may not be mutually exclusive, often trade-offs exist in clinical management where the decision to achieve one goal may come at the expense of another. Integral to this process is a discussion of the possible health outcomes that may result as a consequence of different treatment strategies and establishing an individual treatment plan that best fits each patient's goals.[21] Continued communication

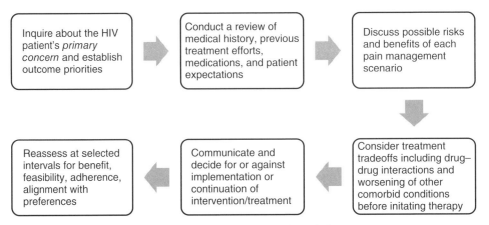

Figure 7.1 Approach to pain management in the setting of multimorbidity.

with the patient and reassessment at established intervals for adherence, benefits, and changes in any preferences is also warranted.

This approach is not necessarily different from the goal-focused patient-centered approach one might apply in any patient; however, in individuals with multimorbidity, the trade-offs may be more pronounced, and systematic utilization of this strategy may allow providers to break down a complex situation into multiple smaller treatment decisions. Strong consideration should be given to both pharmacologic and nonpharmacologic therapies that may be time intensive but carry minimal risk (see Chapter 10).

The algorithm in Figure 7.1 synthesizes the above and offers an approach to managing pain in older adults HIV patients with multimorbidity.

Case studies of chronic pain in the context of multimorbidity and HIV

The following cases highlight the principles, described above, of managing chronic pain in the setting of multimorbidity.

Case examples

Case 1: A 63-year-old HIV patient with a history of hepatitis C with cirrhosis, alcohol and substance abuse, and osteoarthritis involving the knees presents with worsening knee pain, epigastric pain, and 2-day history of dark stools.

- **Past medical hhistory**: HIV infection, hepatitis C coinfection with cirrhosis, alcohol abuse, IV drug use, chronic kidney disease, history of upper GI bleed requiring hospitalization, dyslipidemia, and coronary artery disease.

- **Medications**: Emtricitabine 200 mg, tenofovir 300 mg, efavirenz 600 mg, atorvastatin 20 mg, esomeprazole 40 mg, clopidogrel 75 mg, diclofenac 50 mg BID, and Norco 5/325 p.r.n pain.

Management considerations:

- ∘ **Inquire about the patient's concerns and establish outcome priorities:** The patient's primary concern, despite her multiple comorbidities, is chronic knee pain impairing her mobility. She seeks advice for treatment options for her chronic knee pain.

- ∘ **Review the patient's medical history, previous treatment efforts, medications, and patient expectations:** This patient's pain management is complicated by her comorbid conditions. NSAIDS present a problem because of her previous history of GI bleeding and acetaminophen (in the doses she needs for pain relief) is problematic given her existing liver disease. HCV-infected patients should be cautioned to limit exposure to alcohol and acetaminophen use >2 g/day, which have been shown to contribute to steatosis and fibrosis [22].

◦ **Consider treatment trade-offs including DDIs and worsening of other comorbid conditions before initiating therapy**: This patient is at risk for increased renal toxicity due to the DDI that occurs if diclofenac and tenofovir are used concurrently [23]. Another important point to consider in this patient is the patient's liver disease since diclofenac adds stress to the liver and she is at risk for developing end-stage liver disease (ESLD). ESLD confers a poor prognosis for patients with HIV infection with a 1-year survival around 50–55% [24]. Fortunately, HIV infection is no longer a contraindication to transplantation.

◦ **Communicate and decide for or against implementation or continuation of intervention/treatment**: One potentially helpful treatment for this patient's chronic knee pain is surgery. However, given this patient's history of CAD and liver disease, she may not be a suitable candidate for surgical intervention. Medical management of her knee pain may be limited to physical therapy and opioid analgesics with or without low-dose acetaminophen. Behavioral interventions such as cognitive behavioral therapy and pain self-management have also been shown to improve pain and functional outcomes in individuals with chronic musculoskeletal pain and should be utilized [25]. Given her history of substance use, intensive patient education and close monitoring will be necessary.

◦ **Reassess at selected intervals for benefit, feasibility, adherence, and alignment with preferences**: Given this patient's history of substance abuse and importance of adherence to ART for liver transplant eligibility, close follow-up is warranted. The patient must be aware that her pain condition may not be fully alleviated and that outcomes will be focused on improving function and quality of life.

Case 2: A 55-year-old HIV-infected patient with a 3-year history of peripheral neuropathy presents for an annual follow-up with complaints of increased pain in his upper extremities and worsening depression. He requests to increase his methadone dose as he is not experiencing improvement of his peripheral neuropathy. He also admits that he has not been consistent in his use of his antidepressant medications due to unpleasant side effects. However, he expects complete alleviation of his pain symptoms.

PMH: HIV, hypertension, diabetes mellitus, chronic renal insufficiency, peripheral neuropathy, chronic musculoskeletal pain from a previous MVA, and depression.

Medications: Emtricitabine 200 mg, tenofovir 300 mg, efavirenz 600 mg, methadone 10 mg BID, amlodipine 5 mg, citalopram 20 mg, metformin 850 mg BID, and benazepril/hydrochlorothiazide 5/6.25.

Management considerations:

◦ **Inquire about the patient's concerns and establish outcome priorities**: As with each patient with chronic pain in the context of multimorbidity, outcome priorities must be established. In this case, the patient's primary priority is remission of his chronic peripheral nerve pain. His second concern and priority is alleviation of his worsening depression. A discussion with the patient should focus on how each of his conditions affects his daily function and HIV disease management.

◦ **Review the patient's medical history, previous treatment efforts, medications, and patient expectations**: This patient has several medical conditions that may affect his chronic pain experience. His long-standing diabetes mellitus may directly contribute to worsening of his peripheral neuropathy [26]. Therefore, it will be important to optimize his glucose control. Previous treatment efforts included medical management with methadone 10 mg BID. The patient requests a higher dose of methadone because he believes it may help with his worsening peripheral neuropathy.

○ **Educate the patient about possible treatment options based on his/her outcome priorities**: An important point to discuss with this patient is a treatment plan that manages multimorbidity while also minimizing polypharmacy. In this case, the patient has two medical conditions, depression and peripheral neuropathy that may benefit from a single treatment with duloxetine. Given his general unresponsiveness to opioids, methadone and other opioid analgesics may not be the optimal or sufficient treatment approach because duloxetine may be more effective in addressing both his peripheral neuropathy and depression. Cognitive behavioral therapy has been evaluated in HIV-infected patients with neuropathy with some success and should be considered [27,28] Optimal management of his depression may also improve his overall treatment adherence [29].

○ **Consider treatment trade-offs including DDIs and worsening of other comorbid conditions before initiating therapy**: Methadone metabolism occurs primarily through the cytochrome P450 enzyme system, a system also responsible for the metabolism of many antiretroviral and antidepressant medications. The greatest interactions between methadone and antiretrovirals occur with the nonnucleoside reverse transcriptase inhibitors and the protease inhibitors. Using methadone together with duloxetine may increase the blood levels and effects of both medications.

○ **Communicate and decide for or against implementation or continuation of intervention/treatment**: Based on current literature, gabapentin may be a preferred agent since it has not been shown to have any drug interactions with HIV antiretroviral medications [30]. However, when multiple conditions can be treated with a single agent, one must consider the added benefit of reducing polypharmacy such as better medication adherence and reducing chances for DDIs.

A pain management strategy in this case may be to taper the methadone while initiating and increasing his duloxetine.

○ **Reassess at selected intervals for benefit, feasibility, adherence, and alignment with preferences**: Close follow-up with this patient is necessary, as medication adherence to antidepressant treatment may be important not only to this adherence to ART but also to his pain management. It will be important to educate the patient that the effects of the medication may not be apparent for several weeks.

Summary of cases and conclusion

These cases illustrate the complex treatment decisions faced by providers and patients regarding chronic pain in the setting of multimorbidity. In these situations, there are no "correct" answers. Rather, arriving at a treatment plan requires skilled communication of trade-offs by the physician to the patient and an honest dialogue about patient priorities. For additional strategies regarding communicating about such challenging issues with individuals having chronic pain, see Chapter 3.

References

1 Sackoff, J.E., Hanna, D.B., Pfeiffer, M.R. & Torian, L.V. (2006) Causes of death among persons with AIDS in the era of highly active antiretroviral therapy: New York City. *Annals of Internal Medicine*, **145** (6), 397–406.

2 Palella, F.J. Jr.,, Delaney, K.M., Moorman, A.C. *et al.* (1998) Declining morbidity and mortality among patients with advanced human immunodeficiency virus infection. HIV outpatient study investigators. *The New England Journal of Medicine*, **338** (13), 853–860.

3 Goulet, J.L., Fultz, S.L., Rimland, D. *et al.* (2007) Aging and infectious diseases: do patterns of comorbidity vary by HIV status, age, and HIV severity? *Clinical Infectious Diseases: An Official Publication of the Infectious Diseases Society of America*, **45** (12), 1593–1601.

4 Salter, M.L., Lau, B., Go, V.F., Mehta, S.H. & Kirk, G.D. (2011) HIV infection, immune suppression, and uncontrolled viremia are associated with increased multimorbidity among aging injection drug users. *Clinical Infectious Diseases: An Official Publication of the Infectious Diseases Society of America*, **53** (12), 1256–1264.

5 Kim, D.J., Westfall, A.O., Chamot, E. *et al.* (2012) Multimorbidity patterns in HIV-infected patients: the role of obesity in chronic disease clustering. *Journal of Acquired Immune Deficiency Syndromes*, **61** (5), 600–605.

6 Fortin, M., Hudon, C., Haggerty, J., Akker, M. & Almirall, J. (2010) Prevalence estimates of multimorbidity: a comparative study of two sources. *BMC Health Services Research*, **10**, 111.

7 Merlin, J.S., Westfall, A.O., Raper, J.L. *et al.* (2012) Pain, mood, and substance abuse in HIV: implications for clinic visit utilization, antiretroviral therapy adherence, and virologic failure. *Journal of Acquired Immune Deficiency Syndromes*, **61** (2), 164–170.

8 Hirschhorn, L.R., Kaaya, S.F., Garrity, P.S., Chopyak, E. & Fawzi, M.C. (2012) Cancer and the 'other' noncommunicable chronic diseases in older people living with HIV/AIDS in resource-limited settings: a challenge to success. *AIDS*, **26** (Suppl 1), S65–75.

9 Tate, T., Willig, A.L., Willig, J.H. *et al.* (2012) HIV infection and obesity: where did all the wasting go? *Antiviral Therapy*, **17** (7), 1281–1289.

10 Vincent HK, Seay AN, Montero C, Conrad BP, Hurley RW. & Vincent KR. (2013) Functional pain severity and mobility in overweight older men and women with chronic low-back pain--part I. *American Journal of Physical Medicine and Rehabilitation*, **92** (5), 430–438. dvi:10.1097/PHM.0b013e31828763a0.

11 Justice, A.C. (2010) HIV and aging: time for a new paradigm. *Current HIV/AIDS Reports*, **7** (2), 69–76.

12 Martin, C.P., Fain, M.J. & Klotz, S.A. (2008) The older HIV-positive adult: a critical review of the medical literature. *The American Journal of Medicine*, **121** (12), 1032–1037.

13 Guaraldi, G., Orlando, G., Zona, S. *et al.* (2011) Premature age-related comorbidities among HIV-infected persons compared with the general population. *Clinical Infectious Diseases:*

An Official Publication of the Infectious Diseases Society of America, **53** (11), 1120–1126.

14 Vance, D.E., Wadley, V.G., Crowe, M.G., Raper, J.L. & Ball, K.K. (2011) Cognitive and everyday functioning in older and younger adults with and without HIV. *Clinical Gerontologist*, **34** (5), 413–426.

15 Kilbourne, A.M., Justice, A.C., Rabeneck, L., Rodriguez-Barradas, M., Weissman, S. & Team VP (2001) General medical and psychiatric comorbidity among HIV-infected veterans in the post-HAART era. *Journal of Clinical Epidemiology*, **54** (Suppl 1), S22–8.

16 Hinkin, C.H., Hardy, D.J., Mason, K.I. *et al.* (2004) Medication adherence in HIV-infected adults: effect of patient age, cognitive status, and substance abuse. *AIDS*, **18** (Suppl 1), S19–25.

17 Passmore, P. & Cunningham, E. (2014) Pain assessment in cognitive impairment. *Journal of Pain and Palliative Care Pharmacotherapy*, **28** (3), 305–307. doi:10.3109/15360288.2014.941136

18 Buffum, M.D., Hutt, E., Chang, V.T., Craine, M.H. & Snow, A.L. (2007) Cognitive impairment and pain management: review of issues and challenges. *Journal of Rehabilitation Research and Development*, **44** (2), 315–330.

19 Gudin, J. (2012) Opioid therapies and cytochrome p450 interactions. *J Pain Symptom Manage*, **44** (6 Suppl), S4–S14. doi:10.1016/j.jpainsymman.2012.08.013

20 Guiding principles for the care of older adults with multimorbidity: an approach for clinicians (2012) Guiding principles for the care of older adults with multimorbidity: an approach for clinicians: American Geriatrics Society Expert Panel on the Care of Older Adults with Multimorbidity. *Journal of the American Geriatrics Society*, **60** (10), E1–E25.

21 Fried, T.R., Tinetti, M.E. & Iannone, L. (2011) Primary care clinicians' experiences with treatment decision making for older persons with multiple conditions. *Archives of Internal Medicine*, **171** (1), 75–80.

22 Hezode, C., Zafrani, E.S., Roudot-Thoraval, F. *et al.* (2008) Daily cannabis use: a novel risk factor of steatosis severity in patients with chronic hepatitis C. *Gastroenterology*, **134** (2), 432–439.

23 Madeddu, G., Bonfanti, P., De Socio, G.V. *et al.* (2008) Tenofovir renal safety in HIV-infected patients: results from the SCOLTA Project.

Biomedicine & Pharmacotherapy = Biomedecine & Pharmacotherapie, **62** (1), 6–11.

24 Miro, J.M., Aguero, F., Laguno, M. *et al.* (2007) Liver transplantation in HIV/hepatitis co-infection. *Journal of HIV Therapy*, **12** (1), 24–35.

25 Kroenke, K., Bair, M.J., Damush, T.M. *et al.* (2009) Optimized antidepressant therapy and pain self-management in primary care patients with depression and musculoskeletal pain: a randomized controlled trial. *JAMA, The Journal of The American Medical Association*, **301** (20), 2099–2110.

26 Schutz, S.G. & Robinson-Papp, J. (2013) HIV-related neuropathy: current perspectives. *Hiv/Aids.*, **5**, 243–251.

27 Trafton, J.A., Sorrell, J.T., Holodniy, M. *et al.* (2012) Outcomes associated with a cognitive-behavioral chronic pain management program implemented in three public HIV primary care clinics. *The Journal of Behavioral Health Services & Research*, **39** (2), 158–173.

28 Cucciare, M.A., Sorrell, J.T. & Trafton, J.A. (2009) Predicting response to cognitive-behavioral therapy in a sample of HIV-positive patients with chronic pain. *Journal of Behavioral Medicine*, **32** (4), 340–348.

29 Yun, L.W., Maravi, M., Kobayashi, J.S., Barton, P.L. & Davidson, A.J. (2005) Antidepressant treatment improves adherence to antiretroviral therapy among depressed HIV-infected patients. *Journal of Acquired Immune Deficiency Syndromes*, **38** (4), 432–438.

30 Keswani, S.C., Pardo, C.A., Cherry, C.L., Hoke, A. & McArthur, J.C. (2002) HIV-associated sensory neuropathies. *AIDS*, **16** (16), 2105–2117.

CHAPTER 8

Psychiatric comorbidities among individuals with HIV and chronic pain

Durga Roy[1], C. Brendan Clark[2] and Glenn Treisman[3]

[1] Department of Psychiatry and Behavioral Sciences, Johns Hopkins University, Baltimore, MD, USA

[2] Department of Psychiatry, University of Alabama at Birmingham, Birmingham, AL, USA

[3] Department of Psychiatry and Behavioral Sciences, Department of Internal Medicine, Johns Hopkins University School of Medicine, Broadway, Baltimore, MD, USA

Psychiatric comorbidities are common among individuals with chronic pain. Compounding matters, psychiatric comorbidities are also more common among individuals with HIV than in the general population. Therefore, the provider seeing an HIV-infected patient with chronic pain should be alert to the most common psychiatric comorbidities encountered, screen for them in every patient, and understand how these conditions may impact the patient's chronic pain treatment course.

In this chapter, we discuss the most important psychiatric aspects of managing chronic pain among HIV-infected individuals. Certain psychiatric disorders, especially mood disorders such as Major Depressive Disorder and Bipolar Disorder, anxiety disorders such as Generalized Anxiety Disorder and Posttraumatic Stress Disorder, and psychotic disorders such as Schizophrenia inherently exacerbate chronic pain conditions. In addition, an individual's life experiences can directly influence aspects of chronic pain and its treatment. Substance use disorders, personality, and temperament also directly impact chronic pain treatment; these topics are covered more completely in other chapters.

Psychiatric diseases that exacerbate chronic pain

Several psychiatric diseases have increased prevalence in individuals with HIV, including Major Depressive Disorders, anxiety spectrum disorders including Posttraumatic Stress Disorder, Bipolar Disorder, and Schizophrenia [1]. These comorbidities may predispose individuals to acquiring HIV and are also associated with worse HIV outcomes, including adherence to ART and retention in HIV primary care. Of these comorbidities, depression is the best studied in the context of chronic pain and, thus, will be the focus of our discussion. Our discussion will do its best to differentiate between Major Depressive Disorder (meeting full DSM-V criteria for the disorder), depressive mood referred to as depression (self-report of increased negative mood without the accompanying physical and cognitive impairments found in the disorder), depressive symptoms (meeting partial but not full criteria for Major Depressive Disorder), and demoralization (self-report of depressed mood in response to a stressor or negative life event).

Chronic Pain and HIV: A Practical Approach, First Edition.
Edited by Jessica S. Merlin, Peter A. Selwyn, Glenn J. Treisman and Angela G. Giovanniello.
© 2016 John Wiley & Sons, Ltd. Published 2016 by John Wiley & Sons, Ltd.

Co-occurrence of chronic pain and psychiatric comorbidities among individuals with HIV

At this point, there are no epidemiological studies of the co-occurrence of chronic pain and psychiatric comorbidities in individuals living with HIV. In non-HIV samples, co-occurrence varies greatly based on demographics and pain conditions [2,3]. Literature on chronic pain and concomitant psychiatric illness in individuals with HIV is just now emerging, and recent studies suggest a high degree of psychiatric comorbidity associated with chronic pain in this population. For example, in a cohort of indigent HIV-infected individuals recruited primarily from homeless shelters and food programs, Miaskowski *et al.* found that 43% reported depression, but that report of depression was strongly correlated with self-report of pain severity. Only 9% of the subgroup reporting mild pain also reported depression; however, 43% of the moderate pain subgroup and 48% of the severe pain subgroup reported depression. In another study of 154 HIV-infected individuals recruited as a convenience sample in an ambulatory HIV clinic, one third had a previous history of psychiatric illness, more than half were found to experience 4/6 psychological symptoms queried, and nearly half of all patients experienced at least one psychological symptom at high distress or high frequency. Half of all patients (74, 47.7%) experienced "high distress" or "high frequency" from at least one psychological symptom [33]. In addition, Merlin *et al.* found a high degree of overlap between self-report of pain, symptoms of depression and anxiety, and substance use among individuals with HIV [31].

In addition, Merlin et al. also present a biopsychosocial framework for chronic pain in individuals with HIV. This framework acknowledges that psychosocial stressors such as traumatic events, psychiatric comorbidity, and stigma are common among both individuals with HIV and individuals with chronic pain. This framework suggests that individuals with both HIV and chronic pain may, as a result, have a particularly high burden of these psychosocial stressors.

The relationship between depression and chronic pain

Depression and chronic pain are closely integrated. Depression increases aspects of pain, pain increases aspects of depression, and numerous factors can increase both pain and depression simultaneously. As a result, depressed mood as well as Major Depressive Disorder should be incorporated into any formulation of chronic pain.

Depression often precedes the onset of chronic pain and can increase pain sensitivity [27,28]. While changes in pain sensitivity have been described in Posttraumatic Stress Disorder [4] and Generalized Anxiety Disorder as well as Panic Disorder [5], they are best documented in depression. As many as 60% of patients with Major Depressive Disorder suffer changes in pain perception and processing [6]. Depressive symptoms may be an independent risk factor for the onset of pain syndromes such as neck and back pain [7,8] or fibromyalgia [9] and as much as 16% of the chronic pain population may have preexisting depressive symptoms [10]. Patients with Major Depressive Disorder have significantly more frequent, more intense, and more unpleasant pain complaints than healthy control subjects [11].

Depression not only increases sensitivity to pain, but it can also complicate treatment by interfering with patients' ability to engage in appropriate self-care and cope with daily stress. Depression is associated with changes in sleep, appetite, and energy. The resulting lethargy and apathy can inhibit engagement in treatment, exercise, and other techniques for pain management. Depression has been linked with social impairment and irritability [12,13]. This can cause problems at work as well as in interpersonal relationships [14]. Furthermore, it can lead to disagreements with providers (see Chapter 13, Care of the Difficult Patient). As pain treatment is typically directed toward restoring patients' function, comorbid depression can make pain treatment much more challenging [29].

Individuals with depression are more likely to misuse prescribed opioids than individuals without depression, regardless of history of substance use disorder [15]. Complicating matters further, illicit drug use is a risk factor for the acquisition of human immunodeficiency virus (HIV), and a significant proportion of HIV-infected patients with pain syndromes have a comorbid substance use disorder [32]. Individuals with a history of illicit drug use are also more likely to misuse prescribed opioids [16]. Adding even another layer of complexity, the combination of psychiatric illness including depression, substance use disorder, and HIV (the "triply diagnosed patient") represents a patient population that is overrepresented in ambulatory HIV care due to their symptom severity and chronicity [1]. In these patients, pain is particularly difficult to manage, and opioids may be especially problematic.

Bipolar disorder and schizophrenia with chronic pain in HIV

Bipolar disorder and schizophrenia are both associated with an increased risk of HIV infection [1] and are more common among individuals with HIV than individuals without HIV. There is no published data on the relationship between these disorders and chronic pain in HIV-infected patients. In non-HIV populations, the available literature suggests a strong association between bipolar disorder and chronic pain [17], but not between schizophrenia and chronic pain [18].

Our clinical experience is that these disorders complicate chronic pain management in a variety of ways. These severe psychiatric illnesses are generally associated with poorer medical outcomes, so patients may have more medical comorbidities that contribute to their chronic pain and complicate its management. High rates of traumatic injury in these conditions may increase the likelihood of developing chronic pain. Mood lability, especially in Bipolar Disorder, may affect chronic pain in similar ways to depression as described above. Stigma associated with these severe mental illnesses may make it difficult to fully engage the interdisciplinary team ideally needed to treat these patients' chronic pain. Finally, treatment of psychiatric comorbidity and managing psychiatric

symptoms in these patients is typically a critical first step toward improving patients' pain. This is because patients with poorly controlled bipolar disorder and schizophrenia are less likely to be able to engage in important conversations about the nature of chronic pain, and the role of pharmacologic and nonpharmacologic management including behavioral therapies. However, especially in those with the most severe mental illness, finding appropriate psychiatric treatment settings and achieving long-lasting symptom remission may be a particular challenge.

Life experiences that exacerbate chronic pain conditions

Traumatic, stressful life events are common among HIV-infected individuals. One study of traumatic life events such as death in the family, job loss, divorce, incarceration, and assault found that HIV-infected individuals experienced an average of three such events in the past year [19].

The impact of traumatic life events can be profound. They can result in decreased positive mood and diminished happiness, which is often labeled as depression, but may not encompass the physical (sleep, appetite, and energy) and cognitive (concentration, memory, and focus) deficits that characterize Major Depressive Disorder. Traumatic events that do not lead to major depression, but still cause states of distress are best described as demoralization. The term was popularized by Jerome Frank, one of the fathers of modern psychiatry [20]. He described the way in which psychological losses or injuries produced a state of low mood and diminished optimism that recovered with time, support, and encouragement. Compounding matters, pain also often produces demoralization. HIV and the associated burdens of living with a chronic illness and its stigma often make demoralization worse. Demoralized patients are less health seeking, less engaged in rehabilitation, and more pessimistic. This may affect their ability to recover as well as their adherence to medications. In fact, there is evidence to suggest that traumatic life events among HIV-infected individuals are associated with suboptimal adherence to antiretroviral therapy and retention in HIV primary care [21]. Such demoralization may also lead patients to seek comfort, rather than recovery, as a goal.

Life experience affects the interpretation and experience of pain. Experience "teaches" patients to see things in a particular way. Learned helplessness may result from being forced to endure aversive stimuli, or stimuli that are painful or otherwise unpleasant. Then, the individual becomes unable or unwilling to avoid subsequent encounters with those stimuli, even if they are escapable, presumably because of the learned lack of control over situations that are similar. Chronic pain conditions may represent such aversive stimuli, and patients may falsely believe that they no longer have the ability to change or get better [22].

Patients may also have diverse points of view about medical care, including chronic pain care. Firmly held beliefs based on life experience and culturally derived ideas lead to complications in chronic pain treatment. For example, the belief that all suffering should be relieved is currently partly responsible for the epidemic of opiate use in the United States [23,24]. Other commonly encountered ideas include the belief that natural drugs are inherently better, medications are bad, and the medical profession conducts experiments on patients without their consent. Other factors including poverty, geographic isolation, and lack of community resources barriers lead to medical disenfranchisement. Navigating communication around these complex issues is an important component of HIV care in general, and in the authors' experience, in the care of HIV-infected individuals with chronic pain.

The psychology of each individual is unique and is a result of a unique set of life experiences. There is no simple single way to understand patients, and the domain of life experience may require an extended relationship with a patient to appreciate. Although all patients need a rehabilitative treatment plan to improve their pain and function, each patient needs an individual understanding of how to make the treatment plan work for them, to overcome the barriers they face as a unique individual, and to aid in their recovery.

Identifying and treating psychiatric illness in individuals with HIV

Given the high prevalence of psychiatric comorbidities among HIV-infected individuals with chronic pain, and the importance of these comorbidities in chronic pain management, routine screening is essential. Screening tools that have been used in HIV clinic settings include the PHQ-9 for depression and the GAD-7 for anxiety [25]. A detailed psychiatric and addiction history is also necessary. If the patient's psychiatric diagnosis is unclear, a psychiatrist should be consulted.

Psychiatric comorbidities should be treated aggressively in any individual in whom they are found; this is especially important among individuals with chronic pain. For example, given the close connection between chronic pain and depression described above, treatment of comorbid depression often results in dramatic improvement in patients' pain. We recommend an approach that involves upfront pharmacologic and nonpharmacologic treatment (e.g., cognitive behavioral therapy or supportive psychotherapy) of the psychiatric illness, alongside low-risk, nonopioid analgesics, and physical therapy when indicated (see Chapter 13). Over time, as a relationship between the patient and provider is formed and psychiatric symptoms begin to improve, we also focus on discussing pain self-management strategies and setting achievable goals using motivational interviewing (see Chapter 13). We use opioids cautiously in patients who have poorly controlled psychiatric symptoms as they may exacerbate these symptoms and result in opioid misuse [15].

A proactive approach that focuses on early identification and referral to intervention can eliminate many problems before they develop (e.g., addiction, conflict with providers). Even mild levels of psychological distress can grow into disorders quickly when combined with chronic pain and dysfunctional coping styles [30]. Individuals with a tendency to catastrophize, ruminate on their impairment, and fear that their pain will grow to become intolerable have been shown to develop mental illness as a result of the anxiety and stress produced by these maladaptive thinking patterns [26]. Patients reporting such coping styles should be monitored for increasing distress. Educating nonmentally ill, but psychologically distressed patients on the dangers inherent in the described coping styles can prevent the eventual progression to mental illness.

It is important to note that some patients may not expect such an emphasis on treatment of comorbid psychiatric illness in chronic pain treatment. For a detailed discussion of communication with patients about the close relationship between mood and pain, and the importance of treating both together, see Chapter 13.

Summary

Psychiatric comorbidities play an important role in chronic pain management. Major Depressive Disorder has the most well-described role in complicating chronic pain, but Bipolar Disorder, Schizophrenia, personality, temperament, addictions, and the individual story of the patient all play a profound role in the course of pain management and must be effectively treated in order to help patients recover. In a time of shrinking resources, psychiatric elements are often ignored or undertreated. This leads to increased disability, revolving hospital admissions, increased medical testing, unhelpful treatment, and increasing addictions. The enormous costs of ignoring the psychiatric comorbidity in patients with chronic pain, both in terms of financial losses and losses of human capacity, are beyond measure. It is imperative that we continue to strive toward providing

integrated medical and psychiatric care for our patients, as well as advocating for the resources needed to provide that care.

References

1 Treisman, G.J. & Angelino, A. (2004) *The Psychiatry of AIDS: A Guide to Diagnosis and Treatment*. Johns Hopkins Press.

2 Currie, S.R. & Wang, J.L. (2004) Chronic back pain and major depression in the general Canadian population. *Pain*, **107** (1), 54–60.

3 Miller, L.R. & Cano, A. (2009) Comorbid chronic pain and depression: who is at risk? *The Journal of Pain*, **10** (6), 619–627.

4 Otis, J.D., Keane, T.M. & Kerns, R.D. (2003) An examination of the relationship between chronic pain and post-traumatic stress disorder. *Journal of Rehabilitation Research and Development*, **40** (5), 397–405.

5 Fraenkel, Y.M., Kindler, S. & Melmed, R.N. (1996–1997) Differences in cognitions during chest pain of patients with panic disorder and ischemic heart disease. *Depression and Anxiety*, **4** (5), 217–222.

6 Fava, M., Mallinckrodt, C.H., Detke, M.J., Watkin, J.G. & Wohlreich, M.M. (2004) The effect of duloxetine on painful physical symptoms in depressed patients: do improvements in these symptoms result in higher remission rates? *Journal of Clinical Psychiatry*, **65** (4), 521–530.

7 Carroll, L.J., Cassidy, J.D. & Côté, P. (2003) Factors associated with the onset of an episode of depressive symptoms in the general population. *Journal of Clinical Epidemiology*, **56** (7), 651–658.

8 Reid, M.C., Williams, C.S., Concato, J., Tinetti, M.E. & Gill, T.M. (2003) Depressive symptoms as a risk factor for disabling back pain in community-dwelling older persons. *Journal of American Geriatrics Society*, **51** (12), 1710–1717.

9 McBeth, J. & Silman, A.J. (2001) The role of psychiatric disorders in fibromyalgia. *Current Rheumatology Reports*, **3** (2), 157–164.

10 Croft, P.R., Papageorgiou, A.C., Ferry, S., Thomas, E., Jayson, M.I. & Silman, A.J. (1995)

Psychologic distress and low back pain. Evidence from a prospective study in the general population. *Spine*, **20** (24), 2731–2737.

11 Lautenbacher, S., Spernal, J., Schreiber, W. & Krieg, J.C. (1999) Relationship between clinical pain complaints and pain sensitivity in patients with depression and panic disorder. *Psychosomatic Medicine*, **61** (6), 822–827.

12 Pasquini, M., Picardi, A., Biondi, M., Gaetano, P. & Morosini, P. (2004) Relevance of anger and irritability in outpatients with major depressive disorder. *Psychopathology*, **37** (4), 155–160.

13 Joiner, T.E., Metalsky, G.I., Katz, J. & Beach, S.R. (1999) Depression and excessive reassurance-seeking. *Psychological Inquiry*, **10** (3), 269–278.

14 Segrin, C. (2000) Social skills deficits associated with depression. *Clinical Psychology Review*, **20** (3), 379–403.

15 Grattan, A., Sullivan, M.D., Saunders, K.W., Campbell, C.I. & Von Korff, M.R. (2012) Depression and prescription opioid misuse among chronic opioid therapy recipients with no history of substance abuse. *Annals of Family Medicine*, **10** (4), 304–311.

16 Morasco, B.J. & Dobscha, S.K. (2008) Prescription medication misuse and substance use disorder in VA primary care patients with chronic pain. *General Hospital Psychiatry*, **30** (2), 93–99.

17 Stubbs, B., Eggermont, L., Mitchell, A.J. *et al.* (2015) The prevalence of pain in bipolar disorder: a systematic review and large-scale meta-analysis. *Acta Psychiatrica Scandinavica*, **131** (2), 75–88.

18 Engels, G., Francke, A.L., van Meijel, B. *et al.* (2014) Clinical pain in schizophrenia: a systematic review. *The Journal of Pain*, **15** (5), 457–467.

19 Pence, B.W., Raper, J.L., Reif, S., Thielman, N.M., Leserman, J. & Mugavero, M.J. (2010) Incident stressful and traumatic life events and human immunodeficiency virus sexual transmission risk behaviors in a longitudinal, multisite cohort study. *Psychosomatic Medicine*, **72** (7), 720–726.

20 Frank, J. (1961) *Persuasion and Healing: A Comparative Study of Psychotherapy*. JHU Press.

21 Mugavero, M.J., Raper, J.L., Reif, S. *et al.* (2009) Overload: impact of incident stressful events on antiretroviral medication adherence and virologic failure in a longitudinal, multisite human immunodeficiency virus cohort study. *Psychosomatic Medicine*, **71** (9), 920–926.

22 Samwel, H.J., Evers, A.W., Crul, B.J. & Kraaimaat, F.W. (2006) The role of helplessness, fear of pain, and passive pain-coping in chronic pain patients. *The Clinical Journal of Pain*, **22** (3), 245–251.

23 Berge, K.H. & Burkle, C.M. (2014) Opioid overdose: when good drugs break bad. *Mayo Clinic Proceedings*, **89** (4), 437–439.

24 Hirsch, R.L. (2014) The contribution of patient satisfaction to the opiate abuse epidemic. *Mayo Clinic Proceedings*, **89** (8), 1168.

25 Perry, B.A., Westfall, A.O., Molony, E. *et al.* (2013) Characteristics of an ambulatory palliative care clinic for HIV-infected patients. *Journal of Palliative Medicine*, **16** (8), 934–937.

26 Samwel, H.J., Evers, A.W., Crul, B.J. & Kraaimaat, F.W. (2006) The role of helplessness, fear of pain, and passive pain-coping in chronic pain patients. *Clin J Pain*, **22** (3), 245–251.

27 Blumer, D. & Heilbronn, M. (1982) Chronic pain as a variant of depressive disease: the pain-prone disorder. *Journal of Nervous and Mental Disease*, **170** (7), 381–406.

28 Bravo, L., Mico, J.A., Rey-Brea, R., Pérez-Nievas, B., Leza, J.C. & Berrocoso, E. (2012) Depressive-like states heighten the aversion to painful stimuli in a rat model of comorbid chronic pain and depression. *Anesthesiology*, **117** (3), 613–625.

29 Dworkin, R.H., Richlin, D.M., Handlin, D.S. & Brand, L. (1986) Predicting treatment response in depressed and non-depressed chronic pain patients. *Pain*, **24** (3), 343–353.

30 Lucey, B.P., Clifford, D.B., Creighton, J., Edwards, R.R., McArthur, J.C. & Haythornthwaite, J. (2011) Relationship of depression and catastrophizing to pain, disability, and medication adherence in patients with HIV-associated sensory neuropathy. *AIDS Care*, **23** (8), 921–928.

31 Merlin, J.S., Westfall, A.O. & Raper, J.L. (2012) Pain, mood, and substance abuse in HIV: implications for clinic visit utilization, antiretroviral therapy adherence, and virologic failure. *Journal of Acquired Immune Deficiency Syndromes*, **61** (2), 164–170.

32 Basu, S., Bruce, R.D., Barry, D.T. & Altice, F.L. (2007) Pharmacological pain control for human immunodeficiency virus-infected adults with a history of drug dependence. *Journal of Substance Abuse Treatment*, **32** (4), 399–409.

33 Merlin, J.S., Cen, L., Praestgaard, A. & Turner, M. (2012) Pain and physical and psychological symptoms in ambulatory HIV patients in the current treatment era. *Journal of Pain and Symptom Management*, **43** (3), 638–645.

CHAPTER 9

Comorbid substance use among persons with HIV and chronic pain

Paula J. Lum[1] and R. Douglas Bruce[2,3]

[1] Department of Medicine, University of California, San Francisco, CA, USA
[2] Department of Medicine, Cornell Scott-Hill Health Center, New Haven, CT, USA
[3] Department of Medicine, Yale University, New Haven, CT, USA

Introduction

The unhealthy use of alcohol, tobacco, and other drugs, whether current or in the past, is an important consideration when evaluating and treating individuals with chronic pain. Not only are HIV-infected persons that use drugs disproportionately affected by pain, but their levels of distress and dysfunction are higher compared to those who report no use. For medical providers, the prescription of opioid analgesics and other controlled substances can be challenging because patients with histories of substance use are at increased risk of developing negative, unintended consequences of opioid treatment (e.g., misuse, addiction, and diversion), and feelings of mistrust or uncertainty have led providers historically to undertreat pain in both people who use drugs and people living with HIV. These challenges are best addressed when HIV providers adopt a risk–benefit framework with an attitude of positive regard for their patients with comorbid substance use and chronic pain. When opioid analgesics are indicated for the treatment of chronic pain, a prescribing provider's tasks are to continually assess if the benefits of prescribing outweigh the risks of harm and to take actions to minimize the risks of negative consequences, including not prescribing opioids. At the same time, a skilled clinician will value the inherent worth and potential of her patient, demonstrate

an active interest in understanding a patient's internal perspective, respect a patient's autonomy to choose his own direction, and affirm a patient's strengths and efforts [1]. These tasks, which are of critical importance when caring for persons with substance use histories, occur at the time of first evaluation, treatment initiation, and periodic monitoring throughout the duration of treatment for pain. In this chapter, we examine (1) the wide range of substance use and recommended terminology to describe it, (2) the profound effects of unhealthy substance use on the HIV care cascade, (3) the experience of pain by persons with HIV and substance use problems, (4) the challenges faced by HIV providers caring for patients with co-occurring pain and addiction, and (5) specific advice for evaluating and treating moderate–severe chronic pain in patients living with HIV disease and current or prior substance use disorders.

Understanding the language of substance use

The identification of patients with unhealthy substance use is essential to improve the management of chronic pain. In order to accurately screen and assess patients, providers must understand the nomenclature of substance use behaviors. Confusion about substance use terminology in both the medical community

Chronic Pain and HIV: A Practical Approach, First Edition.
Edited by Jessica S. Merlin, Peter A. Selwyn, Glenn J. Treisman and Angela G. Giovanniello.
© 2016 John Wiley & Sons, Ltd. Published 2016 by John Wiley & Sons, Ltd.

Table 9.1 DSM-5 criteria for substance use disorder.

1 Taking the substance in larger amounts or for longer than you meant to
2 Wanting to cut down or stop using the substance but not managing to
3 Spending a lot of time getting, using, or recovering from use of the substance
4 Cravings and urges to use the substance
5 Not managing to do what you should at work, home, or school because of substance use
6 Continuing to use, even when it causes problems in relationships
7 Giving up important social, occupational, or recreational activities because of substance use
8 Using substances again and again, even when it puts you in danger
9 Continuing to use, even when you know you have a physical or psychological problem that could have been caused or made worse by the substance
10 Needing more of the substance to get the effect you want (tolerance)
11 Development of withdrawal symptoms, which can be relieved by taking more of the substance

The number of criteria above correlates with the severity of the disorder. Two or three symptoms indicate a mild disorder, four or five moderate substance use disorder, and six or more indicate a severe substance use disorder. From the DSM-5, American Psychiatric Association, 2013.

and the public reinforces stigma and too often results in referrals to inappropriate levels of care [2]. Language that describes people who use drugs as "addicts" or "abusers" can undermine a patient–provider encounter and derail a patient's motivation to seek help or treatment. Nonjudgmental terminology, on the other hand, facilitates a more accurate assessment of substance use behaviors and a more appropriate pain treatment plan.

Whether relating to the nonmedical use of a prescribed medication or illicit drug use, the definition of "unhealthy use" or "misuse" extends broadly from a range of drug use behaviors described as "risky" or "problematic" to the maladaptive patterns classified by the American Psychiatric Association's *DSM-IV-TR* as "substance abuse" and "substance dependence" or by the revised *DSM-5* as "substance use disorder" and the chronic brain disease of "addiction." Unfortunately, the two terms "substance dependence" and "physical dependence" often have been mistaken to mean the same thing, resulting in misdiagnoses and inappropriate treatment interventions. While still used frequently in journal articles and the lay press, substance "abuse" and "dependence" were replaced in 2013 with the less hierarchical *DSM-5* term "substance use disorder" designated further as mild, moderate, or severe [3]. Only

2 of 11 diagnostic criteria within a 12-month period are required for a diagnosis of substance use disorder. The number of criteria met correlates with the severity of the disorder (see Table 9.1 for specific criteria). An important exception is the medically supervised use of opioid analgesics or other psychoactive medications for which *tolerance* and *withdrawal* are physiologic adaptations and, therefore, should not be counted as diagnostic criteria for an opioid use disorder.

The medical term "addiction" by comparison refers to a primary, chronic, neurobiological disease, with genetic, psychosocial, and environmental factors influencing its development and manifestations. It is characterized by behaviors that include impaired control over drug use, compulsive use, continued use despite harm, and craving, often involving cycles of relapse and remission (American Society of Addiction Medicine definition of addiction: http://www.asam.org/for-the-public/definition-of-addiction). Individuals diagnosed with the disease of addiction often meet diagnostic criteria for substance dependence (DSM-IV) or moderate–severe substance use disorder (DSM-5). All of these terms can be found in the literature, and we replicate them as they are used by authors in the specific studies in our following discussion.

Epidemiology of substance use in persons living with HIV in the United States

HIV-infected individuals are disproportion-ately affected by alcohol and other drug use. Epidemiological studies show that the rates of heavy drinking among HIV-infected individuals are twice [4] and tobacco use 2–3 times that of the general US population [5]. In the HIV Cost and Service Utilization Study (HCSUS), a 2001 national probability sample of 2864 HIV-infected patients, 40% of patients reported illicit drug use in the prior year [6]. When assessed in a number of different HIV care set-tings, the prevalence of co-occurring substance use disorders also is high: 21% among 1125 patients in North Carolina [7], 26% among 9751 Kaiser Permanente patients [8], and 45% among 1774 patients at the University of Washington [9]. In a more recent convenience sample of 208 patients recruited from the waiting room of a safety net HIV clinic in San Francisco [10], 83% reported using illicit drugs or prescription medications for nonmedical reasons in the prior 3 months and 82% tested positive for at least one of these drugs on concurrent urine toxicology screening.

Unhealthy substance use is also a well-documented risk factor for HIV acquisition [11–13]. Alcohol, heroin, crack cocaine, and amphetamine type substances (ATS) are known to directly or indirectly contribute to HIV risk [14,15]. Heavy alcohol use, for example, is associated with a minimum twofold increase in risk for HIV infection in San Francisco [16], and ATS use among MSM doubles or triples the probability of engaging in high-risk sexual behavior and acquiring sexually transmitted infections, including HIV [17]. Among US adults with AIDS in 2011, the CDC estimated 29% of cases among men and 39% among women were related to drug injection (Cen-ters for Disease Control and Prevention. *HIV Surveillance Report, 2011*; vol. 23. http://www .cdc.gov/hiv/topics/surveillance/resources/ reports/. Published February 2013. Accessed 1/19/15). From the beginning of the epidemic through 2011, more than 358,000 cumulative cases of AIDS in the United States occurred by drug injection (Centers for Disease Control and Prevention. *HIV Surveillance Report, 2011*; vol. 23. http://www.cdc.gov/hiv/topics/surveillance/ resources/reports/. Published February 2013. Accessed 1/19/15), and global estimates of the prevalence and number of people who injected drugs and were living with HIV in 2012 are 13.1% and 1.7 million, respectively (United Nations Office on Drugs and Crime, *World Drug Report 2014*. United Nations publication, Sales No. E.14.XI.7) [18].

Left untreated, substance use disorders are associated with decreases in linkage to and retention in HIV care [19–21], delays in antiretroviral therapy (ART) initiation [22], poorer ART adherence [23,24], and accelerated HIV disease progression [25–28]. Unhealthy substance use also contributes to a myriad of non-AIDS-related health conditions, such as hepatic, renal, and cardiac disease, some can-cers, and destabilizing mental health disorders [12,27,29–32]. Among HIV-infected popula-tions, a significant relationship exists between substance use and morbidity and mortality [12,33–36]. The profound impact that sub-stance use has on people living with HIV/AIDS underscores our recommendation to ask about substance use as part of the every initial medical history and at least annually thereafter.

The experience of pain in persons with HIV and substance use disorders

HIV-infected persons with substance use prob-lems report higher pain severity, higher rates of depression and anxiety, and greater disruption in daily functioning due to pain than do individ-uals without substance use problems [37–39]. In an assessment of 504 ambulatory AIDS patients in New York between 1992 and 1995, persons who reported drug injection as an HIV transmission factor also reported significantly more symptoms and higher rates of symptom distress than persons who reported hetero- or homosexual contact as their transmission factor [37]. HIV-infected persons with substance use disorders also have reported less pain relief from opioid analgesic medications, taking higher doses of medications than prescribed, and increased use of street drugs and opioids to relieve symptoms other than pain [38,40,41].

Addiction and chronic pain share common neurobiological pathways, and it is not surprising that individuals with substance use disorders are also disproportionately affected by pain. Both pain and addiction are impacted greatly by sensory input and by secondary adaptations in the white matter connections between the frontal cortex and the dopamine-rich reward pathways in the midbrain [42]. In the case of addiction, brain circuits involved in reward, motivation, and memory are dysregulated, which manifest as altered impulse control, altered judgment, and the dysfunctional pursuit of rewards [ASAM long definition of addiction, found at http://www.asam.org/for-the-public/definition-of-addiction]. In the treatment of moderate-to-severe pain, the most commonly used opioid analgesics activate μ-opioid receptors, which not only inhibit nociceptive signals along pain-modulating pathways but also can produce an experience of euphoria that reinforces the dopaminergic circuits altered by addiction [43,44]. With chronic opioid use, however, most patients develop physical dependence, which manifests as *tolerance* to both the drug's analgesic and pleasurable effects, *withdrawal* when drug levels are reduced abruptly, and in some cases opioid-induced *hyperalgesia* [45]. Withdrawal-mediated pain can be experienced initially as anxiety and craving and can be observed in patients either coming down from using an illicit short-acting opioid (e.g., heroin) or at the end of dose for short-acting opioids prescribed for pain. Through a state of adaptation to chronic use, the dopaminergic reward circuit is driven more by dysphoria than euphoria [42]. Affected patients characterize their goals more as trying to feel "better" or "normal" than trying to feel "good." While withdrawal and tolerance are expected manifestations of physical dependence, they can sometimes be misinterpreted by medical providers as evidence of drug-seeking behavior or addiction. The point at which pain ends and opioid craving begins may be difficult to know for persons with co-occurring pain and addiction and their providers [43].

Finally, because addiction and chronic pain share common neurobiological pathways, it is also not surprising that affected individuals may seek the experience of pleasure through the nonmedical use of other substances as a strategy to counteract their pain. This is especially true for patients, who have had poor responses to traditional pain modalities or whose requests for more aggressive opioid therapy are disregarded as drug-seeking behavior [42]. In our experience caring for persons living with HIV and addiction, it is not uncommon for patients to report heroin injection to self-manage pain, the use of stimulants such as cocaine or methamphetamine that trigger the release or inhibit the reuptake of dopamine, or consuming sedative hypnotics such as benzodiazepines, barbiturates, and alcohol to temporarily escape their daily discomfort. The extent to which our patients' pursuit of the gray areas between euphoria and analgesia reinforce addictive behaviors, which seem to only further increase their stigmatization and medical neglect, underscores the great need for interdisciplinary programs in which substance use treatment can serve the needs of patients with comorbid chronic pain.

Chronic pain management challenges for HIV clinicians caring for people who use drugs

Growing public health concerns about iatrogenic addiction, increasing rates of fatal opioid analgesic overdose, and the diversion of controlled substances have resulted in greater patient scrutiny and prescriber pharmacovigilance (i.e., attentiveness to one's prescribing and patient behavior related to that prescribing) [46–49]. For HIV providers, many of whom trained in an era of providing hospice care to patients with undertreated pain, managing chronic pain in the modern HIV treatment era is a renewed challenge. Patients no longer need die of their HIV infection, but they and their providers must contend now with aging and with the health consequences of their behaviors and choices.

This challenge is exemplified in the practice of safe opioid prescribing and evaluating behaviors concerning for increased risks of harm to either the individual patient or his community. Studies of populations living with HIV report more concerning behaviors (e.g., lost or stolen prescriptions, taking more than prescribed doses) among patients with substance use histories. Tsao *et al.*[48] examined 2267 HIV-infected patients' self-reports of "aberrant opioid use," defined as using "analgesics or other prescription painkillers without a doctor's prescription, in larger amounts than prescribed, or for a longer period than prescribed" in the preceding 12 months. For patients who were classified as having problem drug use histories, 18% reported aberrant opioid use compared to 9% in patients without a problem drug use history. In a more recent sample of 296 homeless and marginally housed persons living with HIV in which nearly all (91%) reported pain in the prior week, two-thirds met DSM-IV criteria for stimulant or opioid abuse or dependence [50], 37% reported any "opioid analgesic aberrant behavior" and 18.5% reported "major" aberrant behaviors such as selling their prescription pain medications or taking them to get high in the prior 3 months. Aberrant behaviors were reported by significantly more subjects with recent illicit drug use than those without recent use (40% vs 23%, *p* = 0.03). When caring for HIV-infected patients with co-occurring substance use and chronic pain, the HIV clinician's dilemma is not only to predict the risk of concerning behaviors but also to ascertain the differential diagnosis for these behaviors and take prompt action to reduce or eliminate them when they occur.

Specific guidance for managing chronic pain in patients with HIV disease and current or prior substance use histories

Recognizing the high prevalence of substance use among persons living with HIV and the significant impact unhealthy substance use can have on HIV outcomes and chronic pain management, a patient's report of past or current substance use is a strong signal to prioritize this health issue up front. Chronic pain may be more severe, distressing, and difficult to treat in persons with co-occurring HIV disease and substance use. Feelings of anger, frustration, and manipulation may be experienced by patients and providers alike. We believe these experiences are made worse by treatment plans and clinic policies that do not address a patient's individual circumstances and do not treat a patient with positive regard. A tendency to develop cookie-cutter treatment algorithms that overrule a provider's clinical judgment too often result in the "policing" and stigmatization of patient behaviors, which we believe is out of place in a clinical environment. In the remaining sections of this chapter, we offer specific guidance on topics in chronic pain management of particular relevance to HIV-infected patients who use alcohol and other drugs.

1. Evaluate all patients for unhealthy substance use in the initial pain assessment and prior to prescribing opioid analgesics: We recommend that all patients seeking treatment for chronic pain undergo the same evaluation and risk stratification regardless of HIV or other disease status. This initial evaluation includes screening all patients for unhealthy use and assessing patients with positive screens further for substance use disorders and other consequences. Recall that conversations about alcohol and other drug use can be shaming; nonjudgmental language and attitudes are the hallmarks of a skilled HIV provider working with an already heavily stigmatized population. We suggest making a habit of asking permission (*"Would it be okay if we talked about alcohol and other drugs?"*) or headlining the conversation (*"I ask all my patients about alcohol and drugs"*). This approach not only sets the agenda and engages the patient, but it also communicates respect and reduces patient resistance.

Single-question screeners for alcohol and other drugs have been developed and validated for general primary care patient populations and may be applicable to HIV patient populations. The NIAAA single-question alcohol screener elicits the number of heavy drinking days in the past year by asking men under age 65: *"How many times in the past year have you had 5 or more standard drinks in a day?"*[51] (See Table 9.2). A response of one or more is a positive screen. When tested in a primary care clinic of an

Table 9.2   Validated single question screening for unhealthy alcohol and drug use.

Alcohol: *"How many times in the past year have you had 5 (4 for women or men >65 years of age) or more standard drinks in a day?"*
- Validated NIAAA single question screener elicits the number of heavy drinking days in the past year
- What's a standard drink? 12 oz. beer, 5 oz. wine, 1.5 oz. spirits or brandy. Use a standard drink chart (below).
- Scoring: 1 or more = positive screen. At-risk drinking is defined as greater than 1 time in the past year. Almost all people with alcohol use disorders report drinking heavily at least occasionally.

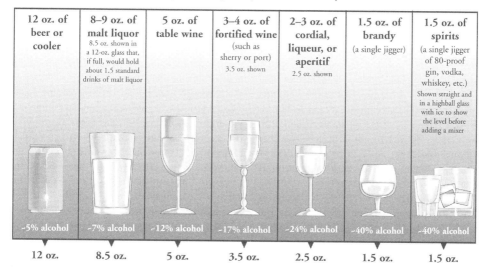

12 oz. of beer or cooler	8–9 oz. of malt liquor 8.5 oz. shown in a 12-oz. glass that, if full, would hold about 1.5 standard drinks of malt liquor	5 oz. of table wine	3–4 oz. of fortified wine (such as sherry or port) 3.5 oz. shown	2–3 oz. of cordial, liqueur, or aperitif 2.5 oz. shown	1.5 oz. of brandy (a single jigger)	1.5 oz. of spirits (a single jigger of 80-proof gin, vodka, whiskey, etc.) Shown straight and in a highball glass with ice to show the level before adding a mixer
~5% alcohol	~7% alcohol	~12% alcohol	~17% alcohol	~24% alcohol	~40% alcohol	~40% alcohol
12 oz.	8.5 oz.	5 oz.	3.5 oz.	2.5 oz.	1.5 oz.	1.5 oz.

Drugs: *"How many times in the past year have you used an illegal drug or used a prescription medication for nonmedical reasons?"*
- To clarify term "nonmedical reasons," ask: *"for instance because of the experience or feeling it caused."*
- Scoring: 1 or more = positive screen: At-risk drug use ≥1 time in the past year.

urban safety net hospital, this one question was 84% sensitive and 78% specific for risky alcohol consumption, and 88% sensitive and 67% specific for a current alcohol use disorder [52]. Similarly, a clinician can use a validated single-question screener for other substance use: *"How many times in the past year have you used an illegal drug or a prescription medication for nonmedical reasons?"* Again, a response of one or more is a positive screen. This single question was 100% sensitive and 73.5% specific for detecting a substance use disorder in an urban safety net clinic [53], although care must be taken, especially with patients that do not use illicit drugs, that the patient correctly understands the meaning of "nonmedical use." Failure to do so could potentially lead to higher

rates of false-positive screening results [54]. The four-item CAGE Adapted to Include Drugs (CAGE-AID) questionnaire may be suited for lifetime but not current substance use [55]. Questions that provide a safe space for accurate responses improve the utility of screening. For example, asking a patient, *"How many times in the past year have you used cocaine?"* is likely to obtain more useful information than *"Do you use cocaine?"* The former question normalizes the behavior, so that a patient is more likely to share confidential information. The latter question places the patient in a position of having to confess or declare a socially undesirable behavior. Thus, message framing is critical to create a patient–provider relationship in which patients are not penalized or shamed for being truthful.

Patients who screen positive for unhealthy use should be further assessed for the patterns and complications of their use, including substance use disorder diagnostic criteria. Assessments can be conducted by HIV clinic staff using well-established validated tools or explored by the provider in the patient interview. The WHO's *Alcohol, Smoking, and Substance Involvement Screening Test (ASSIST)* is a good choice for assessing the risk of health and other problems in patients using alcohol and other classes of drugs [56]. Originally developed as a clinician-administered tool that can be time consuming, the ASSIST demonstrated good test–retest reliability when administered to patients in an audio-guided computer-assisted self-interview (ACASI) format [57]. The *Alcohol Use Disorders Identification Test (AUDIT)* is a 10-item tool for assessing alcohol alone [58]. In a 2013 study of 837 HIV-infected men in the Veterans Aging Cohort Study [59], a three-item version (*AUDIT-C*) performed as well as the AUDIT for identifying risky drinking, alcohol dependence, and unhealthy alcohol use in patients with and without HIV disease [60]. In busy HIV clinics, the AUDIT-C with cutoff scores of three or four is a reasonable alternative to the full AUDIT, and both versions can be self-administered.

A complete substance use history includes a patient's present and past use, as well as a family history of substance use. A family history is critical because 40–60% of the predisposition to addiction has a genetic basis. The clinician should ask about the use of illicit drugs and the nonmedical use of prescribed medications, such as opioids, benzodiazepines, and stimulants; their frequency, quantity, and routes of administration; and elicit any negative aspects using open-ended questions ("*What are some of the not-so-good things for you about smoking crack?*"). Prior treatment experiences, especially successful ones, should be elicited and positively affirmed ("*You've made it to treatment and been successful there before.*"). Opioid-dependent patients that have recently experienced a period of abstinence, either as a result of treatment or incarceration, are at high risk of overdose (due to decreased tolerance), if they relapse or resume prior higher dose opioid analgesics [61]. Thus, an accurate substance use history is critical not only to make correct substance use

diagnoses but also to assess an appropriate level of future risk of harm and to develop a chronic pain treatment plan that partners with patients to reduce that risk and address their current clinical needs. Providers often consider the time required to conduct screening and assessment for unhealthy substance as an obstacle to their implementation in primary care settings; however, the availability of patient-administered questionnaires, team-based care practices, and integrated behavioral health initiatives may result in clinical workflows that allow support staff to help the provider complete these important initial activities.

Through substance use screening and assessment, the clinical team can determine if a patient meets diagnostic criteria for a substance use disorder. Patients diagnosed with substance abuse (DSM-IV) or mild substance use disorder (DSM-5) may benefit from brief counseling interventions during office visits. (See the Table 9.1 for specific DSM diagnostic criteria.) Patients diagnosed with substance dependence (DSM-IV) or moderate–severe substance use disorder (DSM-5) are likely to require higher levels of care including residential detoxification and treatment, intensive outpatient treatment (IOP), individual or group therapy, and/or a trial of medication-assisted therapy (e.g., buprenorphine, methadone, naltrexone, nicotine replacement, and varenicline). For patients in recovery, relapse prevention strategies area important components of a chronic pain treatment plan.

2. Identify and address co-occurring mental illness in patients with substance use disorders: Co-occurring mental illness is prevalent among individuals with substance use disorders and providers should be aware that co-occurring mental illness exacerbate both the substance use disorder and the patient's chronic pain. Untreated mental illness can lead to relapse to substance use and limit the effectiveness of treatments for chronic pain (see Chapter 8 for more information about mental illness in HIV patients with chronic pain).

3. Use a risk–benefit framework to tailor opioid treatment decisions to the individual patient: Substance use screening and assessment inform risk stratification and a clinician's pain treatment plan, including determination of whether the potential benefits of opioid treatment (i.e., to pain severity, function, and quality of life) outweigh the risks of its unintended, negative effects (i.e., misuse, addiction, and diversion). Unhealthy substance use, whether current or in the past, is not an absolute contraindication to opioid treatment for chronic pain. Some patients may be using more of an illicit substance to self-medicate a painful disorder. In these situations, the treatment of pain can help support a substance use treatment plan. Other patients may engage in risky use but do not meet criteria for a substance use disorder. Opioid analgesics can be included in a menu of treatment options for moderate-to-severe pain when (1) a patient's pain significantly impacts function and quality of life, (2) nonopioid medications and nonpharmacologic therapies have been exhausted, and (3) patients agree to have their opioid use closely monitored. Pursuing a trial of opioid therapy requires clinical judgment that considers the severity of substance use (i.e., remote vs. risky use vs. current substance use disorder), the patient's own perception of his or her substance use as problematic or needing to change, and if the patient is engaged in substance use treatment.

Opioid risk screening tools that are administered to patients prior to prescribing any opioid analgesics may assist providers in predicting the development of problematic opioid use. These tools include the SOAPP [62], SOAPP-R [63], ORT[64] and PMQ[65] (self-administered), and the DIRE[66] questionnaires. None of these tools, however, has been evaluated in HIV-infected patient populations, and none has been shown to be superior to another[67,68] or sufficiently reliable to accurately predict addiction prospectively [69]. Given these limitations, these tools may inform but should not be used exclusively to determine whether or not a patient should be prescribed an opioid analgesic for chronic pain. A comprehensive substance use assessment and the clinical judgment of the healthcare provider are required to make that determination.

The initiation of opioid therapy in any patient is always a "time-limited trial." The risk–benefit of safely prescribing controlled substances for chronic pain to persons with substance use histories is dynamic, because patient behavior can change. Providers need to be willing to monitor for these changes and tailor the treatment plan to the individual patient's current condition. While the risks of opioid treatment may initially outweigh the benefits for some patients with co-occurring substance use, providers can offer nonpharmacologic and nonopioid pharmacologic pain management until the risks of the adverse consequences of opioid treatment are mitigated (see Chapters 9, 10, and 11). HIV providers and clinics can take an active role supporting patients to reduce the risk of harm, whether they are referring a patient to residential detoxification and addiction treatment, teaching a family member how to administer naloxone to prevent an overdose, or identifying supportive housing that offers on-site medication management. Patients with co-occurring substance use in whom the benefits of opioids balance or outweigh the risks should receive closer initial monitoring (e.g., smaller quantities of medications dispensed more frequently or weekly pill counts and frequent clinic visits) and an appropriate plan for outpatient treatment or relapse prevention. Clinicians should keep in mind that substance use is often a patient's attempt to reduce suffering, whether physical pain or psychological distress or shame, and this coping mechanism may improve with substance use and mental health treatment as components of an effective chronic pain treatment plan.

Patient–provider opioid agreements are an opportunity to exchange information and set mutual expectations prior to prescribing (see Chapter 12). These treatment agreements are invaluable for discussing (1) the potential benefits and risks of opioid treatment with an individual patient, (2) patient and provider responsibilities in the treatment relationship, (3) the forms of patient monitoring that will be requested to reassess treatment benefits and risk over time, and (4) how concerning behaviors will be addressed. For example, if the risks of prescribing should outweigh the treatment's benefits, the treatment plan will need to be modified to reduce these risks, and an opioid analgesic may need to be tapered and discontinued.

4. Offer patients treatment for active substance use: Individuals with active substance use disorders should be offered appropriate evidence-based treatment. Effective substance use treatment is likely to improve chronic pain management and may have both pharmacological (i.e., medications) and psychosocial (i.e., counseling) components. Some patients are not ready to make a change in their drug use behaviors, and patient-centered counseling at office visits can be used to explore ambivalence, build motivation, and strengthen commitment to change. Providers may find that conversations about behavior change are more productive using the techniques of Motivational Interviewing, "a collaborative conversation style for strengthening a person's own motivation and commitment to change."[1] Partnership, acceptance, compassion, and evocation are the four key aspects underlying the practice of MI (see www.motivationalinterviewing.org). Patient readiness and commitment to change are necessary in order to proceed to a substance use action plan, which may include behavioral therapies, medical management, and/or referral to more specialized treatment. The specific choice depends on what the patient is ready for and what is clinically indicated for his/her substance use severity. Motivational interviewing as an important tool in communicating with patients about challenging topics is also addressed in Chapters 12 and 13.

While a detailed review of treatments for different substance use disorders is beyond the scope of this chapter, HIV providers should recognize the important role that addiction treatment plays in improving both chronic pain and HIV outcomes. Moreover, many addiction treatments can be integrated into the HIV outpatient clinical environment. An extensive literature on this subject matter can be found elsewhere [70–73], and pharmacotherapies are briefly summarized here.

FDA-approved medication-assisted treatment (MAT) for tobacco use disorder includes bupropion, varenicline, and nicotine replacement therapy in multiple formulations. Multiple quit attempts are often required to succeed, and combinations of tobacco cessation medications appear to be more effective than single agents [74].

Medications approved for alcohol use disorder appear to modulate the function of opioid, glutamate, or serotonin neurotransmission. In addition to naltrexone, they include disulfiram and acamprosate [75–77]. Systematic reviews generally agree that compared to placebo, oral naltrexone prevents relapse to heavy drinking after an initial abstinence period and increases the percentage of nondrinking days [78–81]. Naltrexone also was found to be superior to acamprosate, which requires thrice-daily dosing and is contraindicated in patients with renal disease [82]. As an opioid antagonist, however, naltrexone cannot be administered concurrently with opioid analgesics, which may limit its utility in patients with moderate–severe chronic pain. Disulfiram deters alcohol consumption by inhibiting aldehyde dehydrogenase. The buildup of acetaldehyde causes an uncomfortable reaction characterized by flushing, weakness, nausea, tachycardia, and in some instances, hypotension. Disulfiram was found to have a substantial impact on alcohol use (effect size of 0.68), resulting in significantly longer periods of alcohol abstinence in a controlled trial of disulfiram for cocaine dependence in opioid dependent patients maintained on methadone [83]. Disulfiram is thought to be most effective with supervised administration or with highly motivated patients [76]. Topiramate is not FDA approved for alcohol use disorder but has shown efficacy in randomized trials[84] and is included as a treatment of alcohol use disorders by the NIAAA [85]. Topiramate is attractive because it may be used concurrently with opioids, especially for the treatment of neuropathic pain, without the negative reinforcement of disulfiram, and has demonstrated efficacy for alcohol use disorder in patients with posttraumatic stress disorder, which is common in persons living with HIV [86,87].

Currently approved pharmacotherapies for opioid use disorder include opioid agonist therapy with methadone or buprenorphine and naltrexone, an opioid antagonist that reduces dopaminergic reward [88,89]. The benefits of methadone[90,91] and buprenorphine[92–94] in persons living with HIV are well documented. High dropout rates in studies of daily oral naltrexone [95], however, have led to ongoing active investigations of sustained-release formulations of naltrexone that require only once monthly dosing [96–98].

Stimulant use disorders, particularly amphetamine type stimulants, are challenging to treat and behavioral therapies currently are the only evidence-based treatment [99,100]. While promising preliminary results have been reported in small randomized trials combining weekly counseling either with mirtazapine in MSM that reduced methamphetamine use[101] or with naltrexone in treatment seekers that reduced amphetamine relapse[102], these findings have yet have yet to be reproduced in larger samples. In addition, five early trials in either methadone- or buprenorphine-maintained patients suggested the potential efficacy of disulfiram for treating cocaine dependence [83,103–106]. By blocking dopamine beta hydroxylase in the nucleus accumbens, disulfiram may blunt cocaine craving and euphoria. Findings from more recent trials, however, have had mixed results and showed poorer treatment outcomes in women compared to men [107–109].

Urine drug testing (UDT) can be a useful method during either behavioral or medication treatments for documenting use in the prior 2–5 days. As a mutually agreed upon component of counseling or behavioral treatments, UDT may help patients reflect on their frequency or patterns of use and provide patients with concrete, measurable goals to work toward (i.e., increasing the number or ratio of confirmed methamphetamine-negative urine tests in a set time period). UDT can be particularly powerful when combined with contingency management as a means to increase the personal reward/value of appropriate urine toxicology, or when combined with when combined with behavioral interventions such as cognitive behavioral therapy (CBT) [99].

Some patients with chronic pain syndromes struggle with the unhealthy use of multiple substances, which adds complexity to the clinical management of chronic pain. Moreover, some patients may have a greater awareness of one substance use problem and be less concerned by others. For example, a patient with chronic pain may be enrolled in methadone maintenance treatment for a heroin use disorder, yet discount the consequences of smoking a pack of cigarettes daily on her severe COPD and her increased risk of overdose when prescribed additional opioid analgesics. The astute HIV provider casts a wide net when screening for substance use problems and considers the feasibility of addressing multiple disorders simultaneously or prioritizing treatment of one ahead of the other [110]. In a meta-analysis of 19 RCTs [111], Prochaska *et al.* detected a 25% increased likelihood of long-term abstinence from alcohol and illicit drugs when tobacco cessation interventions were provided together with other substance use treatments. Consultation with an addiction medicine specialist is recommended when caring for complex patients with chronic pain and multiple substance use disorders.

5. Choose rational pharmacotherapy when prescribing medications that carry a higher risk of potential harm to patients with substance use histories. If the decision to prescribe opioid analgesics is made, the provider must consider which medication to prescribe. Opioid analgesic potency, for example, does not appear to be associated with increased risk of opioid misuse. In a small study [112], Walsh and colleagues found that the abuse liability profile of hydromorphone, hydrocodone, and oxycodone did not differ substantially when administered in a blinded manner to individuals with a history of prescription misuse. Prescribing the lowest effective opioid analgesic dose can be achieved by exploiting the synergism or additive effects of different medications and their sites of action on the pain pathway. Gilron et al., for example, demonstrated that morphine when combined with gabapentin not only decreased neuropathic pain severity but also required lower doses of each medication than when prescribed alone [113].

The provider also may wish to decide whether extended-release or long-acting (ER/LA) or immediate-release or short-acting (IR/SA) opioid formulations should be prescribed for an HIV-infected patient with co-occurring substance use. For episodic pain, breakthrough pain, and in opioid-naïve patients, IR/SA formulations are appropriate choices; but their brief duration and rapid onset of action also may mimic the bolus effects of illicit drugs on the reward centers in the brain. For patients who have constant pain or have developed opioid tolerance, the more stable drug concentrations achieved by

ER/LA formulations may be preferable with breakthrough pain addressed first by nonopioid modalities. ER/LA opioid analgesics also reduce the fluctuations in the IR/SA dosing cycle that can produce withdrawal-mediated pain at the end of dose. Continuous exposure to ER/LA formulations, however, also could lead to higher opioid tolerance, physical dependence, and hyperalgesia. Because there is continuing debate but insufficient evidence at this time to declare which formulation is safer or more effective [114], we recommend individualizing treatment choices based on the patient's prior experience and current response to the medication. Expanding treatment choices for individual patients with substance use histories also means that nonpharmacological treatments and nonopioid pharmacotherapies need to play a greater role either in combination with opioid analgesics or alone. These other treatments may include physical therapy and weight loss for back pain; capsaicin, anticonvulsants, antidepressants, and cannabinoids for neuropathic pain; cognitive behavioral therapy, and acupuncture (see Chapter 10, Pharmacologic and Nonpharmacologic Therapies).

Finally, with the legalization of cannabis in some municipalities, increasing attention has shifted to the use of cannabinoids for the treatment of specified symptoms or medical conditions. Cannabinoids likely have a role in the modulation of pain [115], and two small randomized trials have demonstrated reductions in HIV-related neuropathic pain severity, especially among patients with prior cannabis exposure [116,117]. However, due consideration must be given to its potential risks of neuropsychiatric adverse effects at higher doses, the harmful effects of smoked forms of cannabis in patients with preexisting severe lung disease, and addiction risk to patients with preexisting cannabis use disorder. The effects of short-term cannabis use may include impaired short-term memory and motor coordination; altered judgment; and in high doses, paranoia and psychosis [118]. Smoke inhalation from any burning plant is hazardous to alveolar tissue, and the long-term pulmonary effects of smoking cannabis are difficult to determine given the high prevalence of tobacco smoking in this population[70] and methodological limitations for estimating

lifetime exposure to marijuana in retrospective studies of its effects on pulmonary function [119]. Moreover, compared to the general population, tobacco use is significantly higher in HIV-infected populations and persons with HIV disease already experience increased pulmonary morbidity and overall mortality due to tobacco use. Whether daily cannabis use contributes to more rapid progression of liver fibrosis in persons with chronic hepatitis C virus coinfection remains controversial [120,121]. Therefore, patients with HIV–HCV coinfection should be informed of this potential association and weigh the risks and benefits before engaging in or continuing cannabinoid use for chronic pain.

6. Regularly monitor patients who are prescribed opioid analgesics and respond promptly to concerning behaviors. Concerning behaviors require thoughtful evaluation and a prompt and measured clinical response. The differential diagnosis includes undertreated pain (as in "pseudoaddiction"), unhealthy substance use, financial gain, coercion by others, or any combination of the above. One important way that such behaviors are often detected is by urine drug screens. It is important, however, to be aware of the utility and limitations of urine drug testing. Immunoassays for amphetamine and methamphetamine, for example, can cross-react with other substances such as bupropion, trazodone, sildenafil, and some synthetic cathinones ("bath salts"), to cause false-positive results (see Chapter 12, Opioid Treatment Agreements and Urine Drug Screens, for a more complete discussion of urine drug screen interpretation). False negatives can occur if the substance is taken infrequently (as with p.r.n. dosing) or in individuals who are fast metabolizers. Confirmatory testing of positive results by liquid/gas chromatography and mass spectroscopy is therefore essential when using urine drug testing in clinical practice to make decisions about continuing to prescribe (see Chapters 10 and 11, Opioid Treatment Agreements and Urine Drug Screens).

Given the limitations of urine drug screening, and a general understanding that a substance use disorder occupies only one end of the spectrum of substance use, we do not recommend abruptly stopping opioid analgesics in patients with unexpected urine drug screen results alone. These results are part of the clinical data that help inform treatment decisions. Other sources of data include additional testing, conversations with the patient, the patient's treatment support (e.g., sponsor, family, and drug treatment counselor), and closer monitoring. On the other hand, a persistent or escalating pattern of concerning behaviors despite prompt, nonconfrontational, face-to-face discussions and more intensive monitoring to minimize their occurrence requires treatment plan modifications. Depending on the working diagnosis for the behavior's etiology, these modifications may include addiction treatment or pain specialist referrals, opioid treatment taper or discontinuation, and/or changing to a nonopioid or nonpharmacologic treatment modality. In perhaps no other patient population is a risk–benefit framework, explicit prescribing agreements, periodic monitoring, and a broad differential more useful for ensuring that the benefits of opioid prescribing outweigh the potential harms and for maintaining the kind of productive patient–provider relationship all persons with HIV deserve. The groundwork laid during the initial evaluation and a clinical relationship that judges the treatment instead of the patient are invaluable in situations when the risks do outweigh the treatment's benefits and either more frequent/intensive monitoring is indicated or pain medications must be tapered off or even discontinued. (See Chapters 10 and 11 for a more detailed discussion of opioid prescribing and decision-making.)

7. Pain management considerations for patients receiving medication-assisted treatment for a substance use disorder. Medication-assisted treatment for addiction can greatly affect chronic pain management decisions. Naltrexone and buprenorphine both have high affinity for the μ-opioid receptor. Naltrexone is contraindicated in patients receiving opioid therapy for chronic pain, and full agonist opioid analgesics are displaced from opioid receptors by buprenorphine. Topiramate and gabapentin may provide dual benefits to patients with neuropathic pain and alcohol use disorders. Methadone for comorbid pain and opioid use disorder deserves special consideration and is discussed separately below.

Because most prescription drug monitoring programs (PDMP) do not currently report data about opioid agonist medications dispensed or administered to patients by licensed opioid treatment programs, HIV primary care providers may not know that their patients are receiving methadone for an opioid use disorder. Part of good clinical practice is to coordinate clinical care, and it is important for the HIV clinician to obtain appropriate releases of information that allow communication between the HIV clinic and the substance use treatment provider or facility. There is also a common misperception among many primary care providers that enrollment in a methadone maintenance treatment programs is sufficient for treating chronic pain. Although once daily dosing of opioid agonist therapy is effective for extinguishing opioid withdrawal and craving, analgesic effects require divided doses [122]. Compared with a once daily effective dose of 80–100 mg for the treatment of opioid use disorder, methadone dosing for chronic pain typically requires smaller doses taken three to four times a day. Methadone clinics do not have the staffing or the infrastructure to dispense this frequently although some clinics will occasionally be willing to split a dose, that is, observe half a dose at the clinic and give the patient the remainder for later that day. Patients receiving opioid agonist therapy for an opioid use disorder need their providers to communicate about and coordinate the prescribing of all controlled substances. A prescriber should insure that the addiction treatment facility is aware of the medication that is prescribed and verify which substances are expected in the urine drug screens.

Conclusion

HIV-infected patients with unhealthy substance use and comorbid chronic pain require special consideration and deserve our full attention. The presence of a substance use disorder does not preclude the use of opioid analgesics or other treatments for chronic pain. As with all medical conditions, an HIV provider should conduct a thorough history and examination and use a risk–benefit framework for determining the most appropriate treatment for that patient. More frequent or intensive monitoring improves safe opioid prescribing when indicated, and not all concerning behaviors require opioid treatment discontinuation. Substance use treatment is likely to improve a patient's experience of pain and reduce the risks of opioid treatment. Learning how to assess a patient's readiness for treatment, enhance motivation for behavior change, and develop action plans with ready patients are valuable behavior-change communication tools that every medical provider can learn. Office-based pharmacotherapies for opioid, tobacco, and alcohol use disorders are available although currently underutilized in HIV clinics. Behavioral treatments are currently the most effective for stimulant use disorders. Team-based care in HIV clinics can reduce some of the obstacles perceived by individual providers in implementing interventions for both chronic pain and substance use problems. Collaboration with pain and addiction medicine specialists can be especially beneficial for complex patients and require signed consents to exchange protected and sensitive health information.

Acknowledgments

The authors wish to acknowledge the contributions of Daniel P. Alford, MD MPH, and the SCOPE of Pain Opioid Risk Evaluation and Mitigation Strategy Continuing Education Program (www.scopeofpain.org) that greatly inform the content of this chapter. We thank them for their championship of a health-oriented, risk-benefit approach to the safe and competent use of opioids for managing chronic pain, and which we have found essential to the care of persons with comorbid substance use.

References

1 Miller, W.R. & Rollnick, S. (2013) *Motivational Interviewing: Helping People hange*, 3rd edn. Guilford Press, New York, NY.

2 Broyles, L.M., Binswanger, I.A., Jenkins, J.A. *et al.* (2014) Confronting inadvertent stigma and pejorative language in addiction scholarship: a recognition and response. *Substance Abuse*, **35**, 217–221.

3 Hasin, D.S., O'Brien, C.P., Auriacombe, M. *et al.* (2013) DSM-5 criteria for substance use disorders: recommendations and rationale. *The American Journal of Psychiatry*, **170**, 834–851.

4 Galvan, F.H., Bing, E.G., Fleishman, J.A. *et al.* (2002) The prevalence of alcohol consumption and heavy drinking among people with HIV in the United States: results from the HIV Cost and Services Utilization Study. *Journal of Studies on Alcohol*, **63**, 179–186.

5 Burkhalter, J.E., Springer, C.M., Chhabra, R., Ostroff, J.S. & Rapkin, B.D. (2005) Tobacco use and readiness to quit smoking in low-income HIV-infected persons. *Nicotine & Tobacco Research*, **7**, 511–522.

6 Bing, E.G., Burnam, M.A., Longshore, D. *et al.* (2001) Psychiatric disorders and drug use among human immunodeficiency virus-infected adults in the United States. *Archives of General Psychiatry*, **58**, 721–728.

7 Pence, B.W., Miller, W.C., Whetten, K., Eron, J.J. & Gaynes, B.N. (2006) Prevalence of DSM-IV-defined mood, anxiety, and substance use disorders in an HIV clinic in the Southeastern United States. *Journal of Acquired Immune Deficiency Syndromes*, **42**, 298–306.

8 DeLorenze, G.N., Satre, D.D., Quesenberry, C.P., Tsai, A.L. & Weisner, C.M. (2010) Mortality after diagnosis of psychiatric disorders and co-occurring substance use disorders among HIV-infected patients. *AIDS Patient Care and STDs*, **24**, 705–712.

9 Tegger, M.K., Crane, H.M., Tapia, K.A., Uldall, K.K., Holte, S.E. & Kitahata, M.M. (2008) The effect of mental illness, substance use, and treatment for depression on the initiation of highly active antiretroviral therapy among HIV-infected individuals. *AIDS Patient Care and STDs*, **22**, 233–243.

10 Rose, C.D., Kamitani, E., Eng, S., Lum, P.J. (2012) Screening and brief intervention for unhealthy substance use in HIV primary care settings is associated with substance use reductions and viral suppression among PLWHIV in San Francisco, CA, USA. Poster presentation THPE606. In: *XIX International AIDS Conference*, Washington, DC.

11 Saitz, R. (2005) Clinical practice. unhealthy alcohol use. *The New England Journal of Medicine*, **352**, 596–607.

12 Braithwaite, R.S., Conigliaro, J., Roberts, M.S. *et al.* (2007) Estimating the impact of alcohol consumption on survival for HIV+ individuals. *AIDS Care*, **19**, 459–466.

13 Samet, J.H., Walley, A.Y. & Bridden, C. (2007) Illicit drugs, alcohol, and addiction in human immunodeficiency virus. *Panminerva Medica*, **49**, 67–77.

14 Morin, S., Myers, J., Shade, S., Koester, K., Maiorana, A. & Rose, C. (2007) Predicting HIV transmission risk among HIV-infected patients seen in clinical settings. *AIDS and Behavior*, **11**. (5 Suppl):S6-16.

15 Kalichman, S.C., Simbayi, L.C., Cain, D. & Jooste, S. (2007) Alcohol expectancies and risky drinking among men and women at high-risk for HIV infection in Cape Town South Africa. *Addictive Behaviors*, **32**, 2304–2310.

16 Colfax, G.N. (2010). In: Coffey, S. (ed),, In this presentation, Dr. Colfax addresses changing strategies for HIV prevention in San Francisco. He gives an overview of the characteristics of the San Francisco Department of Public Health's (SFDPH) HIV Prevention Program and discusses its focus on HIV status awareness, prevention with positives (PWP), primary drivers of HIV (such as substance use), and structural interventions to reduce risk *HIV Prevention in San Francisco: Where Do We Go from Here?* Harder+Company Community Research.

17 Buchacz, K., McFarland, W., Kellogg, T.A. *et al.* (2005) Amphetamine use is associated with increased HIV incidence among men who have sex with men in San Francisco. *AIDS*, **19**, 1423–1424.

18 *World Drug Report*. (2014) United Nations Office of Drugs and Crime.

19 Gardner, E.M., McLees, M.P., Steiner, J.F., Del Rio, C. & Burman, W.J. (2011) The spectrum of engagement in HIV care and its relevance to test-and-treat strategies for prevention of HIV infection. *Clinical Infectious Diseases*, **52**, 793–800.

20 Cunningham WE, Sohler NL, Tobias C, Drainoni M-l, Bradford J, Davis C, *et al.* (2006) Health services utilization for people with HIV infection: comparison of a population targeted for outreach with the U.S. population in care. *Medical Care,* **44** 1038–1047. 1010.1097/1001.mlr .0000242942.0000217968.0000242969.

21 Metsch, L.R., Bell, C., Pereyra, M. *et al.* (2009) Hospitalized HIV-infected patients in the era of highly active antiretroviral therapy. *American Journal of Public Health*, **99**, 1045–1049.

22 Loughlin, A., Metsch, L., Gardner, L., Anderson-Mahoney, P., Barrigan, M. & Strathdee, S. (2004) Provider barriers to prescribing HAART to medically-eligible HIV-infected drug users. *AIDS Care*, **16**, 485–500.

23 Conen, A., Fehr, J., Glass, T.R. *et al.* (2009) Self-reported alcohol consumption and its association with adherence and outcome of antiretroviral therapy in the Swiss HIV Cohort Study. *Antiviral Therapy*, **14**, 349–357.

24 Chander, G., Lau, B. & Moore, R.D. (2006) Hazardous alcohol use: a risk factor for non-adherence and lack of suppression in HIV infection. *Journal of Acquired Immune Deficiency Syndromes*, **43**, 411–417.

25 Samet, J.H., Cheng, D.M., Libman, H., Nunes, D.P., Alperen, J.K. & Saitz, R. (2007) Alcohol consumption and HIV disease progression. *Journal of Acquired Immune Deficiency Syndromes*, **46**, 194–199.

26 Baum, M.K., Rafie, C., Lai, S., Sales, S., Page, B. & Campa, A. (2009) Crack-cocaine use accelerates HIV disease progression in a cohort of HIV-positive drug users. *Journal of Acquired Immune Deficiency Syndromes*, **50**, 93–99.

27 Kalichman, S.C., Simbayi, L.C., Kaufman, M., Cain, D. & Jooste, S. (2007) Alcohol use and sexual risks for HIV/AIDS in sub-Saharan Africa: systematic review of empirical findings. *Prevention Science*, **8**, 141–151.

28 Colfax, G. & Shoptaw, S. (2005) The methamphetamine epidemic: implications for HIV prevention and treatment. *Current HIV/AIDS Reports*, **2**, 194–199.

29 Hahn, J.A., Woolf-King, S.E. & Muyindike, W. (2011) Adding fuel to the fire: alcohol's effect on the HIV epidemic in sub-Saharan Africa. *Current HIV/AIDS Reports*, **8**, 172–180.

30 Jaffe, J.A. & Kimmel, P.L. (2006) Chronic nephropathies of cocaine and heroin abuse: a

critical review. *Clinical Journal of the American Society of Nephrology*, **1**, 655–667.

31 Lange, R.A. & Hillis, L.D. (2001) Cardiovascular complications of cocaine use. *New England Journal of Medicine*, **345**, 351–358.

32 Schütze, M., Boeing, H., Pischon, T. *et al.* (2011) Alcohol attributable burden of incidence of cancer in eight European countries based on results from prospective cohort study. *BMJ*, **342**:d1584.

33 Chesson, H.W., Harrison, P. & Stall, R. (2003) Changes in alcohol consumption and in sexually transmitted disease incidence rates in the United States: 1983–1998. *Journal of Studies on Alcohol*, **64**, 623–630.

34 Colfax, G., Vittinghoff, E., Husnik, M.J. *et al.* (2004) Substance use and sexual risk: a participant- and episode-level analysis among a cohort of men who have sex with men. *American Journal of Epidemiology*, **159**, 1002–1012.

35 Crothers, K., Griffith, T.A., McGinnis, K.A. *et al.* (2005) The impact of cigarette smoking on mortality, quality of life, and comorbid illness among HIV-positive veterans. *Journal of General Internal Medicine*, **20**, 1142–1145.

36 Lifson, A.R., Neuhaus, J., Arribas, J.R. *et al.* (2010) Smoking-related health risks among persons with HIV in the Strategies for Management of Antiretroviral Therapy Clinical Trial. *American Journal of Public Health*, **100**, 1896–1903.

37 Vogl, D., Rosenfeld, B., Breitbart, W. *et al.* (1999) Symptom prevalence, characteristics, and distress in AIDS outpatients. *Journal of Pain and Symptom Management*, **18**, 253–262.

38 Marcus, K.S., Kerns, R.D., Rosenfeld, B. & Breitbart, W. (2000) HIV/AIDS-related pain as a chronic pain condition: implications of a biopsychosocial model for comprehensive assessment and effective management. *Pain Medicine*, **1**, 260–273.

39 Tsao, J.C., Dobalian, A. & Stein, J.A. (2005) Illness burden mediates the relationship between pain and illicit drug use in persons living with HIV. *Pain*, **119**, 124–132.

40 Larue, F., Fontaine, A. & Colleau, S.M. (1997) Underestimation and undertreatment of pain in HIV disease: multicentre study. *BMJ*, **314**, 23–28.

41 Richardson, J.L., Heikes, B., Karim, R., Weber, K., Anastos, K. & Young, M. (2009) Experience of pain among women with advanced HIV disease. *AIDS Patient Care and STDs*, **23**, 503–511.

42 Clark M.R, Treisman G.J. (2011) Chronic pain and addiction. *Basel*; New York: Karger.

43 Savage, S.R., Kirsh, K.L. & Passik, S.D. (2008) Challenges in using opioids to treat pain in persons with substance use disorders. *Addiction Science & Clinical Practice*, **4**, 4–25.

44 Al-Hasani, R. & Bruchas, M.R. (2011) Molecular mechanisms of opioid receptor-dependent signaling and behavior. *Anesthesiology*, **115**, 1363–1381.

45 Garland, E.L., Froeliger, B., Zeidan, F., Partin, K. & Howard, M.O. (2013) The downward spiral of chronic pain, prescription opioid misuse, and addiction: cognitive, affective, and neuropsychopharmacologic pathways. *Neuroscience and Biobehavioral Reviews*, **37**, 2597–2607.

46 Breitbart, W., Passik, S., McDonald, M.V. *et al.* (1998) Patient-related barriers to pain management in ambulatory AIDS patients. *Pain*, **76**, 9–16.

47 Breitbart, W., Rosenfeld, B., Passik, S., Kaim, M., Funesti-Esch, J. & Stein, K. (1997) A comparison of pain report and adequacy of analgesic therapy in ambulatory AIDS patients with and without a history of substance abuse. *Pain*, **72**, 235–243.

48 Tsao, J.C., Stein, J.A. & Dobalian, A. (2007) Pain, problem drug use history, and aberrant analgesic use behaviors in persons living with HIV. *Pain*, **133**, 128–137.

49 Lum, P.J., Little, S., Botsko, M. *et al.* (2011) Opioid-prescribing practices and provider confidence recognizing opioid analgesic abuse in HIV primary care settings. *Journal of Acquired Immune Deficiency Syndromes*, **56** (Suppl 1), S91–97.

50 Hansen, L., Penko, J., Guzman, D., Bangsberg, D.R., Miaskowski, C. & Kushel, M.B. (2011) Aberrant behaviors with prescription opioids and problem drug use history in a community-based cohort of HIV-infected individuals. *Journal of Pain and Symptom Management*, **42**, 893–902.

51 Friedmann, P.D., Saitz, R., Gogineni, A., Zhang, J.X. & Stein, M.D. (2001) Validation

of the screening strategy in the NIAAA "Physicians' guide to helping patients with alcohol problems". *Journal of Studies on Alcohol*, **62**, 234–238.

52 Smith, P.C., Schmidt, S.M., Allensworth-Davies, D. & Saitz, R. (2009) Primary care validation of a single-question alcohol screening test. *Journal of General Internal Medicine*, **24**, 783–788.

53 Smith, P.C., Schmidt, S.M., Allensworth-Davies, D. & Saitz, R. (2010) A single-question screening test for drug use in primary care. *Archives of Internal Medicine*, **170**, 1155–1160.

54 McNeely, J., Halkitis, P.N., Horton, A., Khan, R. & Gourevitch, M.N. (2014) How patients understand the term "nonmedical use" of prescription drugs: insights from cognitive interviews. *Substance Abuse*, **35**, 12–20.

55 Brown, R.L. & Rounds, L.A. (1995) Conjoint screening questionnaires for alcohol and other drug abuse: criterion validity in a primary care practice. *Wisconsin Medical Journal*, **94**, 135–140.

56 Humeniuk, R., Ali, R., Babor, T.F. *et al.* (2008) Validation of the alcohol, smoking and substance involvement screening test (ASSIST). *Addiction* **103**, 1039–47.

57 McNeely, J., Strauss, S.M., Wright, S. *et al.* (2014) Test-retest reliability of a self-administered alcohol, smoking and substance involvement screening test (ASSIST) in primary care patients. *Journal of Substance Abuse Treatment*, **47**, 93–101.

58 Bohn, M.J., Babor, T.F. & Kranzler, H.R. (1995) The alcohol use disorders identification test (AUDIT): validation of a screening instrument for use in medical settings. *Journal of Studies on Alcohol*, **56**, 423–432.

59 Strauss, S.M. & Rindskopf, D.M. (2009) Screening patients in busy hospital-based HIV care centers for hazardous and harmful drinking patterns: the identification of an optimal screening tool. *Journal of the International Association of Physicians in AIDS Care (Chicago, Ill.)*, **8**, 347–353.

60 McGinnis, K.A., Justice, A.C., Kraemer, K.L., Saitz, R., Bryant, K.J. & Fiellin, D.A. (2013) Comparing alcohol screening measures among HIV-infected and -uninfected men. *Alcoholism, Clinical and Experimental Research*, **37**, 435–442.

61 Binswanger, I.A., Stern, M.F., Deyo, R.A. *et al.* (2007) Release from prison – a high risk of death for former inmates. *New England Journal of Medicine*, **356**, 157–165.

62 Akbik, H., Butler, S.F., Budman, S.H., Fernandez, K., Katz, N.P. & Jamison, R.N. (2006) Validation and clinical application of the screener and opioid assessment for patients with pain (SOAPP). *Journal of Pain and Symptom Management*, **32**, 287–293.

63 Butler, S.F., Budman, S.H., Fernandez, K.C., Fanciullo, G.J. & Jamison, R.N. (2009) Cross-validation of a screener to predict opioid misuse in chronic pain patients (SOAPP-R). *Journal of Addiction Medicine*, **3**, 66–73.

64 Webster, L.R. & Webster, R.M. (2005) Predicting aberrant behaviors in opioid-treated patients: preliminary validation of the opioid risk tool. *Pain Medicine*, **6**, 432–442.

65 Adams, L.L., Gatchel, R.J., Robinson, R.C. *et al.* (2004) Development of a self-report screening instrument for assessing potential opioid medication misuse in chronic pain patients. *Journal of Pain and Symptom Management*, **27**, 440–459.

66 Belgrade, M.J., Schamber, C.D. & Lindgren, B.R. (2006) The DIRE score: predicting outcomes of opioid prescribing for chronic pain. *The Journal of Pain: Official Journal of the American Pain Society*, **7**, 671–681.

67 Turk, D.C., Swanson, K.S. & Gatchel, R.J. (2008) Predicting opioid misuse by chronic pain patients: a systematic review and literature synthesis. *Clinical Journal of Pain*, **24**, 497–508.

68 Chou, R., Fanciullo, G.J., Fine, P.G., Miaskowski, C., Passik, S.D. & Portenoy, R.K. (2009) Opioids for chronic noncancer pain: prediction and identification of aberrant drug-related behaviors: a review of the evidence for an American Pain Society and American Academy of Pain Medicine clinical practice guideline. *The Journal of Pain*, **10**, 131–146.

69 Sehgal, N., Manchikanti, L. & Smith, H.S. (2012) Prescription opioid abuse in chronic pain: a review of opioid abuse predictors and strategies to curb opioid abuse. *Pain Physician*, **15**, ES67–92.

70 Bruce, R.D. (2011) Medical Interventions for Addiction. In: Ge, a. (ed), *Neurology of AIDS, 3rd Ed* edn. Oxford University of Press, New York.

71 Bruce, R.D., Kresina, T.F. & McCance-Katz, E.F. (2010) Medication-assisted treatment and HIV/AIDS: aspects in treating HIV-infected drug users. *AIDS*, **24**, 331–340.

72 Altice, F.L., Kamarulzaman, A., Soriano, V.V., Schechter, M. & Friedland, G.H. (2010) Treatment of medical, psychiatric, and substance-use comorbidities in people infected with HIV who use drugs. *Lancet*, **376**, 367–387.

73 Lum, P.J. & Tulsky, J.P. (2006) The medical management of opioid dependence in HIV primary care settings. *Current HIV/AIDS Reports*, **3**, 195–204.

74 Clinical Practice Guideline Treating Tobacco U, Dependence Update Panel L, Staff (2008) A clinical practice guideline for treating tobacco use and dependence: 2008 update. A U.S. Public Health Service report. *American Journal of Preventive Medicine*, **35**, 158–176.

75 Fuller, R.K., Branchey, L., Brightwell, D.R. *et al.* (1986) Disulfiram treatment of alcoholism. A Veterans Administration cooperative study. *JAMA*, **256**, 1449–1455.

76 Fuller, R.K. & Gordis, E. (2004) Does disulfiram have a role in alcoholism treatment today? *Addiction*, **99**, 21–24.

77 Kiritzé-Topor, P., Huas, D., Rosenzweig, C., Comte, S., Paille, F. & Lehert, P. (2004) A pragmatic trial of acamprosate in the treatment of alcohol dependence in primary care. *Alcohol and Alcoholism*, **39**, 520–527.

78 Srisurapanont, M. & Jarusuraisin, N. (2005) Opioid antagonists for alcohol dependence. *Cochrane Database of Systematic Reviews*, **2** CD001867.

79 Kranzler, H.R. & Van Kirk, J. (2001) Efficacy of naltrexone and acamprosate for alcoholism treatment: a meta-analysis. *Alcoholism, Clinical and Experimental Research*, **25**, 1335–1341.

80 Bouza, C., Angeles, M., Munoz, A. & Amate, J.M. (2004) Efficacy and safety of naltrexone and acamprosate in the treatment of alcohol dependence: a systematic review. *Addiction*, **99**, 811–828.

81 Anton, R.F. (2008) Naltrexone for the management of alcohol dependence. *New England Journal of Medicine*, **359**, 715–721.

82 Anton, R.F., O'Malley, S.S., Ciraulo, D.A. *et al.* (2006) Combined pharmacotherapies and behavioral interventions for alcohol dependence: the COMBINE study: a randomized controlled trial. *JAMA*, **295**, 2003–2017.

83 Carroll, K.M., Nich, C., Ball, S.A., McCance, E. & Rounsavile, B.J. (1998) Treatment of cocaine and alcohol dependence with psychotherapy and disulfiram. *Addiction*, **93**, 713–727.

84 Johnson, B.A., Rosenthal, N., Capece, J.A. *et al.* (2007) Topiramate for treating alcohol dependence: a randomized controlled trial. *JAMA, the Journal of the American Medical Association*, **298**, 1641–1651.

85 National Institute on Alcohol Abuse and Alcoholism (U.S.) (2007) Rockville, M.D. (ed), *Helping Patients Who Drink Too Much: A Clinician's Guide: updated 2005 edition*. [Rev. Jan. 2007]. U.S. Dept. of Health and Human Services, National Institutes of Health, National Institute on Alcohol Abuse and Alcoholism.

86 Batki, S.L., Pennington, D.L., Lasher, B. *et al.* (2014) Topiramate treatment of alcohol use disorder in veterans with posttraumatic stress disorder: a randomized controlled pilot trial. *Alcoholism, Clinical and Experimental Research*, **38**, 2169–2177.

87 Guglielmo, R., Martinotti, G., Quatrale, M. *et al.* (2015) Topiramate in alcohol use disorders: review and update. *CNS Drugs* **29**, 383–395.

88 Comer, S.D., Sullivan, M.A., Yu, E. *et al.* (2006) Injectable, sustained-release naltrexone for the treatment of opioid dependence: a randomized, placebo-controlled trial. *Archives of General Psychiatry*, **63**, 210–218.

89 Tetrault, J.M., Tate, J.P., McGinnis, K.A. *et al.* (2012) Hepatic safety and antiretroviral effectiveness in HIV-infected patients receiving naltrexone. *Alcoholism, Clinical and Experimental Research*, **36**, 318–324.

90 Palepu, A., Tyndall, M.W., Joy, R. *et al.* (2006) Antiretroviral adherence and HIV treatment

outcomes among HIV/HCV co-infected injection drug users: the role of methadone maintenance therapy. *Drug and Alcohol Dependence*, **84**, 188–194.

91 Uhlmann, S., Milloy, M.J., Kerr, T. *et al.* (2010) Methadone maintenance therapy promotes initiation of antiretroviral therapy among injection drug users. *Addiction*, **105**, 907–913.

92 Lucas, G.M., Chaudhry, A., Hsu, J. *et al.* (2010) Clinic-based treatment of opioid-dependent HIV-infected patients versus referral to an opioid treatment program: a randomized trial. *Annals of Internal Medicine*, **152**, 704–711.

93 Altice, F.L., Bruce, R.D., Lucas, G.M. *et al.* (2011) HIV treatment outcomes among HIV-infected, opioid-dependent patients receiving buprenorphine/naloxone treatment within HIV clinical care settings: results from a multisite study. *Journal of Acquired Immune Deficiency Syndromes*, **56** (Suppl 1), S22–32.

94 Fiellin, D.A., Weiss, L., Botsko, M. *et al.* (2011) Drug treatment outcomes among HIV-infected opioid-dependent patients receiving buprenorphine/naloxone. *Journal of Acquired Immune Deficiency Syndromes*, **56** (Suppl 1), S33–38.

95 Coviello, D.M., Cornish, J.W., Lynch, K.G., Alterman, A.I. & O'Brien, C.P. (2010) A randomized trial of oral naltrexone for treating opioid-dependent offenders. *American Journal on Addictions*, **19**, 422–432.

96 Goonoo, N., Bhaw-Luximon, A., Ujoodha, R., Jhugroo, A., Hulse, G.K. & Jhurry, D. (2014) Naltrexone: a review of existing sustained drug delivery systems and emerging nano-based systems. *Journal of Controlled Release*, **183**, 154–166.

97 Ahamad, K., Milloy, M.J., Nguyen, P. *et al.* (2015) Factors associated with willingness to take extended release naltrexone among injection drug users. *Addiction Science & Clinical Practice*, **10**, 12.

98 Di Paola, A., Lincoln, T., Skiest, D.J., Desabrais, M., Altice, F.L. & Springer, S.A. (2014) Design and methods of a double blind randomized placebo-controlled trial of extended-release naltrexone for HIV-infected, opioid dependent prisoners

and jail detainees who are transitioning to the community. *Contemporary Clinical Trials*, **39**, 256–268.

99 Colfax, G., Santos, G.M., Chu, P. *et al.* (2010) Amphetamine-group substances and HIV. *Lancet*, **376**, 458–474.

100 Brensilver, M., Heinzerling, K.G. & Shoptaw, S. (2013) Pharmacotherapy of amphetamine-type stimulant dependence: an update. *Drug and Alcohol Review*, **32**, 449–460.

101 Colfax, G.N., Santos, G.M., Das, M. *et al.* (2011) Mirtazapine to reduce methamphetamine use: a randomized controlled trial. *Archives of General Psychiatry*, **68**, 1168–1175.

102 Jayaram-Lindstrom, N., Hammarberg, A., Beck, O. & Franck, J. (2008) Naltrexone for the treatment of amphetamine dependence: a randomized, placebo-controlled trial. *The American Journal of Psychiatry*, **165**, 1442–1448.

103 Carroll, K.M., Fenton, L.R., Ball, S.A. *et al.* (2004) Efficacy of disulfiram and cognitive behavior therapy in cocaine-dependent outpatients: a randomized placebo-controlled trial. *Archives of General Psychiatry*, **61**, 264–272.

104 Carroll, K.M., Nich, C., Ball, S.A., McCance, E., Frankforter, T.L. & Rounsaville, B.J. (2000) One-year follow-up of disulfiram and psychotherapy for cocaine-alcohol users: sustained effects of treatment. *Addiction*, **95**, 1335–1349.

105 George, T.P., Chawarski, M.C., Pakes, J., Carroll, K.M., Kosten, T.R. & Schottenfeld, R.S. (2000) Disulfiram versus placebo for cocaine dependence in buprenorphine-maintained subjects: a preliminary trial. *Biological Psychiatry*, **47**, 1080–1086.

106 Petrakis, I.L., Carroll, K.M., Nich, C. *et al.* (2000) Disulfiram treatment for cocaine dependence in methadone-maintained opioid addicts. *Addiction*, **95**, 219–228.

107 Carroll, K.M., Nich, C., Shi, J.M., Eagan, D. & Ball, S.A. (2012) Efficacy of disulfiram and twelve step facilitation in cocaine-dependent individuals maintained on methadone: a randomized placebo-controlled trial. *Drug and Alcohol Dependence*, **126**, 224–231.

108 DeVito, E.E., Babuscio, T.A., Nich, C., Ball, S.A. & Carroll, K.M. (2014) Gender differences in clinical outcomes for cocaine dependence: randomized clinical trials of behavioral therapy and disulfiram. *Drug and Alcohol Dependence*, **145**, 156–167.

109 Oliveto, A., Poling, J., Mancino, M.J. *et al.* (2011) Randomized, double blind, placebo-controlled trial of disulfiram for the treatment of cocaine dependence in methadone-stabilized patients. *Drug and Alcohol Dependence*, **113**, 184–191.

110 Kalman, D., Kim, S., DiGirolamo, G., Smelson, D. & Ziedonis, D. (2010) Addressing tobacco use disorder in smokers in early remission from alcohol dependence: the case for integrating smoking cessation services in substance use disorder treatment programs. *Clinical Psychology Review*, **30**, 12–24.

111 Prochaska, J.J., Delucchi, K. & Hall, S.M. (2004) A meta-analysis of smoking cessation interventions with individuals in substance abuse treatment or recovery. *Journal of Consulting and Clinical Psychology*, **72**, 1144–1156.

112 Walsh, S.L., Nuzzo, P.A., Lofwall, M.R. & Holtman, J.R. Jr., (2008) The relative abuse liability of oral oxycodone, hydrocodone and hydromorphone assessed in prescription opioid abusers. *Drug and Alcohol Dependence*, **98**, 191–202.

113 Gilron, I., Bailey, J.M., Tu, D., Holden, R.R., Weaver, D.F. & Houlden, R.L. (2005) Morphine, gabapentin, or their combination for neuropathic pain. *New England Journal of Medicine*, **352**, 1324–1334.

114 Pedersen, L., Borchgrevink, P.C., Riphagen, I.I. & Fredheim, O.M. (2014) Long- or short-acting opioids for chronic non-malignant pain? A qualitative systematic review. *Acta Anaesthesiologica Scandinavica*, **58**, 390–401.

115 Woolridge, E., Barton, S., Samuel, J., Osorio, J., Dougherty, A. & Holdcroft, A. (2005) Cannabis use in HIV for pain and other medical symptoms. *Journal of Pain and Symptom Management*, **29**, 358–367.

116 Abrams, D.I., Jay, C.A., Shade, S.B. *et al.* (2007) Cannabis in painful HIV-associated sensory neuropathy: a randomized placebo-controlled trial. *Neurology*, **68**, 515–521.

117 Ellis, R.J., Toperoff, W., Vaida, F. *et al.* (2009) Smoked medicinal cannabis for neuropathic pain in HIV: a randomized, crossover clinical trial. *Neuropsychopharmacology*, **34**, 672–680.

118 Volkow, N.D., Baler, R.D., Compton, W.M. & Weiss, S.R. (2014) Adverse health effects of marijuana use. *The New England Journal of Medicine*, **370**, 2219–2227.

119 Pletcher, M.J., Vittinghoff, E., Kalhan, R. *et al.* (2012) Association between marijuana exposure and pulmonary function over 20 years. *JAMA*, **307**, 173–181.

120 Hezode, C., Roudot-Thoraval, F., Nguyen, S. *et al.* (2005) Daily cannabis smoking as a risk factor for progression of fibrosis in chronic hepatitis C. *Hepatology*, **42**, 63–71.

121 Brunet, L., Moodie, E.E., Rollet, K. *et al.* (2013) Marijuana smoking does not accelerate progression of liver disease in HIV-hepatitis C coinfection: a longitudinal cohort analysis. *Clinical Infectious Diseases*, **57**, 663–670.

122 Basu, S., Bruce, R.D., Barry, D.T. & Altice, F.L. (2007) Pharmacological pain control for human immunodeficiency virus-infected adults with a history of drug dependence. *Journal of Substance Abuse Treatment*, **32**, 399–409.

CHAPTER 10

Pharmacologic and Non-Pharmacologic treatment approaches to chronic pain in individuals with HIV

J. Hampton Atkinson[1,2,3], Shetal Patel[4] and J.R. Keltner[1,2,3]

[1] Psychiatry Service, VA San Diego Healthcare System, San Diego, CA, USA

[2] Department of Psychiatry, University of California, San Diego, CA, USA

[3] HIV Neurobehavioral Research Program, University of California, La Jolla, San Diego, CA, USA

[4] Research Service, VA San Diego Healthcare System, La Jolla Village Drive, San Diego, CA, USA

Introduction

Modern antiretroviral treatments and their dramatic effects on lifespan and overall life quality in HIV populations have revealed another epidemic hidden in our midst: the epidemic of chronic pain. Formerly obscured by the pressing consequences of HIV disease, it is now evident that HIV patients experience the same burdens of chronic pain that affect the general population – chronic back pain, neuropathic pain, fibromyalgia, arthritic conditions, and irritable bowel syndrome (IBS). Drawing primarily upon meta-analyses of published randomized trials, this chapter reviews the evidence base for the efficacy of standard pharmacological and adjunctive treatments (antidepressants, anticonvulsants, cognitive behavioral therapy (CBT), and transcutaneous neurostimulation) for these disorders. It likewise assesses efficacy for acupuncture and complementary and alternative therapies, including "energy" medicine, chiropractic medicine, massage, hypnosis, yoga, biofeedback, and dietary supplementation. By separating possibly "useful" from probably "useless" therapy, this review attempts to guide a rational approach to effective treatment and to describe areas for future research.

At an early stage of the epidemic, chronic pain was identified as an important comorbidity in HIV [1]. It since has remained underdiagnosed and undertreated [2]. Perhaps the grim prognosis of HIV disease in these early years fostered neglect since life expectancy was limited and acute medical crises abounded. With the advent of modern combination antiretroviral therapy (cART) life spans are trending upward, and patients are seeking enhanced quality of life. Physicians now are obligated to reconsider the diagnosis and treatment of the most prevalent conditions found in the general population: chronic back pain, non-HIV neuropathic pain, fibromyalgia, rheumatoid disorders, osteoarthritis, and IBS. Indeed, chronic pain syndromes are recognized now to be so prevalent that they are considered an "evolving epidemic" in HIV disease [3]. Estimates of prevalence of non-HIV-related pain exceed 20%. Impact on life quality is substantial and stands out even in a population with many other burdens beyond pain [2].

This chapter uses a framework of neurobiology and the behavioral sciences to categorize and assess treatment approaches to some of the most frequently encountered non-HIV, non-neoplastic chronic pain syndromes in HIV, with the exception of headaches (see Chapter 5). We

Chronic Pain and HIV: A Practical Approach, First Edition.
Edited by Jessica S. Merlin, Peter A. Selwyn, Glenn J. Treisman and Angela G. Giovanniello.
© 2016 John Wiley & Sons, Ltd. Published 2016 by John Wiley & Sons, Ltd.

reviewed the evidence base for pharmacological interventions, focusing on antidepressants, anticonvulsants, nonsteroidal anti-inflammatory drugs (NSAIDs), acetaminophen, and topical agents. We also reviewed nonpharmacological therapies (cognitive behavioral treatment, exercise regimens, and transcutaneous electrical stimulation) and conclude with the broad category of popular treatments that are classified as complementary or alternative therapies (e.g., acupuncture, bioelectromagnetic fields, biofeedback, chiropractic manipulation, dietary supplements, hypnosis, massage, and yoga).

Because the field of chronic pain treatment is vast, this chapter draws upon meta-analyses and systematic reviews as guides to therapeutic efficacy. Admittedly there are limitations to this method. Conclusions from meta-analyses are obviously constrained by the variable quality of the clinical trials included in the report (e.g., poorly specified inclusion criteria and nonstandardized outcome measures). Methodological weaknesses are reflected by the fact that many reviews are not able to pool data because they lack a standardized outcome measure. Furthermore, an unfortunate price of neglecting pain in HIV is that there is little research specifically studying pain treatment outcomes in HIV-infected individuals experiencing the pain conditions commonly found in the general population. Thirdly, most research identifies pain intensity as the primary outcome. Therefore, meta-analyses and reviews may not address other end points, such as everyday function or quality of life. This is important since some treatments seem to improve function without necessarily reducing pain intensity [4].

In deciding whether to recommend a particular therapy to an individual patient, based on this overview of the literature, it might be recognized that some meta-analyses and reviews set very high standards for declaring efficacy for an intervention (e.g., 50% pain relief or greater). Individual patients might find lesser degrees of pain relief to be meaningful. Finally, for many pain syndromes, the outcome from an intervention seems to follow a U-shaped function rather than a graded response – some patients achieve very good relief whereas others have no discernible benefit [5]. This may make it more difficult to discern efficacy in meta-analyses.

Neurobiologic and behavioral rationales of chronic pain treatment

A complete and adequate explanation of the transition from acute to chronic pain is lacking. It is generally agreed that persisting pain often involves interplay of neurobiologic mechanisms and "cognitive" or "behavioral" factors. Treatment approaches roughly map onto these mechanisms. Classical theory holds that monoamines such as norepinephrine and serotonin have a role in pain neurotransmission and that disruption in these systems is reflected by a transition to chronic pain. Evidence over the last decade indicates that although monoamine function is obviously important, the transition from acute to chronic pain may be associated with neuroinflammation, neuronal loss, and broad structural and functional abnormalities in the central nervous system [6]. Antidepressants have long been considered an important treatment in chronic pain based on their property of enhancing monoamine neurotransmission by inhibiting the reuptake of serotonin and noradrenaline at neural synapses. This property is thought to facilitate the action of inhibitory pain pathways descending from the dorsal raphe (serotonergic) or locus coeruleus (noradrenergic) to block the transmission of "painful" sensory stimuli from the periphery at the level of the dorsal horn of the spinal cord. But these agents have other complex effects on neurotransmitter receptors or enzymes. One theory is that antidepressants in part exert therapeutic effects by downregulating some postsynaptic receptors (e.g., β-adrenergic receptors and 5HT2a receptors), enhancing 5HT1a receptor transmission, and decreasing firing of autoinhibitory monoamine neurons. Other evidence suggests antidepressants may have neuroprotective effects and promote neurogenesis and synaptic connectivity. Some antidepressants have effects on cholinergic transmission, acid-sensing sodium and calcium channels, glutamate and N-methyl-D-aspartate (NMDA) receptors, sigma 1 and 2 receptors, and histone acetylation [7]. They are widely used, but their efficacy has come under question, and they cannot be considered generally effective across all chronic pain diagnoses.

Behavioral theory conceptualizes chronic pain as a perception influenced by psychological, behavioral, and environmental factors. In this view, chronic pain may be summarized as a self-reinforcing, malignant cycle consisting of an initial injury or pain-associated illness, which can raise fears of subsequent reinjury or harm, generalized fear of movement, restricted activity, physical deconditioning, and withdrawal from rewarding activities, resulting in demoralization or depression, and an organization of life around pain avoidance and reliance on medical care for pain relief. Behavioral medicine therapies attempt to take the focus off pain relief as an exclusive goal, and instead promote self-efficacy and self-management skills to progressively enhance activity, improve coping skills to reduce anxiety, demoralization or depression, and set goals for rewarding activity despite pain [4]. These approaches can be generally applied in diverse chronic pain syndromes. Furthermore, this type of intervention is short term, usually deliverable in once weekly sessions over a period of approximately 8 weeks, with the express intent of preparing patients to practice the skills learned to become self-sufficient. Different "brands" of behavioral medicine therapy exist (e.g., cognitive, operant, and respondent) and their relative contributions to outcomes are a subject of research. But in clinical practice, interventions usually consist of an amalgam of these varieties. The scientific rationale for the other traditional nonpharmacological therapies such as physical exercises and transcutaneous neurostimulation resides in part on effects on inhibiting pain transmission at the level of the spinal cord [8].

Complementary and alternative (CAM) therapies were originally defined as treatments not generally taught or delivered in Western medical institutions. This categorization is now somewhat more relaxed since several of these therapies have moved into established institutional medicine, based in part on competition in the healthcare marketplace to attract patients.

The scientific basis for some of these treatments is unclear. For example, the traditional theory of acupuncture asserts that stimulation of specific points on the skin (e.g., by needling or heat) is to correct body "imbalances [8]." These therapies are widely used in the general population and have a loyal following in HIV settings [9]. The evidence base assessing efficacy is growing, but additional studies are needed to clarify the proper role of these treatments.

Establishing goals for treatment outcomes

The usual outcomes targeted for treatment are pain intensity, pain interference (e.g., with sleep), everyday physical functioning, life quality, and mood. Pain relief is what most clinicians automatically aim to achieve. Evidence suggests that reducing pain intensity by approximately 30% translates on average to a significantly improved quality of life [10].

On the other hand, substantial pain relief may not be possible in some chronic pain states, and other outcomes should be considered. Furthermore, it appears that patients find the usual research outcomes focusing on pain intensity lacking and seek more from treatment [11]. This is consistent with evidence that, even with clear-cut reduction of pain, it does not follow that function improves without the addition of specific therapy to improve mobility, or manage daily activities [4]. If clinicians and patients expand the definition of successful treatment to include return of function or enhanced life quality, rather than focusing exclusively on reduced pain intensity, then treatment selection may involve cognitive behavioral or other therapies as the main intervention. It is essential that the clinician and patient agree on primary and secondary end points and on the degree of improvement desired. Such discussions establish expectations, define "success," set realistic goals (e.g., complete elimination of pain is unlikely), and facilitate a multidisciplinary, collaborative approach to care since there is usually no single answer. Such discussions may be viewed as "preparing the patient for treatment" but are just as easily seen as preparing the clinician for the collaborative care of the patient, by understanding the individual's attitudes, expectations, and goals, which may include outreach to a wide range of interventions.

Interventions and efficacy in selected chronic pain states

Pharmacological approaches: antidepressants, anticonvulsants, and other agents

Meta-analyses document the efficacy of selected antidepressants and anticonvulsants/mood stabilizers for several specific pain syndromes. The practical implication is that treatment success is more likely if specific classes of antidepressants and anticonvulsants are chosen to target specific pain diagnoses, rather than assuming that all of these agents are equally analgesic for all chronic pain conditions [12].

The most extensive evidence documents the efficacy of tricyclic antidepressants (TCA) and the anticonvulsants gabapentin and pregabalin for neuropathic pain (e.g., painful diabetic neuropathy, postherpetic neuralgia, and traumatic nerve injury) [12,13]. Here the number-needed-to-treat (NNT) with TCA for an efficacious outcome range from 1.5 to 3.6. There is less evidence for the newer, second-generation antidepressants, but these agents (e.g., duloxetine and venlafaxine) are generally more tolerable and may be equally efficacious. Mechanistically, the tricyclics and duloxetine and venlafaxine may be characterized as having effects either predominantly on the norepinephrine transporter or "balanced" effects on the norepinephrine and serotonin transporters (although venlafaxine has effects on norepinephrine transporters only with daily dosages ≥150 mg daily) [7]. There is less literature on the more selective serotonin reuptake inhibitors (SSRIs); in general, these agents have not been found to be as efficacious as the tricyclics for neuropathic pain, with the possible exception of citalopram and paroxetine [12–15]. In the case of tricyclics, the dosage range for an analgesic effect usually is lower than for an antidepressant effect (e.g., 25–100 mg daily); the

effective doses for duloxetine and venlafaxine are the standard antidepressant doses.

Finally, oral NSAIDS are not effective for neuropathic pain, but topical NSAIDS may be helpful for peripheral neuropathic pain such as herpes zoster or postherpetic neuralgia [16]. Topical lidocaine may be effective for peripheral neuropathic pain and allodynia (a painful sensation evoked by a stimulus that is not normally painful) [17].

Evidence of efficacy of antidepressants in chronic nonneuropathic pain syndromes is more mixed. For example, tricyclic agents are widely prescribed for chronic back pain, whereas some meta-analyses substantiate their efficacy[18] more recent ones question their utility [19]. On the other hand, multisite trials report potential efficacy for duloxetine [20]. There is no evidence that the SSRIs are effective in chronic back pain. Evidence is also mixed regarding the other agents. An early influential review noted that oral NSAIDS were ineffective for chronic low back pain [21], but in recent years other reviews suggest that oral NSAIDS effectively manage nonneuropathic low back pain [22,23]. Acetaminophen is still considered first-line treatment for chronic low back pain [22]. Topical NSAIDS are not effective for chronic low back pain [24], but topical lidocaine may be effective [22].

Fibromyalgia may also respond to selected antidepressants with reductions in pain and overall symptom burden [25]. In general, the tricyclics and second-generation antidepressants with noradrenergic and serotonergic effects may be efficacious (i.e., serotonin noradrenaline reuptake inhibitors [SNRIs] such as duloxetine and milnacipran). Positive outcomes included improved patient ratings of pain intensity, sleep, and overall well-being. The NNT is estimated at around 4. The role of SSRIs in general is less clear, with reports that fluoxetine can be efficacious but that citalopram and paroxetine are not. Doses for all agents are in the range used to treat major depression [12]. On the other hand, oral NSAIDS are not effective for the management of fibromyalgia [25].

IBS is another potentially antidepressant-responsive syndrome, as judged by a systematic review and meta-analysis including nine studies comparing TCAs to placebo, and five trials using SSRIs. Tricyclics were beneficial with an overall NNT of 4. Doses were generally in the low-to-middle range used in other pain syndromes (e.g., amitriptyline 10 mg and desipramine 150 mg daily). Several SSRIs (citalopram, fluoxetine, and paroxetine) were efficacious, with an NNT of 3.5. In this instance, efficacious doses were in the range used to treat major depression (e.g., citalopram 20–40 mg, fluoxetine 20–40 mg, and paroxetine 20–40 mg). Depression and anxiety symptoms often accompany IBS, but improvement in pain symptoms was not correlated with scores on depression, suggesting that treatment exerted an analgesic effect independent of an antidepressant or antianxiety effect [26].

Finally, antidepressants are occasionally considered for use in rheumatoid arthritis as analgesics, but little evidence supports their efficacy [27]. Oral NSAIDS are effective for rheumatoid arthritis pain [28], but acetaminophen is not [29]. Oral NSAIDS, acetaminophen, and topical NSAIDS are all effective for osteoarthritis pain [12,30,31].

In terms of anticonvulsants, gabapentin and pregabalin demonstrate efficacy in painful diabetic neuropathy and postherpetic neuralgia. Other anticonvulsants, such as carbamazepine and valproate, are often used if these first-line treatments fail, but there is no strong evidence they are reliably effective [32].

There is one small study ($N = 150$) suggesting efficacy for gabapentin in fibromyalgia and seven trials ($N \sim 3000$ patients) of pregabalin. In both cases, about 50% of patients experienced a 30% or greater decrease in pain intensity. The efficacious dose was 2400 mg daily for gabapentin and 300–600 mg daily for pregabalin. The NNT was 5 for gabapentin and 8 for pregabalin. The time to response was about 30 days, similar to what is seen for antidepressants [12,33]. The durability of efficacy was examined for responders to pregabalin: at 6-month follow-up about one in three patients continued to experience more than 30% pain relief [34]. There are no other known trials testing the efficacy of other anticonvulsants in fibromyalgia [33].

In summary, these psychotropic agents can be a mainstay of pain treatment, which, compared to opioids, offers advantages in terms of tolerability, safety, and absence of potential for abuse or addiction. Many chronic pain syndromes are complicated by comorbid depressive or anxiety disorders. In these instances, a TCA or SNRI antidepressant at the standard antidepressant dosage range may alleviate the depressive disorder. In addition, SSRIs at standard doses may be effective for depression and anxiety (e.g., generalized anxiety disorder). If the clinician wishes to treat both conditions simultaneously, the choice of which psychotropic to select would depend on the pain syndrome and the coexisting psychiatric disorder. For example, from the evidence cited above, it appears that psychotropics with strong noradrenergic actions may be more likely to be effective for neuropathic pain than an SSRI, so the choice might be duloxetine, an agent that could address both pain and depression. If the person has an SSRI-responsive condition such as IBS and either major depression or generalized anxiety disorder, the choice would be an SSRI-like citalopram or sertraline.

Nonpharmacological approaches
Behavioral therapies
Behavioral therapies, of which CBT is the best researched, are widely used to treat chronic pain syndromes. The most thoroughly studied conditions are chronic back pain and diffuse musculoskeletal pain syndromes, with over 30 randomized trials (about 3500 patients) contributing to the evidence base of respectable quality overall [35]. The results show moderate improvement in terms of pain relief, improved function, and life quality in the short term (e.g., 12 weeks) compared to usual care. There are no head-to-head comparisons of CBT to pharmacotherapy for chronic pain, but it appears that CBT may be just as successful and have fewer adverse effects. In addition, a separate body of evidence suggests that behavioral medicine therapy is effective for depression and depressive symptoms [36]. This is important since a sizable proportion of chronic pain patients experience depressive symptoms or have a frank major depressive disorder.

With regard to other conditions, there is evidence from over 20 randomized trials of fibromyalgia (enrolling over 2000 patients) that CBT compared to wait list control or usual care is of some benefit in terms of reduction in pain and improvement in function [37]. The role of CBT for treatment of pain in IBS is inconclusive, owing to the sparse literature (six studies) and low methodological quality of the research [26].

In summary, behavioral therapy can be important to overall treatment outcome and is likely applicable in many chronic pain states but has only been extensively studied in relatively few syndromes. A barrier to its widespread application is the scarcity of trained experts in mental health to deliver the intervention, which means this one-on-one treatment is often unavailable to low-income patients or those living outside metropolitan areas. Fortunately, the principles of this approach, termed "self-management skills training" or "pain self-management," can be administered by nonmental health clinicians to help patients use techniques such as setting goals for activities, relaxation exercises, and self-monitoring to determine physical and emotional antecedents and consequences of pain. Research is underway to adapt behavioral therapies to interactive mobile smart phones ("mobile health or mHealth") to help deliver the key therapeutic ingredients, and chronic pain syndromes are an obvious treatment target for this approach [38]. Group treatment approaches are also becoming more widespread. These innovations may enhance accessibility and applicability of this valuable resource.

Exercise therapy

Aerobic exercise (e.g., biking, swimming, and walking) and specific exercise therapy (e.g., for strengthening and flexibility) have been studied for chronic back pain and compared to usual care and various physiotherapy treatments (e.g., hot packs, massage, traction, and ultrasound). There was strong evidence that exercise therapy was superior to usual care, but that exercise therapy and conventional physiotherapy were equally effective. It is uncertain whether any specific type of exercises (strengthening, flexion, and extension) is more therapeutic than another. Exercises appear to be useful within an overall program geared toward returning individuals to everyday activity and

function and may improve mood and a sense of well-being [39].

Transcutaneous electrical stimulation (TENS)

Transcutaneous electrical stimulation is a standard component in the multimodal treatment of musculoskeletal conditions, particularly chronic low back pain. TENS units deliver electrical stimulation to underlying peripheral nerves via electrodes placed on the skin surface, near the source of maximal pain [40]. The use of TENS is based on the Gate Control Theory, conceptualized by Melzack and Wall [41], which posits that the stimulation of large diameter (A-β), primary sensory nerve fibers activates inhibitory interneurons in the substantia gelatinosa of the spinal cord dorsal horn and blocks the transmission of nociceptive ("pain") signals from small diameter A-δ and C fibers. Overall, TENS is postulated to "close the gate" and dampen the perception of pain. TENS applications used in clinical care differ in frequency, amplitude, pulse width, and waveform, with the two most common application being either conventional TENS (the stimulus produces a comfortable tingling sensation) or acupuncture-like TENS (the stimulator elicits muscle twitching). The devices in most of the controlled studies were worn from 20 to 60 min daily [42].

Given its widespread use, it is surprising that its efficacy is not more convincingly established. Only four higher quality-controlled randomized trials (approximately 600 patients) were included in a recent qualitative review. The results of placebo-controlled studies (in which the sham TENS device did not deliver an electrical current to the skin surface electrodes) indicated that verum TENS did not reliably reduce low back pain intensity, did not reduce disability, and did not improve work status [42].

TENS has also been studied for knee osteoarthritis. A recent systematic review examined 18 randomized trials (approximately 800 patients) in which verum TENS was compared to sham TENS or no treatment controls. The quality of the studies was rated as poor, and the results were inconclusive [43]. It does not appear that TENS can be recommended for painful knee osteoarthritis.

Complementary and alternative therapies (CAM)

The National Institutes of Health National Center for Complementary and Alternative Medicine classifies these therapies into four groups: energy medicine, mind–body medicine, manipulative body-based medicine, and biologically based medicine [8,44]. Acupuncture is categorized separately. CAM therefore covers a wide range from biofeedback and bioelectromagnetic-based ("energy") therapies, to hypnosis, meditation, yoga, and vitamin supplementation. Authoritative reviews note that the diverse CAM literature is difficult to summarize according to a single metric of quality of the individual clinical trials and recommends that a broad rating of efficacy is most feasible and clinically useful at this point. The five levels of efficacy for each modality are as follows: (1) not empirically supported (anecdotal reports only); (2) possibly efficacious (standardized outcomes used but without randomized assignment to a control condition); (3) probably efficacious (based on studies using wait list control, within- or between-subject replication designs); (4) efficacious (trials with randomized assignment to investigational therapy or to standard of care, alternative treatment, or sham [placebo], with rigorous inclusion criteria, specified outcome measures, and appropriate data analysis); (5) efficacious and specific (at least two independent randomized studies document statistical superiority of the treatment compared to a credible control) [8].

Acupuncture

Acupuncture is a component of Traditional Chinese Medicine (TCM), which aims to address the principle that illness results from an imbalance of "energy flow." By stimulating specific anatomical sites (acupuncture points) along specific "energy pathways" (meridians) acupuncture restores proper flow and the resulting harmonious balance is reflected in a return to health [44]. Some authorities argue that attempting to isolate the procedure of acupuncture from its basis in the diagnostic milieu of TCM, and to apply it in randomized trials of patients diagnosed using the nomenclature of Western medicine will invariably underestimate its efficacy [8]. Conventional explanations of the effects of acupuncture suggest it may activate the endogenous opioid and catecholamine neurotransmitter systems (e.g., there is evidence in humans that acute acupuncture analgesia is blocked by naltrexone) [45]. Functional magnetic resonance imaging during acupuncture reveals activation of insula, dorsolateral prefrontal cortex, and midbrain, areas known to be involved in the anticipation and experience of pain. These findings suggest that diverse brain regions, as well as opioid and dopaminergic mechanisms associated with analgesic and reward systems may be involved in the response to acupuncture [44].

Randomized trials of acupuncture have been conducted for various chronic pain conditions. Higher quality trials compare traditional or verum acupuncture with sham needling (i.e., insertion of acupuncture needles superficially and in sites unrelated to traditional points specified by meridians) and a standard-of-care or a no treatment group. Treatment is delivered typically in two weekly sessions for 5 weeks or longer. In terms of chronic low back pain, several studies (comprising >1000 patients) indicate that verum and sham acupuncture are equivalent in efficacy and statistically superior in reducing pain intensity and improving function to standard of care (e.g., medications and exercise) at 6-month follow-up. [46,47] Although these reviews conclude that both acupuncture and needling are efficacious, a notable flaw is that the studies reviewed failure to control for the nonspecific effects of therapist contact time, which is intensive in both acupuncture groups but limited in usual care. The positive results on long-term follow-up, however, may overweigh this weakness and support the conclusion that acupuncture and needling are probably efficacious for chronic low back pain [46].

Research on the efficacy of acupuncture for other pain conditions raises some of the same questions regarding specificity of effects. For example, results from a meta-analysis using acupuncture for fibromyalgia (seven studies) suggested that verum acupuncture and sham acupuncture were equivalent, particularly if methodological issues such as unblinding were accounted for, leading to the judgment that acupuncture could not be recommended for fibromyalgia. One problem with this conclusion is that there were no "usual care" controls to take into account the possible therapeutic effects of both verum and sham acupuncture [48]. A recent meta-analysis of the efficacy of acupuncture for knee osteoarthritis based on 11 studies of "better quality" (almost 900 patients) concluded that pain relief afforded by acupuncture was superior to effects of sham acupuncture, muscle strengthening exercises, weight loss, aerobic exercise, and no intervention. It was reported that acupuncture may provide a "minimal clinically important," short-term (weeks to months) relief for patients with low intensity pain. The conclusions were that acupuncture could be considered in a multidisciplinary treatment plan for pain in knee osteoarthritis [49]. Results for rheumatoid arthritis are based on a few low-quality studies. Acupuncture does not appear to benefit pain, function, number of swollen-tender joints, erythrocyte sedimentation rates, or C-reactive protein. The evidence at this time therefore cannot support use of acupuncture for rheumatoid arthritis [50].

A recent systematic review surveyed 25 trials (including >1500 patients) of acupuncture for diabetic painful neuropathy. The review noted that there were reports of efficacy, but concluded the evidence base was inconclusive because of serious methodological problems in the conduct of the trials. Even the seven highest quality studies lacked a sham acupuncture control. These trials were further weakened by failures to specify neuromedical diagnostic criteria, predetermined outcome criteria, procedures for randomization and blinding, or describing dropouts or using an intent-to-treat analysis. It appears more work needs to be done before acupuncture could be recommended for painful diabetic neuropathy [51].

Finally with regard to safety, reviews have reported that adverse effects of acupuncture are infrequent, but that there are some reports of infection and death (e.g., from pneumothorax and cardiac tamponade) resulting from this technique [52].

Energy medicine

This type of intervention is based on the use of electromagnetic fields to perturb the "energy fields" that are hypothesized to surround and integrate with the patient's body. Treatment is delivered continuously or intermittently either by wearable, battery-powered devices or by fixed, clinic-based generators. Four randomized trials (a total of 230 patients) comparing sham to verum pulsed electromagnetic field generators indicate that this intervention is probably efficacious in terms of pain relief and improvement in function for knee osteoarthritis. A variation of this type of intervention delivers low-level (subsensory threshold) electric current to the skin. One randomized trial suggested efficacy in fibromyalgia and another one reported efficacy in reducing pain due to spinal cord injury compared to sham treatment. Although there is no proof of "energy fields," the reviews remark that the positive evidence for efficacy, the lack of apparent adverse effects, and the simple, inexpensive nature of the therapy warrant its consideration for clinical care and further research [8].

Therapeutic touch, Reiki, and Qigong/Qi therapies posit that pain and disease are based on the concept of spiritual or vital energy "imbalances." These can be addressed by a therapist's laying on of hands (Reiki), by a master practitioner's spiritual energy without touching (therapeutic touch), or by adjusting energy or vital force (Qi) by the practitioner's presence or by specifically training the patient to coordinate movement, breathing, and meditation ("Gong," means training). There is little evidence that therapeutic touch, Reiki, or Qigong benefits the chronic pain syndromes covered in this review (although tension headaches may benefit from touch therapy) [8].

Mind–Body medicine

This broad category of methods includes meditation, hypnosis, yoga, and biofeedback [8].

Meditation

Meditation is defined as the individual's regulation of mental attention and awareness of their internal and external states and experiences. Some types of meditation focus on specific techniques (e.g., visual images, repetition of focusing words, phrases, or breathing); others such as mindfulness meditation move away from a focus on specifics to foster a detached observation of pain and its associated thoughts and feelings [8]. The usual treatment targets have been low back pain or musculoskeletal pain, fibromyalgia, and IBS. The literature is weakened by small sample sizes, high attrition, short-term follow-up, and results that have been mixed. As a result, meditation is not viewed as a pain intervention to be recommended routinely, but rather an adjunct to patients who are oriented to seek supportive approaches for relieving stress or anxiety [8,53].

Hypnosis

Hypnosis or guided imagery is acquired, skill-based intervention. Hypnosis involves a therapist guiding the patient to respond to therapeutic suggestion of comfort and relaxation to reduce pain, with the patient being taught to self-induce this state by using cues (e.g., deep breaths and eyelid closure) [8,54,55]. Imagery interventions train patients to imagine an internal reality (e.g., visiting a pleasant tropical isle) in the absence of an external stimulus. The intent of these therapies is to change the patient's perception of pain in terms of its sensory, cognitive, and emotional impact by way of the therapists' suggestion or by use of the patient's imagination [54,55]. Its use in pain management usually includes relaxation or calming followed by suggestions about altering how pain is experienced (e.g., "warm" rather than "stabbing") or interpreting it as less threatening, to reduce its impact and the patient's sense of vulnerability. Skill building involves sessions with a hypnotist; often the therapist audio records a hypnosis induction for the patient to practice at home. The goal of treatment if for the patient to learn to use self-hypnosis in everyday life on a long-term basis to achieve a target goal [8,55,56]. Some patients become more adept than others in learning and using hypnosis. Hypnosis therefore heavily relies on a patient's "talent" rather than a hypnotist's ability to induce a "trance." The clinical trial literature on hypnosis is difficult to interpret given that sampling may

be subject to certain biases (e.g., recruitment of treatment "failures" who see hypnosis as a "last chance"; or conversely enrollment of individuals invested in positive outcomes from hypnosis). Induction techniques are not standardized or are only briefly described. The success and depth of induction may not be ascertained. There is some evidence for the efficacy of hypnosis compared to standard of care or no treatment, in relief of chronic back pain, osteoarthritis, and fibromyalgia pain, but the benefits may not surpass those from progressive muscle relaxation [8,54–56]. Evidence from four randomized trials suggest short-term pain benefits for IBS [57,58]. The evidence seems to point toward efficacy for hypnosis in terms of pain relief, in selected disorders, but the literature is weak. On the other hand, hypnosis is benign having few adverse effects and provides an improved overall sense of well-being with reduced anxiety and stress [8].

Yoga

Yoga is a philosophical, spiritual, and lifestyle (e.g., diet) system from which specific postures, movements, breathing, and meditation techniques have been extracted and distilled for application in randomized trials for chronic pain. There are many different styles of yoga (e.g., Hatha, Iyengar, and Viniyoga), but little research compares the relative efficacy of these different approaches. The duration of yoga interventions in the clinical trials literature varies from daily sessions for 1 week to twice weekly sessions delivered over 24 weeks. Yoga is usually compared to education, standard of care, or physical therapy control conditions. A recent meta-analysis addressing chronic low back pain included 10 randomized trials (over 950 patients). There was strong evidence of short-term effects (3–12 weeks) and moderate evidence for longer-term effects (up to 26 weeks) on reducing pain intensity and back-related disability. There was no evidence of serious adverse effects. The authors concluded that yoga could be recommended in the care of chronic back pain and that additional research was needed to understand the relative contributions of physical postures, breathing, or meditation to overall effects [59].

Separately one randomized 8-week trial suggested that yoga was superior to wait list control in reducing pain, fatigue, depressed mood, and catastrophic thinking in patients with fibromyalgia [60]. Another trial of yoga for IBSs compared to a wait list control showed positive short-term effects on pain [61]. There were only two randomized trials of yoga for rheumatoid arthritis; one was rated to be of low quality and the other showed no benefit on pain or disability [62]. Thus, although reviews suggest that yoga may be efficacious in some conditions, it is noted that most samples recruited were better educated, more likely to be employed, healthier, and less disabled than the usual chronic pain patient. The relevance and impact of nonspecific factors thought to be important in pain outcomes (e.g., positive expectancy, attention, and physical conditioning) have not been controlled for adequately in the comparison interventions [63,64]. On the other hand, the novelty and body-centered focus of yoga lends itself to a subset of HIV-infected individuals who may find benefit from this method.

Biofeedback

Biofeedback relies on auditory or visual electronic display of autonomic function (e.g., muscle tension, heart rate, breathing, sweating, and brain waves) to train individuals to reduce muscle contraction or heart rate and to decrease pain and anxiety. This method is one of the most comprehensively studied and is so established in headache syndromes that it is considered to be standard rather than a CAM approach [8]. Data also supports efficacy of biofeedback in chronic musculoskeletal pain including low back pain [65]. Seven controlled studies suggest efficacy in fibromyalgia, but follow-up analyses indicated electromyographic feedback of muscle tension but not electroencephalographic feedback of brain waves reduced pain intensity. The mechanism of success in musculoskeletal conditions is thought to be based on the training of patients to recognize and reverse muscle tension that was otherwise out of their awareness [8,66].

In summary, biofeedback is generally thought to be efficacious in chronic musculoskeletal pain and headache syndromes (these disorders are not covered in the present review) and is thought to be effective in helping reduce anxious symptoms associated with these chronic pain states [8]. Its disadvantage is the need for specialized equipment. There appear to be no safety concerns [67].

Manipulative body-based medicine

This approach consists of spinal manipulative therapy (SMT, also called chiropractic manipulation) and massage therapy of soft tissue.

Spinal manipulative therapy – Chiropractic manipulation

SMT involves passive movements of joints and associated tissues (ligaments, tendons, and cartilage) termed "mobilization," along with "manipulation" or more forceful thrusting movements of joints at or beyond their physiologic range, to reduce pain. As applied to chronic low back pain it aims to separate spine facet joint surfaces, relax paraspinal muscles, and reduce intervertebral disc pressure. Since most of these effects are thought to be short-lived, the mechanisms for longer-term benefits are unclear [8].

Studies of SMT compare verum to sham spinal manipulation, to no treatment, to usual care or its various commonly employed components, including medication, exercise, TENS, heat, bed rest, and traction. Two recent large-scale systematic reviews reach different interpretations of the data in chronic back pain, perhaps reflecting the different postures of the review teams, one of which consisted of specialists in SMT. One recent summary surveying 26 randomized trials (over 6000 patients) suggested that SMT had a small, statistically significant, short-term effects of reducing pain and disability compared to other treatments (e.g., exercise or physiotherapy), but that these results were unlikely to be clinically relevant. On the other hand, SMT had statistically significant effects on pain intensity and function when added to other standard treatments. But the reviewers questioned if the costs of this care supported the results [68]. The other review team concluded that SMT reduced pain and improved function in chronic low back pain, but not in cases of pain radiating to the leg or for those with sciatica or radiculopathy. Combining SMT with a program of graded exercise or activity was thought to be beneficial for chronic back pain [69]. A review of the effect of mobilization and manipulation on chronic neck pain showed short-term reductions in pain intensity compared to usual care control [70]. In summary, SMT may be on par with conventional or usual care approaches to treat chronic back pain and may be considered possibly or probably efficacious, but of uncertain cost-benefit [71].

Massage therapy

The therapeutic effects of massage therapy are hypothesized to be based on the gate control theory, increase in serotonin neurotransmission, and enhancement in restorative sleep. The gate control theory mechanism is based on myelinated pressure receptors in the skin and soft tissues, which are thought to transmit impulses from massage faster than pain fibers, thereby closing the gate to pain sensations. In addition, therapeutic effects are attributed to the notion that soft tissue massage increases serotonin centrally and that by promoting relaxation it also enhances deep sleep, which reduces substance P, a neurotransmitter associated with pain. There are many brands of massage therapy (e.g., Rolfing, Swedish, Shiatsu, and Thai), and some techniques employ specific massage at traditional acupuncture points (acupressure). Only a few studies examine efficacy in head-to-head comparisons, and these seem to indicate rough equivalence across styles. Studies employing experienced therapists seem to be more likely to yield positive results [8].

As might be expected, most research was focused on chronic back pain and fibromyalgia. In these trials, massage has been compared to wait list controls, sham treatment (e.g., lasers), strengthening exercises, progressive muscle relaxation, acupuncture, and physiotherapy. Follow-up ranges from very short term (immediate postintervention effects), up to 3 months, or beyond 3 months for outcomes on pain intensity and everyday function. In these studies, massage outperforms sham treatment at all follow-up points, is superior to spinal manipulation immediately posttreatment for pain relief, and is superior to back exercises in short term (up to 3 months) but not thereafter.

Massage and progressive muscle relaxation therapies seem to be equivalent for short- and long-term follow-up. Finally, massage outperforms self-education in back pain over short term but not at 1 year. The literature on acupressure massage has been judged as uninterpretable because of the low quality of most studies [72].

Studies in fibromyalgia are divided on efficacy of massage therapy. At 6-month follow-up, one showed benefits in pain reduction compared to no treatment control, but another showing no effect compared to usual care [8,73]. This is in line with some other complementary and alternative approaches for various pain syndromes in which these therapies are superior to no treatment, but are not necessarily more efficacious than standard back pain treatments.

Most reviews summarize the role of massage therapy as efficacious for chronic back pain, but possibly not for fibromyalgia and other chronic musculoskeletal conditions. This judgment considers the fact that it is difficult to blind these studies and that few trials attempt to control for the nonspecific effects of therapist contact time. Successful outcome may rely on the expertise of the massage therapist. Cost is a consideration with any treatment delivered by specialists. Otherwise, there appear to be few adverse effects other than immediate posttreatment muscle stiffness and soreness.

Biologically based CAM
Dietary supplementation

Dietary supplements are often suggested as alternative treatments for chronic pain, particularly for back pain and knee osteoarthritis: these include vitamins, minerals, amino acids, enzymes, glandular extracts, and herbal preparations (excluding cannabis). The best studied of these are vitamins and glucosamine, an amino sugar necessary in the building of cartilage. There are plausible connections between the need for supplementation and pain but the mechanisms of therapeutic effects are mostly speculative. If simple supplementation relieved pain, this approach might be a cost-effective and a widely adopted intervention [8]. For example, vitamin D deficiency is implicated in the prevalence of several chronic pain conditions and is probably the most extensively studied vitamin in pain treatment. Four randomized studies of acceptable quality were reviewed, including about 300 patients with rheumatoid conditions or diffuse musculoskeletal pain. There was no consistent evidence that vitamin D supplementation reduced pain intensity, but the firmness of this conclusion is uncertain because of the poor overall research quality and the small number of patients enrolled [74]. Some research suggests that vitamin E supplements may have protective effects, reducing the risk of painful chemotherapy-associated neuropathies [75]. Glucosamine and chondroitin sulfate, whether alone or in combination, have been extensively studied. They have been examined in 25 trials including almost 5000 patients [76]. Mechanistically, glucosamine is thought to have anti-inflammatory effects by counteracting interleukin-1, suppressing oxide synthesis, or inhibiting the cyclo-oxygenase-2 pathway [8]. A summary of placebo controlled clinical trials indicated that glucosamine 1500 mg appeared to reduce pain (by 10–20%), improve function, and slow radiologic progression in knee osteoarthritis patients over a 3-year follow-up. It was also noted that glucosamine preparations vary widely in concentrations and that many of the negative trials were conducted with low-quality (i.e., low concentration) supplements. It was unclear from this research whether chondroitin sulfate added therapeutic value. Glucosamine had an adverse effect profile similar to placebo and appears to be safe, and although some concerns were raised that it might interfere with glucose metabolism in diabetic populations, this has not been evident in clinical care [76].

Other supplements have been studied to a lesser degree. α-lipoic acid (ALA), an antioxidant abundant in certain vegetables and widely available as an over-the-counter supplement, is thought to be neuroprotective. It is approved in Europe for painful diabetic neuropathy. Evidence from meta-analyses suggests that infusions of ALA 600 mg daily for 3 weeks are effective and safe. Its drawbacks are the need for administration by IV infusion, gastrointestinal adverse effects, and pruritus [77]. Similarly, there is some evidence from randomized trials in painful diabetic neuropathy for efficacy of acetyl-L-carnitine, a compound naturally produced by the body and available as an over-the-counter dietary supplement, in doses of 1000 mg three times daily by mouth [75].

Used judiciously, it may be that dietary supplements, such as other symptomatic treatments described above, offer benefits in selected painful conditions. This approach could be important as the HIV population ages and becomes vulnerable to osteoarthritis. HIV-infected persons also are at risk for neuropathic pain (e.g., from HIV or diabetes) and are likely to develop neoplastic illness, that if treated with chemotherapy or radiotherapy may induce residual neuropathic pain.

Summary

Chronic pain and its treatment is a vast discipline, which could only partly be addressed in this chapter. By its very definition, the problem is intractable and treatment-resistant. Patient expectations and beliefs can strongly influence the outcome of our interventions [8]. Clinicians also may have high expectations. The history of pain treatment has been likened to a succession of therapeutic fads, each one driven by a cycle of clinicians' high expectations, disappointment over the uncertain benefits of the preceding therapies, and failure to use evidence to attempt to distinguish useful from useless therapy [78]. The aim of this chapter was to describe an evidence base for treatment of some of the major pain syndromes, one that patients and their clinicians could use in discussions and decision-making.

References

1 Breitbart, W., McDonald, M.V., Rosenfeld, B. *et al.* (1996) Pain in ambulatory AIDS patients. I: Pain characteristics and medical correlates. *Pain*, **68**, 243–249.

2 Miaskowsk, C., Penko, J.M., Guzman, D., Mattson, J.E., Bangsberg, D.R. & Kushel, M.B. (2001) Occurrence and characteristics

of chronic pain in a community-based cohort of indigent adults living with HIV infection. *Journal of Pain*, **12**, 1004–1016.

3 Wiebe, L.A., Phillips, T.J., Li, J.M., Allen, J.A. & Shetty, K. (2011) Pain in HIV: an evolving epidemic. *Journal of Pain*, **12**, 619–624.

4 Turk, D.C. & Monarch, E.S. (2002) Biopsychosocial perspective on chronic pain. In: Turk, D.C. & Gatchel, R.J. (eds), *Psychological Approaches to Pain Management: A Practitioner's Handbook*, 2nd edn. Guilford, New York, pp. 3–29.

5 Moore, R.A., Derry, S., McQuay, H.J. *et al.* for the ACTINPAIN writing group of the IASP Special Interest Group (SIG) on Systematic Reviews in Pain Relief. (2010) Clinical Effectiveness: an approach to clinical trial design more relevant to clinical practice, acknowledging the importance of individual differences. *Pain*, **149**, 173–176.

6 Apkarian, A.V., Bushnell, M.C., Treede, R.D. & Zubieta, J.K. (2005) Human brain mechanisms of pain perception and regulation in health and disease. *European Journal of Pain*, **9**, 463–484.

7 Stahl, S.M. (2012) *Stahl's Essential Psychopharmacology: The Prescriber's Guide*, 4th edn. Cambridge University Press, Cambridge, UK.

8 Tan, G., Craine, M.H., Bair, M.J. *et al.* (2007) Efficacy of selected complementary and alternative medicine interventions for chronic pain. *Journal of Rehabilitation Research and Development*, **44**, 195–222.

9 Fairfield, K.M., Eisenberg, D.M., Davis, R.B., Libman, H. & Phillips, R.S. (1998) Patterns of use, expenditures, and efficacy of complementary and alternative therapies in HIV-infected patients. *Archives of Internal Medicine*, **158**, 2257–2263.

10 Farrar, J.T., Young, J.P., LaMoreaux, L., Werth, J.L. & Poole, R.M. (2001) Clinical importance of changes in chronic pain intensity measured on an 11-point numerical pain rating scale. *Pain*, **94**, 149–158.

11 Turk, D.C., Dworkin, R.H., Revicki, D. *et al.* (2008) Identifying important outcome domains for chronic pain clinical trials: an IMMPACT survey of people with pain. *Pain*, **137**, 276–285.

12 Kroenke, K., Krebs, E.E. & Bair, M.J. (2009) Pharmacotherapy of chronic pain: a synthesis

of recommendations from systematic reviews. *General Hospital Psychiatry*, **31**, 206–213.

13 Dworkin, R.H., O'Connor, A.B., Backonja, M. *et al.* (2007) Pharmacologic management of neuropathic pain: evidence-based recommendations. *Pain*, **132**, 237–251.

14 Sindrup, S.H., Bjerre, U., Deigaard, A., Brosen, K., Aes-Jorgensen, T. & Gram, L.F. (1992) The selective serotonin inhibitor citalopram relieves the symptoms of diabetic neuropathy. *Clinical Pharmacology and Therapeutics*, **52**, 547–552.

15 Sindrup, S.H., Gram, L.F., Broen, K., Esboj, O. & Morgensen, D.F. (1990) The selective serotonin reuptake inhibitor paroxetine is effective in the treatment of diabetic neuropathy symptoms. *Pain*, **42**, 135–144.

16 Vo, T., Rice, A.S. & Dworkin, R.H. (2009) Non-steroidal anti-inflammatory drugs for neuropathic pain: how do we explain continued widespread use? *Pain*, **143**, 169–171.

17 Derry, S., Wiffen, P.J., Moore, R.A. & Quinlan, J. (2014) Topical lidocaine for neuropathic pain in adults. *Cochrane Database of Systematic Reviews*, **7** Art. No.: CD010958. doi:10.1002/14651858.CD010958.pub2

18 Salerno, S.M., Browning, R. & Jackson, J.L. (2002) The effect of tricyclic antidepressant treatment on chronic back pain: a meta-analysis. *Archives of Internal Medicine*, **169**, 19–24.

19 Kuijpers, T., van Middelkoop, M., Rubinstein, S.M. *et al.* (2011) A systematic review on the effectiveness of pharmacological interventions for chronic non-specific low-back pain. *European Spine Journal*, **20**, 40–50.

20 Skljarevski, V., Desaiah, D., Liu-Seifert, H. *et al.* (2010) Efficacy and safety of duloxetine in patients with chronic low back pain. *Spine*, **35**, E578–585.

21 van Tulder, M.W., Scholten, R.J., Koes, B.W. & Deyo, R.A. (2000) Nonsteroidal anti-inflammatory drugs for low back pain: a systematic review within the framework of the Cochrane Collaboration Back Review Group. *Spine*, **25**, 2501–2513.

22 Morlion, B. (2011) Pharmacotherapy of low back pain: targeting nociceptive and neuropathic pain components. *Current Medical Research and Opinion*, **27**, 11–33.

23 Chung, J.W., Zeng, Y. & Wong, T.K. (2013) Drug therapy for the treatment of chronic non-specific low back pain: systematic review and meta-analysis. *Pain Physician*, **16**, E685–704.

24 Haroutiunian, S., Drennan, D.A. & Lipman, A.G. (2010) Topical NSAID therapy for musculoskeletal pain. *Pain Medicine*, **11**, 535–549.

25 Claw, D.J. (2014) Fibromyalgia: a clinical review. *JAMA*, **311**, 1547–1555.

26 Ford, A.C., Talley, N.J., Schoenfeld, P.S., Quigley, E.M.M. & Moayyedi, P. (2009) Efficacy of antidepressants and psychological therapies in irritable bowel syndrome: systematic review and meta-analysis. *Gut*, **58**, 367–378.

27 Richards, B.L., Whittle, S.L. & Buchbinder, R. (2011) Antidepressants for pain management in rheumatoid arthritis. *Cochrane Database of Systematic Reviews*, **11** Art. No.: CD008920. doi:10.1002/14651858.CD008920.pub2

28 Hochberg, M.C. (2002) New directions in symptomatic therapy for patients with osteoarthritis and rheumatoid arthritis. *Seminars in Arthritis and Rheumatism*, **32**, 4–14.

29 Hazlewood, G., van der Heijde, D.M. & Bombardier, C. (2012) Paracetamol for the management of pain in inflammatory arthritis: a systematic literature review. *Journal of Rheumatology. Supplement*, **90**, 11–16.

30 Dworkin, R.H., Peirce-Sandner, S., Turk, D.C. *et al.* (2011) Outcome measures in placebo-controlled trials of osteoarthritis: responsiveness to treatment effects in the REPORT database. *Osteoarthritis and Cartilage*, **19**, 483–492.

31 Klinge, S.A. & Sawyer, G.A. (2013) Effectiveness and safety of topical versus oral nonsteroidal anti-inflammatory drugs: a comprehensive review. *The Physician and Sportsmedicine*, **41**, 64–74.

32 Moore, R.A., Wiffen, P.J., Derry, S., Toelle, T. & Rice, A.S.C. (2014) Gabapentin for chronic neuropathic pain and fibromyalgia in adults. *Cochrane Database of Systematic Reviews*, **4** Art. No.: CD007938. doi:10.1002/14651858. CD007938.pub3

33 Wiffen, P.J., Derry, S., Moore, R.A. *et al.* (2013) Antiepileptic drugs for neuropathic pain and fibromyalgia – an overview of Cochrane reviews. *Cochrane Database of Systematic Reviews*, **11** Art. No.: CD010567. doi:10.1002/14651858.CD010567.pub2

34 Siler, A.C., Gardner, H., Yanit, K., Cushman, T. & McDonagh, M. (2011) Systematic review of the comparative effectiveness of antiepileptic drugs for fibromyalgia. *Journal of Pain*, **12**, 407–415.

35 Henschke, N., Ostelo, R.W.J.G., van Tulder, M.W. *et al.* (2010) Behavioural treatment for chronic low back pain. *Cochrane Database of Systematic Reviews*, **7** CD002014. doi:10.1002/14651858.CD002014.pub3

36 Shinohara, K., Honyashiki, M., Imai, H. *et al.* (2013) Behavioural therapies versus other psychological therapies for depression. *Cochrane Database of Systematic Reviews*, **10** Art. No.: CD008696. doi:10.1002/14651858.CD008696.pub2

37 Bernardy, K., Klose, P., Busch, A.J., Choy, E.H.S. & Häuser, W. (2013) Cognitive behavioural therapies for fibromyalgia. *Cochrane Database of Systematic Reviews*, **9** Art. No.: CD009796. doi:10.1002/14651858. CD009796.pub2

38 Kaplan, R.M. & Stone, A.A. (2013) Bringing the laboratory and clinic to the community: mobile technologies for health promotion and disease prevention. *Annual Review of Psychology*, **64**, 471–498.

39 van Tulder, M., Malmivaara, A., Esmail, R. & Koes, B. (2000) Exercise therapy for low back pain: a systematic review within the framework of the Cochrane Collaboration Back Review Group. *Spine*, **25**, 2784–2736.

40 Deyo, R.A., Walsh, N.E., Martin, D.C., Schoenfield, L.S. & Ramamurthy, S. (1990) A controlled trial of transcutaneous electrical stimulation (TENS) and exercise for chronic low back pain. *New England Journal of Medicine*, **322**, 1627–1634.

41 Melzack, R. & Wall, P.D. (1965) Pain mechanisms: a new theory. *Science*, **150**, 971–979.

42 Khadilkar, A., Odebiyi, D.O., Brosseau, L. & Wells, G.A. (2008) Transcutaneous electrical nerve stimulation (TENS) versus placebo for chronic low-back pain. *Cochrane Database of Systematic Reviews*, **4** Art. No.: CD003008. doi:10.1002/14651858.CD003008.pub3

43 Rutjes, A.W.S., Nüesch, E., Sterchi, R. *et al.* (2009) Transcutaneous electrostimulation for

osteoarthritis of the knee. *Cochrane Database of Systematic Reviews*, **4** Art. No.: CD002823. doi:10.1002/14651858.CD002823.pub2

44 Dhanani, N.M., Caruso, T.H. & Carinci, A.J. (2011) Complementary and alternative medicine for pain: an evidence-based review. *Current Pain and Headache Reports*, **15**, 39.

45 Mayer, D. & Rafii, A. (1977) Antagonism of acupuncture in man by the narcotic antagonist naltrexone. *Brain Research*, **121**, 368–372.

46 Furlan, A.D., van Tulder, M., Cherkin, D. *et al.* (2005) Acupuncture and dry-needling for low back pain: An updated systematic review within the framework of the Cochrane Collaboration. *Spine*, **30**, 944–963.

47 Haake, M., Muller, H.H., Schade-Brittinger, C. *et al.* (2007) German Acupuncture Trials (GERAC) for chronic low back pain: randomized, multicenter, blinded, parallel-group trial with 3 groups. *Archives of Internal Medicine*, **167**, 1892–1898.

48 Langhorst, J., Klose, P., Musial, F., Imich, D. & Hauser, W. (2010) Efficacy of acupuncture in fibromyalgia syndrome – a systematic review with a meta-analysis of controlled clinical trials. *Rheumatology*, **49**, 778–788.

49 Corbett, M.S., Rice, S.J.C., Madurasinghe, V. *et al.* (2013) Acupuncture and other physical treatments for the relief of pain due to osteoarthritis of the knee: network meta-analysis. *Osteoarthritis and Cartilage*, **21**, 1290–1298.

50 Urruela, A.M. & Suarez-Almazor, M.E. (2012) Acupuncture in the treatment of rheumatic diseases. *Current Rheumatology Reports*, **14**, 589–597.

51 Chen, W., Yang, G.-y., Liu, B., Manheimer, E. & Liu, J.-P. (2013) Manual acupuncture for treatment of diabetic peripheral neuropathy: a systematic review of randomized controlled trials. *PLoS One*, **8**, e73764.

52 Ernst, E. & Zhang, J. (2011) Cardiac tamponade caused by acupuncture: a review of the literature. *International Journal of Cardiology*, **149**, 287–289.

53 Grossman, P., Niemann, L., Schmidt, S. & Walach, H. (2004) Mindfulness-based stress reduction and health benefits. *A meta-analysis. Journal of Psychosomatic Research*, **57**, 35–43.

54 Bernardy, K., Fuber, N., Klose, P. & Hauser, W. (2011) Efficacy of hypnosis/guided imagery in fibromyalgia syndrome – a systematic review and meta-analysis of controlled trials. *BMC Musculoskeletal Disorders*, **12**, 133.

55 Elkins, G., Jensen, M.P. & Patterson, D.R. (2007) Hypnotherapy for the management of chronic pain. *International Journal of Experimental and Clinical Hypnosis*, **55**, 275–287.

56 Jensen, M. & Patterson, D.R. (2006) Hypnotic treatment of chronic pain. *Journal of Behavioral Medicine*, **29**, 95–124.

57 Webb, A.N., Kukuruzovic, R., Catto-Smith, A.G. & Sawyer, S.M. (2007) Hypnotherapy for treatment of irritable bowel syndrome. *Cochrane Database of Systematic Reviews*, **4** Art. No.: CD005110. doi:10.1002/14651858.cd005110.Pub2

58 Shen Y-H, A. & Nahas, R. (2009) Complementary and alternative medicine for treatment of irritable bowel syndrome. *Canadian Family Physician*, **55**, 143–148.

59 Cramer, H., Lauche, R., Haller, H. & Dobos, G. (2013) A systematic review and meta-analysis of yoga for low back pain. *Clinical Journal of Pain*, **29**, 450–460.

60 Carson, J.W., Carson, K.M., Jones, K.D., Bennett, R.M., Wright, C.L. & Mist, S.D. (2010) A pilot randomized controlled trial of the yoga of awareness program in the management of fibromyalgia. *Pain*, **151**, 530–539.

61 Kuttner, L., Chambers, C.T., Hardial, J., Israeel, D.M., Jacobson, K. & Evans, K. (2006) A randomized trial of yoga for adolescents with irritable bowel syndromes. *Pain Research and Management*, **11**, 217–223.

62 Cramer, H., Lauche, R., Langhorst, J. & Dobos, G. (2013) Yoga for rheumatic diseases: a systematic review. *Rheumatology (Oxford)*, **52**, 2025–2030.

63 Bussing, A., Osterman, T., Ludke, R. & Michaelsen, A. (2012) Effects of Yoga interventions on pain and pain-associated disability: a meta-analysis. *Journal of Pain*, **13**, 1–9.

64 Saad, M. & De Medeiros, R. (2013) Complementary therapies for fibromyalgia syndrome – a rational approach. *Current Pain and Headache Reports*, **17**, 354–361.

65 Flor, H. & Birbaumer, N. (1993) Comparison of the efficacy of electromyographic biofeedback, cognitive-behavioral therapy, and conservative medical interventions in the

treatment of chronic musculoskeletal pain. *Journal of Consulting and Clinical Psychology*, **61**, 653–658.

66 Glombiewski, J.A., Bernardy, K. & Hauser, W. (2013) Efficacy of EMG-and EEG-biofeedback in fibromyalgia syndrome: a meta-analysis and a systematic review of randomized clinical trials. *Evidence-based Complementary and Alternative Medicine*, **1–11** 962741.

67 Arena, J.G. & Blanchard, E.B. (2013) Biofeedback training for chronic pain disorders: a primer. In: Turk, D.C. & Gatchel, R.J. (eds), *Psychological Approaches to Chronic Pain Management: A Practitioner's Handbook*, 2nd edn. Guilford Press, New York, NY, pp. 138–158.

68 Rubinstein, S.M., van Middelkoop, M., Assendelft, W.J.J., de Boer, M.R. & van Tulder, M.W. (2011) Spinal manipulative therapy for chronic low-back pain. *Cochrane Database of Systematic Reviews*, **2** Art. No.: CD008112. doi:10.1002/14651858.CD008112.pub2

69 Lawrence, D.J., Meeker, W., Branson, R. *et al.* (2008) Chiropractic management of low back pain and low back-related leg complaints. A literature synthesis. *Journal of Manipulative and Physiological Therapeutics*, **31**, 659–674.

70 Gross, A., Miller, J., D'Sylva, J. *et al.* (2010) Manipulation or mobilisation for neck pain. *Cochrane Database of Systematic Reviews*, **1** Art. No.: CD004249. doi:10.1002/14651858.CD004249.pub3

71 Cherkin, D.C., Sherman, K.J., Deyo, R.A. & Shekelle, P.G. (2003) A review of the evidence for the effectiveness, safety, and cost of acupuncture, massage therapy, and spinal manipulation for back pain. *Annals of Internal Medicine*, **138**, 898–906.

72 Furlan, A.D., Imamura, M., Dryden, T. & Irvin, E. (2008) Massage for low back pain. *Cochrane Database of Systematic Reviews*, **4** Art. No.: CD001929. doi:10.1002/14651858.CD001929.pub2.

73 Terry, R., Perry, R. & Ernst, E. (2012) An overview of systematic reviews of complementary and alternative medicine for fibromyalgia. *Clinical Rheumatology*, **31**, 55–66.

74 Straube S, Derry S, Moore RA, McQuay HJ. Vitamin D for the treatment of chronic painful conditions in adults. *Cochrane Database of Systematic Reviews* 2010; **1**: Art. No.: CD007771. DOI: 10.1002/14651858.CD007771.pub2.

75 Lee, F.H. & Raja, S.N. (2011) Complementary and alternative medicine in chronic pain. *Pain*, **152**, 28–30.

76 Towheed, T., Maxwell, L., Anastassiades, T.P. *et al.* (2005) Glucosamine therapy for treating osteoarthritis. *Cochrane Database of Systematic Reviews*, **2** Art. No.: CD002946. doi:10.1002/14651858.CD002946.pub2

77 Zeigler, D., Nowak, H., Kempler, P., Vargha, P. & Low, P.A. (2004) Treatment of symptomatic diabetic polyneuropathy with the antioxidant alpha-lipoic acid: a meta-analysis. *Diabetic Medicine*, **21**, 114–121.

78 Deyo, R.A. (1983) Conservative therapy for low back pain: distinguishing useful from useless therapy. *Journal of the American Medical Association*, **250**, 1057–1062.

CHAPTER 11

Potential benefits and harms of prescription opioids in HIV

William C. Becker and E. Jennifer Edelman

Department of Internal Medicine, Yale University School of Medicine, New Haven, CT, USA

Epidemiology of opioid prescribing to HIV-infected patients

While opioids have become a mainstay of pain management for HIV-infected patients and are commonly prescribed, only a limited number of studies have examined the epidemiology of opioid prescribing specifically to HIV-infected patients [1–7]. Depending on the characteristics of the population studied, the prevalence of opioid receipt has ranged from 8% to 57% [1–3,5,6]. For example, one study of HIV-infected patients receiving care through the Veterans Affairs Healthcare System found that in a 1-year time span, approximately one third of patients received one or more opioid prescriptions. Further, among these patients, 31% received them on a long-term basis, defined as at least 90 consecutive days allowing for a 30-day gap between fill/refill [2]. In addition to having a pain-associated condition, patients most likely to receive long-term opioids included older, white patients, those with hepatitis C coinfection and those receiving concomitant antiretroviral therapy (ART) treatment [2]. Other studies have found that HIV-infected patients who were female, had greater comorbidities, and had a substance use history, including prior injection drug use, and anxiolytic use were also more likely to receive long-term opioids [3–5,7]. Among patients receiving long-term opioids, the mean daily morphine equivalent dose ranged from approximately 40 mg to

90 mg with short-acting formulations being the most commonly prescribed [2,3,7]. Opioid prescribing to HIV-infected patients in some studies remained stable from the late 1990s to mid-late 2000s [3,5], while it increased in others [8]. In comparison, opioid prescribing in the general population has continued to rise dramatically [3,9].

Indications for opioids

Guideline-recommended indications for opioids

While there is a strong consensus supporting the use of opioids for moderate-to-severe acute and cancer-related pain, use of opioids in chronic noncancer pain remains controversial [10,11]. For the general population, the most widely cited and perhaps the most widely used guidelines came from the American Pain Society-American Academy of Pain Medicine (APS-AAPM), published in 2009 [12]. These guidelines did not identify specific noncancer conditions as appropriate targets for opioids; rather, they more generally recommended that clinicians may consider a trial of opioid therapy as an option if chronic noncancer pain is moderate or severe, pain is having an adverse impact on function or quality of life, and the potential therapeutic benefits are likely to outweigh potential harms. This was considered a strong recommendation based on low-quality evidence. The "therapeutic trial" concept also incorporated close follow-up and

Chronic Pain and HIV: A Practical Approach, First Edition.
Edited by Jessica S. Merlin, Peter A. Selwyn, Glenn J. Treisman and Angela G. Giovanniello.
© 2016 John Wiley & Sons, Ltd. Published 2016 by John Wiley & Sons, Ltd.

discontinuation of therapy if benefit was lacking or harm apparent.

As data on safety and efficacy continue to evolve, expert groups have advised more selective use of opioids in noncancer pain. "Think twice before prescribing long-term opioids for axial low back pain, headache and fibromyalgia" was one of the principles emerging from the National Summit on Opioid Safety in 2012 [13]. Nonetheless, the most recent Federation of State Medical Boards model policy for the use of opioid analgesics stated, "The medical record should document the presence of one or more recognized medical indications for prescribing an opioid analgesic [14]," but did not further enumerate what those indications are.

While consensus guidelines specific to the management of chronic pain with opioids in HIV-infected patients are lacking, one review on the subject highlighted that given the potential for medication interactions and a variety of other potential complicating factors, "The (HIV-infected patient with chronic pain) should have an adequate trial of nonopioid pain relievers and other treatment modalities before opioids are considered [15]." Similarly, a review on pain treatment among HIV-infected patients with histories of substance use disorders emphasized the need to use adequate doses of nonopioid pharmacologic treatments and incorporation of nonpharmacologic modalities before considering a trial of opioids [16].

Mechanisms of opioid action and clinical pharmacology

Opioid analgesics act through a family of G-protein coupled receptors ubiquitous throughout the central and peripheral nervous system [17]. Most of the clinically important effects of opioids – for example, analgesia, sedation, and respiratory depression – are mediated primarily through activity at the μ-receptor subtype [18]. As such, opioids are classified by their effect on the μ-receptor: full μ agonists, such as morphine and oxycodone, cause maximal biologic response; partial agonists, such as buprenorphine, have a submaximal effect; and antagonists, such as naloxone, occupy the receptor but produce no response. Affinity for the μ-receptor can be thought of as the strength of an opioid's bond with the receptor. Antagonists tend to have greater affinity than partial agonists, which tend to have a greater affinity than full agonists. This phenomenon can be observed clinically in response to naloxone in a patient who has overdosed on a full agonist (i.e., precipitated opioid withdrawal). Potency can be thought of as the strength of a given biologic response; relative analgesic potency of full agonist opioids has been studied and published as equianalgesic tables [19].

Other clinically important pharmacologic considerations of opioids include their onset of action and duration of action. Both of these factors are determined primarily by formulation: intravenous opioids have relatively rapid onset and short duration of action, while oral compounds have a slower onset and longer duration of action. Besides formulation, lipophilicity of an opioid affects how quickly it crosses the blood–brain barrier, which mediates analgesia but also neurocognitive effects [17]. In addition, some opioids have active metabolites, leading to a longer duration of action, especially in patients with impaired renal or hepatic function [20].

Activation of μ-receptors inhibits release of inflammatory mediators, transmission of pain signals along peripheral C-fibers and postsynaptic tracts and also activates descending pain-inhibitory tracts [21]. These diverse analgesic properties make opioids uniquely effective in the treatment of acute pain, where inflammatory pain predominates. However, the transition from acute to chronic pain is marked by neuronal plasticity resulting in central sensitization [22], with active inflammation generally playing a lesser role. This may in part explain the diminished efficacy of opioids for chronic pain, discussed in the upcoming sections.

Potential benefit of opioids

Despite increasing rates of opioid prescribing, evidence supporting the use of opioids for noncancer pain is modest. Two systematic reviews of opioids for chronic back pain found few trials, all of relatively short duration, with small effect sizes favoring opioids over placebo but not consistently over nonsteroidal anti-inflammatory drugs (NSAIDs) [23,24]. For osteoarthritis of the knee or hip, a Cochrane review found a pooled standardized mean difference (SMD) favoring opioids in terms of improved pain control (SMD −0.36, 95% CI −0.47 to −0.26) and function (SMD −0.33, 95% CI −0.45 to −0.21) in 10 studies with a median follow-up of 4 weeks. However, the authors concluded that the comparatively high rates of adverse events in the opioid treatment groups precluded them from recommending opioids as a routine treatment [25]. Another Cochrane review examined the evidence for long-term opioid use including not only randomized controlled trials (RCTs) but also nonrandomized trials and pre–post studies, in a variety of pain conditions examining outcomes at 6 months or longer and concluded, "Despite the identification of 26 treatment groups with nearly 4800 participants, the evidence regarding the effectiveness of long-term opioid therapy in chronic noncancer pain was too sparse to draw firm conclusions [26]." They found some benefit of opioids in study completers, but completers were a small proportion of the overall sample [26]. Importantly, no long-term studies included functional outcomes, which expert consensus groups, such as the Initiative on Methods, Measurement, and Pain Assessment in Clinical Trials (IMMPACT), have determined should be one of the primary outcomes if not the primary outcome of pain clinical trials [27].

There is a paucity of literature examining the long-term effectiveness of opioids on pain among HIV-infected patients in the current treatment era. One study followed 127 HIV-infected patients with chronic pain, most commonly caused by neuropathy (40%), back pain (32%), and arthritis/arthralgias/avascular necrosis (16%), for a median of 5.2 years. In multivariable analysis, opioid analgesics were negatively associated with decreasing pain (adjusted odds ratio 0.24 [95% CI 0.09, 0.62]). The authors suggested several potential explanations for these findings, including selection bias; overreporting of pain in order to be prescribed opioids; opioid-induced hyperalgesia (OIH)-(i.e., increased pain sensitivity); and lack

of long-term opioid efficacy. Of note, they concluded that studies of long-term pain management ought to include longer follow-up periods and that nonpharmacological approaches to pain management should be prioritized [28]. In addition, future studies evaluating the long-term effect of prescription opioids for various pain conditions are warranted.

Potential harms of opioids

There has been increasing attention to the potential harms associated with opioids in recent years [12,29], leading to a number of helpful resources for providers [12,30].

Unintentional overdose and death
Of greatest concern with regard to opioid risk is the dramatic increase of unintentional overdose and death in recent years [31–34]. Studies of the general population indicate that the highest rates of overdose, including fatal overdose, occur among patients with substance use disorders and mental illness. Moreover, overdose risk increases incrementally with increasing opioid dose [32–34]. For instance, one study found that patients with chronic noncancer pain receiving 100 mg morphine equivalents or more per day had an 8.9-fold increased risk of overdose compared to those patients prescribed less than 20 mg morphine equivalents per day [32]. While data specifically examining the risk of prescription opioid–related overdose in HIV-infected patients are lacking, a recent systematic review found that among individuals who use drugs, those with HIV infection had a 74% increased risk of overdose than those without HIV [35], suggesting that they may be more susceptible to prescription opioid–induced overdose.

Injury
Due to their effects on the central nervous system, including dizziness and sedation [30], questions have been raised regarding the relationship between opioids and risk of injury. Recent evidence suggests that drivers prescribed opioids may be more likely to experience road trauma, with those receiving a daily morphine equivalent dose between 100 and

199 mg experiencing a 42% increased odds of road trauma compared to those receiving 1–19 mg [36]. While other factors may have contributed to the findings, prescription opioids have similarly been found to be associated with other injuries, including falls and fractures, in a dose-dependent manner in older populations [37–40]. Notably, the effects of opioids on bone health are likely multifactorial in etiology, relating to their effects on the endocrine system as well as direct effects on bone metabolism [41].

While few studies have examined these questions in HIV-infected populations, one study of HIV-infected patients aged 45–65 years found that opioids were associated with an increased odds of falling (AOR 3.4 [95% CI 1.4, 8.1]) [42]. As HIV-infected patients may be particularly vulnerable to falls and fractures [43] due to their increased prevalence of bone disease [44], extra precautions to minimize injury should be taken among HIV-infected patients prescribed opioids.

Medical complications

Recent data suggest that opioids may be associated with an increased risk for a number of comorbidities, many of which occur more commonly in HIV-infected patients [45–47].

Cardiovascular disease: An analysis of Medicare beneficiaries found that individuals initiating opioids had an increased relative risk of a cardiovascular event (HR 1.77 [95% CI 1.39, 2.24]) compared to those initiating nonselective NSAIDS [48]. Additional studies have similarly documented an association between opioids and myocardial infarction [49,50], but further investigation in this area is needed. This extends the potential cardiovascular complications of opioids beyond the well-recognized arrhythmogenic potential of methadone [51,52].

Respiratory changes: In addition to respiratory depression, opioids may cause changes in breathing patterns during sleep with increases in episodes of central sleep apnea, ataxic breathing, and hypoxemia; however, these studies have generally been small with varied findings based on opioid type [53–56]. Future investigations to determine the potential mechanisms and clinical relevance of these findings in the

general population and HIV-infected patients are indicated.

Endocrine dysfunction: Data consistently indicate that opioids impact endocrine function [41,57]. Opioids directly impact the hypothalamic–pituitary–gonadal axis at multiple levels, resulting in decreased levels of sex hormones [41]. As a result, patients may experience a variety of symptoms, including decreased sexual function and libido, amenorrhea, infertility, musculoskeletal complaints and mood disorders, fatigue and potentially increased pain [41]. Opioids also appear to modulate the hypothalamic–pituitary–adrenal axis, impacting multiple hormones, such as cortisol and dehydroepiandrosterone (DHEA) [41]. HIV itself is frequently associated with endocrine dysfunction, including hypogonadism [58,59], and the long-term benefits and risks of the associated treatments, such as testosterone replacement therapy, remain to be determined. Providers should be mindful of these potential risks with opioids.

Bowel dysfunction: Gastrointestinal complaints are the most commonly experienced type of adverse effects associated with opioids and often persist with ongoing opioid exposure [12]. Opioid-induced bowel dysfunction, most commonly manifesting as constipation [60], may also present as gastroesophageal reflux disease, nausea, vomiting, or chronic abdominal pain [61]. The need to adopt preventive strategies [62] to minimize the risk of opioid-induced bowel dysfunction for an HIV-infected patient will depend on the presence of antiretroviral or HIV disease-related gastrointestinal complaints, which often include diarrhea [63].

Hyperalgesia: OIH may lead to a paradoxical increase in pain severity and should be differentiated from opioid tolerance given the different approaches to treatment [64]. The presence of OIH should be considered when there has been an observed decrease in the effectiveness of opioid therapy without disease progression, especially if pain complaints change to include unexplained pain, diffuse allodynia (i.e., pain from a typically nonpainful stimulus) that is not explained by the original condition, or there is increasing pain with opioid dose escalation. Treatment may include a combination of decreasing opioids with possible taper or consideration of switch to nonopioid agents targeting central sensitization (e.g., gabapentinoids, serotonin–norepinephrine reuptake inhibitors, or *N*-methyl-d-aspartate receptor modulators) [65].

Nonmedical use and opioid use disorders: Given the increased prevalence of substance use disorders among HIV-infected patients, nonmedical use of opioids and the development of opioid use disorders may be of particular concern and has been examined in several recent studies [66–68] (See Chapter 9 for a detailed discussion of this topic).

HIV-specific concerns

Antiretroviral nonadherence: As optimizing adherence to ART is key to its success and substance use is known to impact medication adherence, researchers have hypothesized that the use of prescription opioids may impact antiretroviral adherence. One analysis of 258 HIV-infected patients from the Research in Access to Care in the Homeless (REACH) cohort did not find an association between receipt of prescription opioids and incomplete ART adherence (defined as <90%) (AOR 1.40 [95% CI 0.99, 1.97]), though opioid analgesic misuse was associated with incomplete ART adherence (AOR 1.47 [95% CI 1.06, 2.03]) [69].

Immunosuppression and HIV progression: Of particular concern with HIV-infected patients are preclinical and clinical data indicating that opioids impact the immune system, mediated directly by opioid receptors on immune cells and indirectly through the hypothalamic–pituitary axis [70–72]. Observational data demonstrate that people who inject opioids (e.g., heroin) are at an increased risk of infectious complications consistent with dysfunction of various aspects of the immune system [73]. One recent study of older adults found that prescription opioids were associated with an increased risk of pneumonia [74].

Similarly, preclinical data reveal that opioids influence HIV progression as they have been found to promote growth of HIV in cell cultures; [75] induce lymphocyte apoptosis; and increase expression of HIV-entry coreceptors CCR5 and CXCR [72,76,77]. As results from animal [78] and human studies [79] are conflicting and limited, important questions regarding the clinical relevance of these effects are currently unanswered.

Drug–drug interactions

Since most opioids (e.g., codeine, hydrocodone, oxycodone, methadone, tramadol, and fentanyl) undergo Phase I metabolism, typically involving oxidation by the cytochrome (CYP) P450 enzymes, drug–drug interactions occur with other medications that are substrates, inducers, or inhibitors of these enzymes [80]. For instance, concomitant use of a CYP450 3A4 inhibitor, such as particular antibiotics (e.g., macrolides) or antiretroviral agents, may lead to increased opioid levels. Select protease inhibitors (e.g., boosted lopinavir) and nonnucleoside reverse transcriptase inhibitors (e.g., efavirenz and nevirapine) may precipitate opioid withdrawal by decreasing methadone levels [81]. In contrast, boosted lopinavir has been shown to increase oxycodone levels, possibly requiring dose adjustment [81].

Other opioids (i.e., morphine, oxymorphone, tapentadol, and hydromorphone) undergo Phase II metabolism by uridine diphosphate glucuronosyltransferase, which does not typically lead to clinically significant drug–drug reactions [80]. The majority of opioids are ultimately renally eliminated. Consideration of a patient's underlying hepatic and renal function, as well as the potential for drug–drug interactions or additive side effects (e.g., sedation by combining benzodiazepines and opioids; increased QTc prolongation by combining macrolides or certain antiretroviral agents [e.g., rilpivirine] and methadone) are necessary for optimizing safe opioid prescribing [80,81].

Considerations in prescribing

Meta-analyses reveal modest or equivocal efficacy of opioids and a myriad of adverse effects in the use of chronic noncancer pain. However, carefully monitored opioid therapy at relatively low doses can benefit some patients who can demonstrate safe use as part of a multimodal pain treatment plan. Multimodal treatment – incorporating physical activity (e.g., physical therapy, structured exercise, and yoga), behavioral treatments (e.g., relaxation training, biofeedback, and cognitive behavioral therapy), and rational pharmacotherapy in the setting of promoting patient self-care, self-efficacy, and healthy behavior – is the standard of pain management called for by the Institute of Medicine [82].

If initiating a "therapeutic trial," clinicians must be mindful of the potency, onset of action, and half-life of the medications they prescribe with respect to each individual patient's potential for an adverse event related to opioids. As discussed above, increasingly recognized patient factors, including comorbid conditions (e.g., advanced age [48], sleep-disordered breathing [83], and substance use disorders) and concomitant prescriptions (e.g., benzodiazepines, anticonvulsants, muscle relaxants, and the presence of polypharmacy [84]) should also impact clinicians' decisions on choice of formulation, starting dose, speed of titration, and ceiling dose. Given the increased risk for adverse events in patients with such comorbid factors, it may be prudent to start with lower doses of shorter acting medications until patients can demonstrate safe use. For patients with around-the-clock pain, transition to a long-acting formulation, with concomitant reduction in short-acting medication, is reasonable, although benefit of long-acting formulations compared to short-acting ones has not been consistently demonstrated [85]. As with any high-risk medication, clear communication about goals and expectations of treatment is essential. As discussed in Chapter 12, these are some of the core components of recommended opioid treatment agreements. In addition, the use of opioids should be used with caution in patients with a history of addiction (see Chapter 9) [86].

Opioid dosing thresholds and referral: Some state legislatures have proposed or enacted legislation indicating the maximum daily opioid doses above which referral to a pain specialist is mandated [87]. Professional societies, however, have not made this part of treatment guidelines, perhaps due to the lack of empiric data supporting specific dosage cutoffs and the relative scarcity of pain specialists who prescribe medications.

Considering opioid type and formulation: Prescribers should be aware of the unique pharmacologic properties of methadone, increasingly prescribed for pain. As methadone is responsible for a disproportionate amount of adverse events, including overdose and death, prescribers should take special caution when selecting this opioid for pain. Methadone is a highly lipophilic molecule with a long and variable half-life, predisposing it to accumulation within fat stores [17]. Subsequently, patients face increased risks for toxic effects long after the analgesic effect has worn off. Rapid dose escalation in an attempt to achieve adequate analgesia may result in high risk of inadvertent overdose. In addition, methadone can prolong the QT interval and periodic electrocardiogram monitoring is recommended [88]. Given the increased presence of liver dysfunction in HIV-infected patients, prescribers should be mindful when choosing opioids coformulated with other analgesics, particularly acetaminophen, to minimize the potential for unintentional hepatotoxicity [89]. The US Food and Drug Administration (FDA) has now implemented a 325 mg limit for acetaminophen in pills coformulated with opioids [90].

In summary, opioids represent an important option for pain treatment for some HIV-infected patients. Before initiating a trial of opioid medications, careful consideration of the patient's underlying comorbidities, medications and potential for adverse events, and treatment goals should be reviewed. Measures to optimize safe prescribing, including the use of treatment agreements, urine toxicology testing, and surveillance through prescription drug monitoring program, should be routinely adopted (see Chapter 12).

References

1 Miaskowski, C., Penko, J.M., Guzman, D., Mattson, J.E., Bangsberg, D.R. & Kushel, M.B. (2011) Occurrence and characteristics of chronic pain in a community-based cohort of indigent adults living with HIV infection. *Journal of Pain*, **12** (9), 1004–1016.
2 Edelman, E.J., Gordon, K., Becker, W.C. *et al.* (2013) Receipt of opioid analgesics by

HIV-infected and uninfected patients. *Journal of General Internal Medicine*, **28** (1), 82–90.

3 Silverberg, M.J., Ray, G.T., Saunders, K. *et al.* (2012) Prescription long-term opioid use in HIV-infected patients. *Clinical Journal of Pain*, **28** (1), 39–46.

4 Koeppe, J., Armon, C., Lyda, K., Nielsen, C. & Johnson, S. (2010) Ongoing pain despite aggressive opioid pain management among persons with HIV. *Clinical Journal of Pain*, **26** (3), 190–198.

5 Koeppe, J., Lichtenstein, K., Armon, C. *et al.* (2011) Factors associated with initiation of prolonged analgesic use among patients in the HIV Outpatient Study (HOPS). *Clinical Journal of Pain*, **27** (8), 699–706.

6 Ruiz, M., Armstrong, M., Ogboukiri, T. & Anwar, D. (2014) Patterns of pain medication use during last months of life in HIV-infected populations: the experience of an academic outpatient clinic. *The American Journal of Hospice & Palliative Care*, **31** (8), 793–796.

7 Onen, N.F., Barrette, E.P., Shacham, E., Taniguchi, T., Donovan, M. & Overton, E.T. (2012) A review of opioid prescribing practices and associations with repeat opioid prescriptions in a contemporary outpatient HIV clinic. *Pain Practice*, **12** (6), 440–448.

8 Becker, W.C., Gordon, K., Edelman, E.J. *et al.* (2015) Trends in any and high-dose opioid analgesic receipt among aging patients with and without HIV. *AIDS and Behavior*.[Epub ahead of print]

9 Kenan, K., Mack, K. & Paulozzi, L. (2012) Trends in prescriptions for oxycodone and other commonly used opioids in the United States, 2000–2010. *Open Medicine*, **6** (2), e41–47.

10 Alexander, G.C., Kruszewski, S.P. & Webster, D.W. (2012) Rethinking opioid prescribing to protect patient safety and public health rethinking opioid prescribing. *JAMA*, **308** (18), 1865–1866.

11 Von Korff, M., Kolodny, A., Deyo, R.A. & Chou, R. (2011) Long-term opioid therapy reconsidered. *Annals of Internal Medicine*, **155** (5), 325–328.

12 Chou, R., Fanciullo, G.J., Fine, P.G. *et al.* (2009) Clinical guidelines for the use of chronic opioid therapy in chronic noncancer pain. *Journal of Pain*, **10** (2), 113–130.

13 Gerlach L. (2012) *National summit on opioid safety: a "hair-on-fire" situation* [WWW document]. URL http://nwrpca.org/health-center-news/267-national-summit-on-opioid-safety-a-hair-on-fire-situation.html [accessed on 26 January 2014].

14 Federation of State Medical Boards. (2013) *Model policy on the use of opioid analgesics in the treatment of chronic pain* [WWW document]. URL http://www.fsmb.org/pdf/pain_policy_july2013.pdf [accessed on 8 April 2014].

15 Krashin, D.L., Merrill, J.O. & Trescot, A.M. (2012) Opioids in the management of HIV-related pain. *Pain Physician*, **15** (3 Suppl), ES157–168.

16 Basu, S., Bruce, R.D., Barry, D.T. & Altice, F.L. (2007) Pharmacological pain control for human immunodeficiency virus-infected adults with a history of drug dependence. *Journal of Substance Abuse Treatment*, **32** (4), 399–409.

17 Inturrisi, C.E. (2002) Clinical pharmacology of opioids for pain. *Clinical Journal of Pain*, **18** (4 Suppl), S3–13.

18 Trescot, A.M., Datta, S., Lee, M. & Hansen, H. (2008) Opioid pharmacology. *Pain Physician*, **11** (2 Suppl), S133.

19 Shaheen, P.E., Walsh, D., Lasheen, W., Davis, M.P. & Lagman, R.L. (2009) Opioid equianalgesic tables: are they all equally dangerous? *Journal of Pain and Symptom Management*, **38** (3), 409–417.

20 Lötsch, J. (2005) Opioid metabolites. *Journal of Pain and Symptom Management*, **29** (5), 10–24.

21 Pasternak, G.W. (1993) Pharmacological mechanisms of opioid analgesics. *Clinical Neuropharmacology*, **16** (1), 1–18.

22 Woolf, C.J. & Salter, M.W. (2000) Neuronal plasticity: increasing the gain in pain. *Science*, **288** (5472), 1765–1768.

23 Deshpande, A., Furlan, A., Mailis-Gagnon, A., Atlas, S. & Turk, D. (2007) Opioids for chronic low-back pain. *Cochrane Database of Systematic Reviews*, **18** (3).CD004959

24 Martell, B.A., O'Connor, P.G., Kerns, R.D. *et al.* (2007) Systematic review: opioid treatment for chronic back pain: prevalence, efficacy, and association with addiction. *Annals of Internal Medicine*, **146** (2), 116–127.

25 Nuesch, E., Rutjes, A.W., Husni, E., Welch, V. & Juni, P. (2009) Oral or transdermal opioids

for osteoarthritis of the knee or hip. *Cochrane Database of Systematic Reviews*, **7** (4).CD003115

26 Noble, M., Treadwell, J.R., Tregear, S.J. *et al.* (2010) Long-term opioid management for chronic noncancer pain. *Cochrane Database of Systematic Reviews*, **20** (1).CD006605

27 Dworkin, R.H., Turk, D.C., Farrar, J.T. *et al.* (2005) Core outcome measures for chronic pain clinical trials: IMMPACT recommendations. *Pain*, **113** (1–2), 9–19.

28 Koeppe, J., Lyda, K., Johnson, S. & Armon, C. (2012) Variables associated with decreasing pain among persons living with human immunodeficiency virus: a longitudinal follow-up study. *Clinical Journal of Pain*, **28** (1), 32–38.

29 Chapman, C.R., Lipschitz, D.L., Angst, M.S. *et al.* (2010) Opioid pharmacotherapy for chronic non-cancer pain in the United States: a research guideline for developing an evidence-base. *The Journal of Pain*, **11** (9), 807–829.

30 Baldini, A., Von Korff, M. & Lin, E.H. (2012) A review of potential adverse effects of long-term opioid therapy: a practitioner's guide. *Primary Care Companion for CNS Disorders*, **14** (3).PCC. 11m01326

31 Hall, A.J., Logan, J.E., Toblin, R.L. *et al.* (2008) Patterns of abuse among unintentional pharmaceutical overdose fatalities. *JAMA*, **300** (22), 2613–2620.

32 Dunn, K.M., Saunders, K.W., Rutter, C.M. *et al.* (2010) Opioid prescriptions for chronic pain and overdose: a cohort study. *Annals of Internal Medicine*, **152** (2), 85–92.

33 Bohnert, A.S., Valenstein, M., Bair, M.J. *et al.* (2011) Association between opioid prescribing patterns and opioid overdose-related deaths. *JAMA*, **305** (13), 1315–1321.

34 Gomes, T., Mamdani, M.M., Dhalla, I.A., Paterson, J.M. & Juurlink, D.N. (2011) Opioid dose and drug-related mortality in patients with nonmalignant pain. *Archives of Internal Medicine*, **171** (7), 686–691.

35 Green, T.C., McGowan, S.K., Yokell, M.A., Pouget, E.R. & Rich, J.D. (2012) HIV infection and risk of overdose: a systematic review and meta-analysis. *AIDS*, **26** (4), 403–417.

36 Gomes, T., Redelmeier, D.A., Juurlink, D.N., Dhalla, I.A., Camacho, X. & Mamdani, M.M. (2013) Opioid dose and risk of road trauma in Canada: a population-based study. *JAMA Internal Medicine*, **173** (3), 196–201.

37 O'Neil, C.K., Hanlon, J.T. & Marcum, Z.A. (2012) Adverse effects of analgesics commonly used by older adults with osteoarthritis: focus on non-opioid and opioid analgesics. *The American Journal of Geriatric Pharmacotherapy*, **10** (6), 331–342.

38 Miller, M., Sturmer, T., Azrael, D., Levin, R. & Solomon, D.H. (2011) Opioid analgesics and the risk of fractures in older adults with arthritis. *Journal of American Geriatrics Society*, **59** (3), 430–438.

39 Saunders, K.W., Dunn, K.M., Merrill, J.O. *et al.* (2010) Relationship of opioid use and dosage levels to fractures in older chronic pain patients. *Journal of General Internal Medicine*, **25** (4), 310–315.

40 Li, L., Setoguchi, S., Cabral, H. & Jick, S. (2013) Opioid use for noncancer pain and risk of fracture in adults: a nested case–control study using the general practice research database. *American Journal of Epidemiology*, **178** (4), 559–569.

41 Brennan, M.J. (2013) The effect of opioid therapy on endocrine function. *American Journal of Medicine*, **126** (3 Suppl 1), S12–18.

42 Erlandson, K.M., Allshouse, A.A., Jankowski, C.M. *et al.* (2012) Risk factors for falls in HIV-infected persons. *Journal of Acquired Immune Deficiency Syndromes*, **61** (4), 484–489.

43 Womack, J.A., Goulet, J.L., Gibert, C. *et al.* (2011) Increased risk of fragility fractures among HIV infected compared to uninfected male veterans. *PLoS One*, **6** (2).e17217

44 Cotter, A.G. & Mallon, P.W. (2011) HIV infection and bone disease: implications for an aging population. *Sexual Health*, **8** (4), 493–501.

45 Triant, V.A. (2012) HIV infection and coronary heart disease: an intersection of epidemics. *Journal of Infectious Diseases*, **205** (Suppl 3), S355–361.

46 Gingo, M.R., Morris, A. & Crothers, K. (2013) Human immunodeficiency virus-associated obstructive lung diseases. *Clinics in Chest Medicine*, **34** (2), 273–282.

47 Wren, A. (2013) How best to approach endocrine evaluation in patients with HIV in the era of combined antiretroviral therapy? *Clinical Endocrinology*, **79** (3), 310–313.

48 Solomon, D.H., Rassen, J.A., Glynn, R.J., Lee, J., Levin, R. & Schneeweiss, S. (2010) The comparative safety of analgesics in older adults with arthritis. *Archives of Internal Medicine*, **170** (22), 1968–1976.

49 Li, L., Setoguchi, S., Cabral, H. & Jick, S. (2013) Opioid use for noncancer pain and risk of myocardial infarction amongst adults. *Journal of Internal Medicine*, **273** (5), 511–526.

50 Carman, W.J., Su, S., Cook, S.F., Wurzelmann, J.I. & McAfee, A. (2011) Coronary heart disease outcomes among chronic opioid and cyclooxygenase-2 users compared with a general population cohort. *Pharmacoepidemiology and Drug Safety*, **20** (7), 754–762.

51 Krantz, M.J., Martin, J., Stimmel, B., Mehta, D. & Haigney, M.C. (2009) QTc interval screening in methadone treatment. *Annals of Internal Medicine*, **150** (6), 387–395.

52 Raffa, R.B., Burmeister, J.J., Yuvasheva, E. & Pergolizzi, J.V. Jr., (2012) QTc interval prolongation by d-propoxyphene: what about other analgesics? *Expert Opinion on Pharmacotherapy*, **13** (10), 1397–1409.

53 Walker, J.M., Farney, R.J., Rhondeau, S.M. *et al.* (2007) Chronic opioid use is a risk factor for the development of central sleep apnea and ataxic breathing. *Journal of Clinical Sleep Medicine*, **3** (5), 455–461.

54 Yue, H.J. & Guilleminault, C. (2010) Opioid medication and sleep-disordered breathing. *The Medical Clinics of North America*, **94** (3), 435–446.

55 Radke, J.B., Owen, K.P., Sutter, M.E., Ford, J.B. & Albertson, T.E. (2014) The effects of opioids on the lung. *Clinical Reviews in Allergy and Immunology*, **46** (1), 54–64.

56 Guilleminault, C., Cao, M., Yue, H.J. & Chawla, P. (2010) Obstructive sleep apnea and chronic opioid use. *Lung*, **188** (6), 459–468.

57 Smith, H.S. & Elliott, J.A. (2012) Opioid-induced androgen deficiency (OPIAD). *Pain Physician*, **15** (3 Suppl), ES145–156.

58 Rochira, V., Zirilli, L., Orlando, G. *et al.* (2011) Premature decline of serum total testosterone in HIV-infected men in the HAART-era. *PLoS One*, **6** (12).e28512

59 Zona, S., Guaraldi, G., Luzi, K. *et al.* (2012) Erectile dysfunction is more common in young to middle-aged HIV-infected men than in HIV-uninfected men. *The Journal of Sexual Medicine*, **9** (7), 1923–1930.

60 Bell, T.J., Panchal, S.J., Miaskowski, C., Bolge, S.C., Milanova, T. & Williamson, R. (2009) The prevalence, severity, and impact of opioid-induced bowel dysfunction: results of a US and European Patient Survey (PROBE 1). *Pain Medicine*, **10** (1), 35–42.

61 Ketwaroo, G.A., Cheng, V. & Lembo, A. (2013) Opioid-induced bowel dysfunction. *Current Gastroenterology Reports*, **15** (9), 344.

62 Swegle, J.M. & Logemann, C. (2006) Management of common opioid-induced adverse effects. *American Family Physician*, **74** (8), 1347–1354.

63 Wilcox, C.M. & Saag, M.S. (2008) Gastrointestinal complications of HIV infection: changing priorities in the HAART era. *Gut*, **57** (6), 861–870.

64 Raffa, R.B. & Pergolizzi, J.V. Jr., (2013) Opioid-induced hyperalgesia: is it clinically relevant for the treatment of pain patients? *Pain Management Nursing*, **14** (3), e67–83.

65 Lee, M., Silverman, S.M., Hansen, H., Patel, V.B. & Manchikanti, L. (2011) A comprehensive review of opioid-induced hyperalgesia. *Pain Physician*, **14** (2), 145–161.

66 Barry, D.T., Goulet, J.L., Kerns, R.K. *et al.* (2011) Nonmedical use of prescription opioids and pain in veterans with and without HIV. *Pain*, **152** (5), 1133–1138.

67 Robinson-Papp, J., Elliott, K., Simpson, D.M. & Morgello, S. (2012) Problematic prescription opioid use in an HIV-infected cohort: the importance of universal toxicology testing. *Journal of Acquired Immune Deficiency Syndromes*, **61** (2), 187–193.

68 Vijayaraghavan, M., Penko, J., Bangsberg, D.R., Miaskowski, C. & Kushel, M.B. (2013) Opioid analgesic misuse in a community-based cohort of HIV-infected indigent adults. *JAMA Internal Medicine*, **173** (3), 235–237.

69 Jeevanjee, S., Penko, J., Guzman, D., Miaskowski, C., Bangsberg, D.R. & Kushel, M.B. (2014) Opioid analgesic misuse is associated with incomplete antiretroviral adherence in a cohort of HIV-infected indigent adults in San Francisco. *AIDS and Behavior*, **18** (7), 1352–1358.

70 McCarthy, L., Wetzel, M., Sliker, J.K., Eisenstein, T.K. & Rogers, T.J. (2001) Opioids, opioid

receptors, and the immune response. *Drug and Alcohol Dependence*, **62** (2), 111–123.

71 Sacerdote, P. (2008) Opioid-induced immuno-suppression. *Current Opinion in Supportive and Palliative Care*, **2** (1), 14–18.

72 Sacerdote, P., Franchi, S. & Panerai, A.E. (2012) Non-analgesic effects of opioids: mechanisms and potential clinical relevance of opioid-induced immunodepression. *Current Pharmaceutical Design*, **18** (37), 6034–6042.

73 Roy, S., Ninkovic, J., Banerjee, S. *et al.* (2011) Opioid drug abuse and modulation of immune function: consequences in the susceptibility to opportunistic infections. *Journal of Neuroimmune Pharmacology*, **6** (4), 442–465.

74 Dublin, S., Walker, R.L., Jackson, M.L. *et al.* (2011) Use of opioids or benzodiazepines and risk of pneumonia in older adults: a population-based case–control study. *Journal of American Geriatrics Society*, **59** (10), 1899–1907.

75 Peterson, P.K., Sharp, B.M., Gekker, G., Portoghese, P.S., Sannerud, K. & Balfour, H.H. Jr., (1990) Morphine promotes the growth of HIV-1 in human peripheral blood mononuclear cell cocultures. *AIDS*, **4** (9), 869–873.

76 Li, Y., Merrill, J.D., Mooney, K. *et al.* (2003) Morphine enhances HIV infection of neonatal macrophages. *Pediatric Research*, **54** (2), 282–288.

77 Donahoe, R.M. & Vlahov, D. (1998) Opiates as potential cofactors in progression of HIV-1 infections to AIDS. *Journal of Neuroimmunology*, **83** (1–2), 77–87.

78 Donahoe, R.M. (2004) Multiple ways that drug abuse might influence AIDS progression: clues from a monkey model. *Journal of Neuroimmunology*, **147** (1–2), 28–32.

79 Ninkovic, J. & Roy, S. (2013) Role of the mu-opioid receptor in opioid modulation of immune function. *Amino Acids*, **45** (1), 9–24.

80 Gudin, J. (2012) Opioid therapies and cytochrome p450 interactions. *Journal of Pain and Symptom Management*, **44** (6 Suppl), S4–14.

81 Panel on Antiretroviral Guidelines for Adults and Adolescents. Guidelines for the use of antiretroviral agents in HIV-1-infected adults and adolescents. Department of Health and Human Services. Available at http://www.aidsinfo.nih.gov/ContentFiles/AdultandAdolescentGL.pdf [accessed on 23 October 2015].

82 Committee on Advancing Pain Research Care IoM. *Relieving Pain in America: A Blueprint for Transforming Prevention, Care, Education, and Research*: National Academies Press;(2011). 030921484X.

83 Wang, D. & Teichtahl, H. (2007) Opioids, sleep architecture and sleep-disordered breathing. *Sleep Medicine Reviews*, **11** (1), 35–46.

84 Edelman, E.J., Gordon, K.S., Glover, J., McNicholl, I.R., Fiellin, D.A. & Justice, A.C. (2013) The next therapeutic challenge in HIV: polypharmacy. *Drugs and Aging*, **30** (8), 613–628.

85 Argoff, C.E. & Silvershein, D.I. (2009) A comparison of long- and short-acting opioids for the treatment of chronic noncancer pain: tailoring therapy to meet patient needs. *Mayo Clinic Proceedings*, **84** (7), 602–612.

86 Reid, M.C., Engles-Horton, L.L., Weber, M.B., Kerns, R.D., Rogers, E.L. & O'Connor, P.G. (2002) Use of opioid medications for chronic noncancer pain syndromes in primary care. *Journal of General Internal Medicine*, **17** (3), 173–179.

87 Okie, S. (2010) A flood of opioids, a rising tide of deaths. *New England Journal of Medicine*, **363** (21), 1981–1985.

88 Krantz, M.J., Martin, J., Stimmel, B., Mehta, D. & Haigney, M.C.P. (2009) QTc interval screening in methadone treatment. *Annals of Internal Medicine*, **150** (6), 387–395.

89 Edelman, E.J., Gordon, K.S., Lo Re, V. 3rd,, Skanderson, M., Fiellin, D.A. & Justice, A.C. (2013) Acetaminophen receipt among HIV-infected patients with advanced hepatic fibrosis. *Pharmacoepidemiology and Drug Safety*, **22** (12), 1352–1356.

90 US Food and Drug Administration. (2014) *All manufacturers of prescription combination drug products with more than 325 mg of acetaminophen have discontinued marketing* [WWW document]. URL http://www.fda.gov/Drugs/DrugSafety/InformationbyDrugClass/ucm390509.htm [accessed on 10 April 2014].

CHAPTER 12

Safer opioid prescribing in HIV-infected patients with chronic pain

Joanna Starrels[1] and Jennifer McNeely[2,3]

[1] Department of Medicine, Albert Einstein College of Medicine, Bronx, NY, USA

[2] Department of Population Health, New York University School of Medicine, New York, NY, USA

[3] Department of Medicine, Division of General Internal Medicine, New York University School of Medicine, New York, NY, USA

Introduction

HIV-infected individuals suffer disproportionately from chronic pain, and many are prescribed opioid analgesics [1,2]. Given the public health threat of opioid analgesic misuse, addiction, and overdose, clinicians who prescribe opioids must take precautions to ensure that the opioids they prescribe will be used as safely as possible. HIV-infected patients have higher prevalence of comorbid substance use and mental health problems than the general population, which places these patients at increased risk for opioid misuse and its negative consequences [3,4]. Balancing the risks and benefits of opioid treatment in this patient population can be particularly challenging. For example, HIV and comorbid medical conditions increase the prevalence of chronic pain as well as the risk for fatal opioid overdose [5,6]. These challenges are likely to increase with aging of the HIV-infected population.

In this chapter, we describe strategies that providers can use to assess and reduce the risks of misuse, addiction, and overdose ("opioid use problems") among patients who are prescribed opioids for chronic pain conditions. The strategies we address here are (1) judicious use of opioids, (2) risk assessment, (3) written treatment agreements, (4) urine drug testing, and (5) prescription monitoring programs (PMPs). We then provide guidance to prescribers for responding to high-risk use, and incorporating

practice modifications to implement safer opioid prescribing strategies in diverse practice settings.

The strategies outlined here are considered best practices, based on current guidelines, expert consensus, and existing evidence [7–12]. It is important to note that the evidence and guidelines are rapidly evolving and the recommendations here should not be considered comprehensive or sufficient. Providers should follow the policies and recommendations of their state medical boards and other governing agencies. We believe that implementing strategies for safer opioid prescribing should be done systematically for all patients and have included a brief section describing practice modifications that may facilitate safer opioid prescribing.

Judicious use of opioids for chronic pain

Given the risks of opioid misuse discussed elsewhere in this book (see Chapter 11), the World Health Organization and others recommend prescribing opioids for chronic pain only when other treatments have failed or are contraindicated [12]. When opioid analgesics are prescribed for chronic pain, they should be part of a multimodal approach individualized for each patient, which typically includes both nonpharmacologic treatments such as physical therapy or meditation, as well as adjunctive

Chronic Pain and HIV: A Practical Approach, First Edition.
Edited by Jessica S. Merlin, Peter A. Selwyn, Glenn J. Treisman and Angela G. Giovanniello.
© 2016 John Wiley & Sons, Ltd. Published 2016 by John Wiley & Sons, Ltd.

pharmacotherapies such as anti-inflammatory medications or neuropathic agents. Given emerging evidence that use of high-dose opioids is associated with increased risk for overdose death [13,14], it is prudent to use the lowest effective dose and to raise the dose slowly if necessary. Providers should be aware that opioid doses higher than 100 morphine-equivalent dose units (MEDUs) per day (i.e., 100 mg of morphine or 60 mg of oxycodone) are associated with a sevenfold increase in overdose death, compared to patients prescribed 20 or fewer MEDU [14]. These data have prompted some experts, as well as policymakers in Washington State, to promote a maximum dose prescribed outside of pain management specialty settings [15]. Caution must also be taken if prescribing opioids to patients with medical comorbidities or who use medications or substances that increase the risk of overdose, including patients with obstructive sleep apnea, or who take benzodiazepines or drink alcohol [16].

Risk assessment

Risk assessment principles: Every patient is at some risk for developing opioid use problems. The risk is particularly high in HIV-infected cohorts because the primary risk factor for opioid misuse is also a major risk factor for HIV infection (i.e., prior or current drug use). Studies have found that the prevalence of opioid misuse in HIV-infected cohorts is as high as 47–62% [17–20]. Assessing risk for opioid misuse should be performed when opioids are initially considered and in an ongoing manner throughout treatment with opioids.

Assessing risk requires data collection from multiple sources, including patient self-report, review of medical records and pharmacy data, drug testing, and contacting previous providers. Decisions about whether to prescribe or continue to prescribe opioids for a patient are not based solely on the assessment of risk, but on weighing the risks and benefits at each point in time. Therefore, *risk assessment is a dynamic process*. Patients with no baseline risk factors may develop problem opioid use, whereas those with multiple risk factors may never

misuse their opioid medications. In addition to baseline risk factors described in what follows, ongoing risk assessment considers any red flag behaviors that could indicate misuse. Some examples of such behaviors are unsanctioned dose escalation, reporting lost or stolen prescriptions, obtaining opioid medications from other sources, or unhealthy use of alcohol or other drugs. When a provider identifies that a patient has increased risk for misuse or its consequences, the provider should intensify monitoring or adjust the treatment plan to minimize risk while maximizing the effectiveness of pain management [7]. Unfortunately, there is no simple algorithm for this. Both the pattern and severity of behaviors must be considered (i.e., running out early on one occasion is not as severe as selling prescribed medication or forging a prescription). Further, patients' individual needs and local resources must be considered.

Examples of behaviors that indicate potential opioid misuse.

Medication overuse (unsanctioned dose
   escalation, running out early)
Concurrent alcohol or drug use
Drug test results inconsistent with prescribed or
   reported use
Refusal to provide specimen for drug testing
Seeking or obtaining controlled substances
   from additional sources
Reporting lost or stolen prescriptions or
   medication
Unwillingness to try alternative treatments
   for pain
Sharing or selling prescribed medications
Prescription forgery or stealing

Initial assessment: The initial risk assessment takes time, and when possible, it is best to devote most or all of a visit to this. The goal is to assess risk factors for opioid use problems, including personal and family history of substance use problems, and mental health problems (see Chapters 7 and 8). Understanding a patient's risk for substance use problems is critical to determining how intensely the patient should be monitored and which providers or treatment programs should be included in the treatment plan, and it may guide decisions about the conditions under which opioid treatment would be considered appropriate. Risk assessment is equally important in patients who may already be on chronic opioids but are newly entering your care. This represents an opportunity to identify factors that could have been overlooked by the prior provider and also to set expectations of treatment (see Written treatment agreements).

Components of the initial risk assessment include obtaining (1) substance use screening and history; (2) mental health screening and history; (3) family history of substance use problems; (4) medical record review of pain conditions, treatments, and evidence of opioid misuse; (5) review of prescription and pharmacy data (e.g., using PMP data); and (6) drug testing, most frequently using urine. With patients' consent, collateral history from a patient's family member or friend may be helpful.

Substance use history should include use of tobacco, alcohol, illicit and prescription drugs, using a standardized and validated screening tool. While there are a number of options to choose from, for alcohol we recommend the Alcohol Use Disorders Identification Test (AUDIT-C), which is a three-item questionnaire that is easy to administer and accurately detects hazardous use as well as more severe alcohol problems [21]. For assessment of drug use, many medical settings choose to use the 10-item Drug Abuse Screening Test (DAST-10), which is a relatively short questionnaire that provides an overall "drug" risk level [22]. However, there may be advantages to using a slightly longer but more specific assessment tool, such as the Alcohol, Smoking, and Substance Involvement Screening Test (ASSIST) or National Institute of Drug Abuse (NIDA)-Modified ASSIST, which identifies the risk level of each substance a patient uses (e.g., cocaine and sedatives), integrates alcohol and tobacco screening, and identifies lifetime as well as past year use [23,24]. Several opioid risk screening tools have been developed that aim to stratify patients into low, moderate, and high risk based on the presence of known risk factors [25–29]. There is currently no gold standard for risk stratification; the Opioid Risk Tool is one instrument that has been shown to correlate to the development of opioid misuse behaviors [30]. Mental health screening should include screening for depression and anxiety, for example, using the Patient Health Questionnaire (PHQ-2 and PHQ-9) and Generalized Anxiety Disorder scale (GAD-7) [31].

Prescribing opioids at the time of the first visit with a patient requesting opioids should be avoided in most cases. Rather, a complete risk assessment should be conducted during and following that visit. Exceptions include patients who are transferring care from a colleague and for whom medical records can be reviewed during the visit, and patients for whom previous prescriptions have been verified, through the pharmacy or online PMP. Because opioid withdrawal causes considerable distress, it is sometimes appropriate to prescribe a short supply (e.g., 1 week) to continue verified opioid prescriptions while reviewing records if the previous prescriber is not available.

Ongoing monitoring: Every patient on chronic opioid therapy has risk for misuse, addiction, and overdose, and should be regularly monitored. "Periodic Review" is recommended by the Federation of State Medical Boards and others [7,10]. This involves the provider reassessing patients' progress in terms of both benefits and risks of opioid misuse, during routine visits. The frequency of visits depends on the clinical scenario, and a consensus panel recommended these visits occur at least every 3–6 months, and more frequently for higher risk patients [7]. A review of the risks and benefits of opioids includes addressing each of the "5 A's": (1) how well the patient's pain is being controlled (Analgesia), (2) how well the patient is able to function and perform important physical tasks (Activity), (3) whether the patient is having side effects from the medications (Adverse effects), (4) whether there is evidence of misuse or overuse (Aberrant drug-related behaviors), and (5) the patient's mood and emotional well-being (Affect) [32]. The "5 A's" have been operationalized in a progress note template called the Pain Assessment and Documentation Tool [33]. In this chapter, we focus on assessing for red flag behaviors (Aberrant drug-related behaviors); the other four "A's" are described elsewhere in this book.

Though information from drug testing and PMPs (described below) are useful for gathering objective data about patients' use of prescribed medications and other substances, patients' self-report is critical for truly understanding the risk of opioid misuse. Because patients may perceive an incentive to omit or modify what they report, we have found that asking questions in an open-ended and nonjudgmental way yields the richest information. For example, we recommend asking, "Tell me how you're taking your medication," and "How have you been coping with the pain?" rather than, "Have you taken more than prescribed?" See Chapter 3 for further recommendations about effective communication with patients with chronic pain.

Written treatment agreements

It is essential to educate patients about the risks of opioid medications and about how to use them safely. It is also important that providers communicate with patients about their expectations for how patients will use their pain medications and which conditions they would consider risky enough to taper or discontinue medications. Many experts and some guidelines advocate formalizing these points in written documents called opioid treatment agreements, plans, or contracts [9,12]. We prefer the terms treatment agreement or treatment plan as it should be considered by the provider and patient to be a communication tool rather than a legal document. The strength of the recommendation to use treatment agreements varies among guidelines, from "may consider" to "must" use [11].

Currently, evidence about the outcomes of treatment agreement use is limited. Only observational studies have been conducted, which have found modest reductions in opioid misuse behaviors following multicomponent opioid safety interventions that include use of written treatment agreements [34]. Studies of other outcomes, such as the effect of agreements on addiction, overdose, therapeutic alliance, and retention in care have not been conducted. However, agreements do seem to

help providers, and those who use agreements have reported greater self-efficacy, preparedness, and satisfaction managing patients with chronic pain, compared to providers who do not use agreements [35–38].

We believe that the lack of consensus about recommendations to use agreements stems in part from variation in the form and content of existing agreements, and differences in how they are framed and delivered. Currently, no standard agreement exists, and while some aim to be patient-centered, the tone of others can be punitive or off-putting to patients. Further, while we believe they should be presented as a communication tool to describe the providers' approach and expectations, some providers may present them as a binding contract and patients who need pain medicine may feel coerced into signing. In sum, we agree with Fishman *et al.* that agreements "can be used or abused [39]." We encourage providers to use an agreement but recommend that they (1) use it for all patients to avoid stigmatization; (2) make sure the agreement is readable to your patients (i.e., at an appropriate literacy level and in their language); (3) make it bilateral, for example, describe not only what the patient is expected to do, but what the provider is expected to do; (4) take the time to review it with patients to ensure that they understand and have their questions answered; (5) make it patient-centered and goal-directed, such that patients' individualized functional goals are included and decisions about continuing opioids depend on benefits to the patient as well as risks that may arise; and (6) use it to guide, not dictate, care.

Some guidelines recommend obtaining written informed consent prior to initiating opioid medications for chronic pain [7,10]. Consistent with other informed consent, this should include explanation of the risks and benefits of opioid use. This is an important discussion for all patients, and currently there is variation in how this should be performed and documented. Some providers include this as part of the written treatment agreement, others use a separate document, and others discuss and document without a patient signature. Make sure your practices are consistent with guidelines and policies within your state and other regulatory agencies.

There are a wide variety of opioid treatment agreements available online, which vary in quality. We have included an opioid treatment agreement at the end of this chapter that we believe includes all of the important elements discussed in this chapter. This low-literacy opioid treatment agreement was initially developed by Dr Lorraine Wallace [53]. The version included here was adapted by Drs Jessica Merlin and Joanna Starrels specifically for the 1917 HIV Clinic at the University of Alabama at Birmingham, where it is currently in use.

Urine drug testing (UDT)

In the past decade, urine drug testing has been increasingly adopted and recommended for use in patients who are prescribed long-term opioids or other controlled substances. The goals of drug testing for patients prescribed controlled substances are twofold: first, to confirm that patients are taking the prescribed medication; and second, to identify nondisclosed use of other substances that could interact with or increase the risk of prescribed medications. Though evidence that routine drug testing reduces opioid misuse is scant, substantial evidence exists that drug testing identifies undisclosed substance use and nonuse of prescribed drugs more accurately than relying on patient self-report or observing patient behaviors [40–42]. Guidelines vary about how often and for whom drug testing is recommended, but generally experts recommend testing patients at baseline and randomly throughout treatment, at least every 6 months and more frequently when risk is elevated [7,15]. Expectations regarding drug testing should be discussed with the patient in advance, preferably as part of the treatment agreement. Use of drug testing uniformly for all patients who are prescribed long-term opioids may minimize stigma associated with drug testing [32].

Several different types of drug testing are available, including tests that use blood, saliva, or hair. With current assays, urine has several advantages in that it is widely available; inexpensive; easy to obtain; the window of detection for most opioids reflects recent use (within the last 1–2 days); and results are not impacted, as those for saliva are, by local factors such as smoking or mouthwash [43]. Among urine drug tests, there are also several options, including point-of-care tests, lab-based immunoassay tests, and confirmatory mass spectrometry tests that use gas or liquid chromatography. Each has advantages and limitations, and it is essential that providers who order these tests know the test characteristics and limitations of their specific tests.

Interpreting urine drug test results is more complicated than most providers realize. Studies have found that most providers are not proficient at interpreting urine drug test results accurately, which can impact clinical care of patients in negative ways [44,45]. For example, we are aware of many examples where a provider has decided to discontinue opioids for a patient after concluding that the patient was not taking and may be selling their medication, based on assuming a negative opiate screen indicated that the urine specimen contained no opioids. However, urine drug "screens" that most providers use are immunoassay tests, which are sensitive for detecting only certain substances within a drug class, and report a result as "negative" if the substance is present but the concentration is below the lab's cutoff value. Therefore, a patient who takes low doses of oxycodone, for example, may repeatedly screen negative for "opiates" on immunoassay tests. And synthetic opioids such as methadone, meperidine, and fentanyl will not be detected by immunoassay tests for "opiates." In addition to these false negative test results, providers must also recognize that other substances and even over-the-counter medications can cross-react with immunoassay panels and cause false positive results for some controlled substances [46]. Confirmatory tests (e.g., gas chromatography and mass spectrometry (GC/MS)) are more expensive and less widely available but are much more sensitive and specific for individual medications within a drug class. However, providers interpreting GC/MS results still must take care to interpret results correctly and be aware of opioid metabolic pathways. For example, because oxycodone is metabolized to oxymorphone, a patient who is taking oxycodone is expected to have oxymorphone in their urine [47]. See Table 12.1 for a guide to ordering and interpreting urine drug test results, and other resources that are available [47,48]. We also encourage providers to be familiar with and communicate with their lab, as test methods, protocols, and characteristics vary.

Prescription monitoring programs

PMPs are databases of prescription fills for controlled substances. Currently, they are administered at the state level, and though the majority of states have a program, they

Table 12.1 Quick Guide to Urine Drug Testing.

Quick guide to urine drug testing

RESULTS

Legend:
⊕ Should be +
+ Might be +
F Potential false +

DRUGS TAKEN	Amphetamines	Barbiturates	Benzodiazepines	Buprenorphine	Cocaine	Methadone	Opiates	Oxycodone	PCP	Cannabis	Buprenorphine, norbup.	Codeine, norcodeine	Fentanyl	Hydrocodone	Hydromorphone	Meperidine, normep.	Methadone	Morphine	Oxycodone	Oxymorphone	Heroin (6-MAM)	Common detection time
Prescription opioids											(EIA) Screening ←							GCMS Confirmatory →				
Buprenorphine				⊕							⊕											1–6 days
Codeine							⊕					⊕		+				+				1–3 days
Fentanyl													⊕									24 h
Hydrocodone							⊕							⊕	+							1–3 days
Hydromorphone							+								⊕							1–3 days
Meperidine																⊕						2–3 days
Methadone						⊕											⊕					1–3 days[2]
Morphine							⊕								+			⊕				1–3 days[2]
Oxycodone							+	⊕											⊕	+		24 h
Oxymorphone								⊕												⊕		24 h[2]
Illicit drugs																						
Amphetamines	⊕																					1–3 days
Barbiturates		⊕																				24 h[2]
Benzodiazepines			+*																			3 days[2]
Cocaine					⊕																	1–4 days[2]
Heroin							⊕											+			+	1–3 days[2]
PCP									⊕													1–3 days[2]
Cannabis										⊕												1–3 days[2]
Other																						
Poppy seeds[4]							F					F						F				
Other medications[5]	F	F	F	F		F	F	F	F	F												

[1] Sensitivity of opiate screen to semi-synthetic opioids varies by lab. Generally, hydrocodone > hydromorphone > oxycodone. Higher dose is more likely to yield a + opiate screen. Consider confirmatory test, especially to confirm negative for rx'd drug.
[2] Chronic use may result in longer detection times. 6-MAM is pathognomonic for heroin use, detection time is 12–24 h.
[3] Benzodiazepine screen likely positive if alprazolam or diazepam taken, likely negative if clonazepam, lorazepam. Varies by lab.
[4] Heavy poppy seed ingestion (3+ bagels) may test positive for opiates – repeat off poppy seeds.
[5] Some commonly used medications reported to cause false + results on screening assays are below – order confirmatory test.
Amphetamine: buproprion, SSRIs, chlorpromazine, mexiletine, pseudoephedrine, decongestants, ranitidine, trazodone, labetalol
Barbiturate: ibuprofen, naproxyn, phenytoin.   Benzodiazepine: sertraline, oxaprozin.
Buprenorphine: tramadol, other opioids.   Cocaine: none confirmed. Coca leaves or dental use cause rare true +.
Methadone: diphenhydramine, doxylamine, clomipramine, chlorpromazine, quetiapine, thioridazine, tramadol, verapamil. Opiate: dextromethorphan, diphenhydramine, fluoroquinolones, quinine, rifampin.
Oxycodone: naloxone, see list for "opiates."   PCP: dextromethorphan, diphenhydramine, ibuprofen, tramadol, venlafaxine.
Cannabis: dronabinol, efavirenz, PPIs. Note that ibuprofen does NOT cause false + using modern tests (previously did).

vary widely in terms of data available and accessibility. Most are available online and prescribers can access them in order to review their patients' medication fills. Increasingly, it is recommended that prescribers review PMP data for patients for whom they prescribe controlled substances, and some states, such as Kentucky and New York, now mandate their use. Prescribers must comply with state and federal law regarding when to review PMP data. We recommend using the PMP even when it is not mandated, as valuable information may be obtained.

PMP data is useful to verify a patient's medications, previous prescribers, dates of recent prescriptions, and in some cases, dose prescribed. For new patients transferring care, it is confirmation that these medications have been dispensed for the patient previously. It is also useful for prescribers to know when their prescriptions were filled in order to calculate medication requirements and assess adherence, and to identify if a patient has received controlled substances without their knowledge from another provider. Data about the effectiveness of PMPs is limited, but some studies suggest that PMP data is useful for providers in clinical decision-making, improves their confidence [49], decreases medically unnecessary prescriptions, reduces number of individuals obtaining opioids from multiple sources, and reduces the rate of poison control calls for opioid analgesic exposure (vs states without PMPs) [50]. Studies have not yet been conducted to rigorously evaluate the effect of PMPs on the important but more distal effects, such as clinical outcomes of opioid dependence and overdose. One epidemiologic study found no difference in opioid overdose in states with and without PMPs [51]. Drawbacks to PMPs are that they include in-state prescriptions only, do not include medications that are received at a drug treatment program (i.e., methadone treatment), and can vary widely in terms of comprehensiveness and timeliness with which prescriptions are reported [49].

Responding to high-risk use

How should a prescriber respond to misuse of prescribed opioids? Though it depends on the patient, provider, and practice environment, there are general principles and strategies that provide guidance. First, it is important to consider that red flag behaviors have a differential diagnosis, and prescribers should seek to understand what happened and why before deciding on a response. These red flag behaviors may be red herrings; they don't always indicate risk (e.g., the patient may indeed have lost the prescription), and there are degrees of risk. A high-risk situation such as untreated alcohol dependence requires a different response than occasional marijuana use. Patterns of red flag behaviors, such as repeatedly escalating doses and running out early, indicate higher risk than a single episode. In every situation, the risks of the opioids need to be weighed against the benefits to the patient. Discontinuing opioids may be warranted in a patient who does not seem to be benefiting from them, when there is little or no evidence of misuse; whereas continuing them may be indicated for a patient who benefits greatly from them, even if there is occasional or low-grade misuse. This risk-benefit assessment must be made by clinicians on a case-by-case basis.

Appropriate response to the first instance of a low-grade or "yellow flag" behavior includes discussing your concern with the patient, reviewing the terms of the treatment agreement, communicating guidelines for safe use, and reminding the patient that you consider using illicit drugs or running out early to indicate risk. It is appropriate to increase monitoring – for example, to see the patient more frequently, perform UDT or check PMP more often, engage other providers, refer to specialists, and expand nonopioid treatment strategies. If red flag behaviors continue or a pattern of such behaviors emerges, the prescriber must consider alternative treatments and may decide to taper opioids or transfer the patient to a higher level of care.

In some cases, the decision may be made to taper or discontinue opioids after even a single episode of a high-grade red flag behavior.

Clinical decision-making does not end here. The provider must decide how quickly to taper or whether to discontinue abruptly, whether referrals to other providers or prescribing other medications is indicated, and which additional treatments the patient can be offered.

When a clinician decides that the risks outweigh the benefits and that discontinuing opioids is warranted, it is usually appropriate to taper the medications to reduce opioid withdrawal symptoms. Exceptions, for whom opioids may be discontinued abruptly, include patients who are identified to have multiple, undisclosed opioid prescribers, have forged a prescription, or are confirmed to be selling their medications. Opioid withdrawal, though not fatal, is extremely uncomfortable. The appropriate rate of tapering is ill-defined and depends on the patient. Some guidelines suggest reducing the dose by 10–25% per week; in many patients without acute risks, a slower taper is indicated and better tolerated [7].

If the clinician is concerned that the patient might have an opioid use disorder (i.e., addiction), the patient must be referred for evaluation and treatment by an addiction treatment specialist. There are safe and effective treatments for opioid use disorder, including medication-assisted treatment with methadone or buprenorphine. Primary care or infectious disease specialists can be trained and waivered to prescribe buprenorphine to their patients for treatment of opioid use disorder. Doing so can present an opportunity to control risk while maintaining the therapeutic relationship and providing effective treatment. Clinicians who are not equipped to treat opioid use disorder should be aware of local resources for referring patients.

Clinicians often have concerns that disagreements or decisions to taper opioids will lead patients to drop out of care. This is of particular concern among HIV treatment providers who work hard to engage and retain their patients in care, to maximize treatment of their HIV infection and achieve or maintain viral suppression [52]. It is true that some patients will terminate the relationship with a clinician because of disagreements over opioids; however, it is important to separate the goals of managing HIV and treating pain. If you do need to discontinue opioids for a patient, commit to continuing to manage their HIV and to treating their pain in alternative ways.

Putting these strategies into practice

Standardize care: To ensure that all patients receive equitable treatment and to minimize the risks of opioid misuse across your practice, the optimal approach is to apply the same standards of care to all patients. Larger group practices should have protocols and policies about using treatment agreements, urine drug testing, and refilling opioid prescriptions.

Keep abreast of current research and guidelines: Because we are in the midst of an epidemic of opioid addiction and overdose, new research, recommendations, and regulations are in flux. We recommend identifying a pain champion at your practice who will stay on top of new developments and educate other clinicians.

Engage a multidisciplinary staff: It takes time to implement these strategies, and primary medical providers are not always the best people to complete them. When possible, engage social workers, counselors, or psychologists, particularly those trained in chronic pain and substance use, and nurses or health educators to engage patients in behavioral and self-management strategies for pain management.

References

1 Dobalian, A., Tsao, J.C. & Duncan, R.P. (2004) Pain and the use of outpatient services among persons with HIV: results from a nationally representative survey. *Medical Care*, **42** (2), 129–138.

2 Edelman, E.J., Gordon, K., Becker, W.C. et al. (2013) Receipt of opioid analgesics by HIV-infected and uninfected patients. *Journal of General Internal Medicine*, **28** (1), 82–90.

3 Chander, G., Himelhoch, S. & Moore, R.D. (2006) Substance abuse and psychiatric disorders in HIV-positive patients: epidemiology and impact on antiretroviral therapy. *Drugs*, **66** (6), 769–789.

4 Klinkenberg, W.D. & Sacks, S. (2004) Mental disorders and drug abuse in persons living with HIV/AIDS. *AIDS Care*, **16** (Suppl 1), S22–42.

5 Green, T.C., McGowan, S.K., Yokell, M.A., Pouget, E.R. & Rich, J.D. (2012) HIV infection and risk of overdose: a systematic review and meta-analysis. *AIDS*, **26** (4), 403–417. doi:410.1097/QAD.1090b1013e32834f32819b 32836

6 Wang, C., Vlahov, D., Galai, N. *et al.* (2005) The effect of HIV infection on overdose mortality. *AIDS*, **19** (9), 935–942.

7 Chou, R., Fanciullo, G.J., Fine, P.G. *et al.* (2009) Clinical guidelines for the use of chronic opioid therapy in chronic noncancer pain. *The Journal of Pain*, **10** (2), 113–130.

8 Chou, R., Fanciullo, G.J., Fine, P.G., Miaskowski, C., Passik, S.D. & Portenoy, R.K. (2009) Opioids for chronic noncancer pain: prediction and identification of aberrant drug-related behaviors: a review of the evidence for an American Pain Society and American Academy of Pain Medicine clinical practice guideline. *The Journal of Pain*, **10** (2), 131–146.

9 Trescot, A.M., Boswell, M.V., Atluri, S.L. *et al.* (2006) Opioid guidelines in the management of chronic non-cancer pain. *Pain Physician*, **9** (1), 1–39.

10 Federation of State Medical Boards of the United States (2013) *Model policy on the use of opioid analgesics in the treatment of chronic pain* [WWW document]. URL http://cms.fsmb.org/ Media/Default/PDF/FSMB/Advocacy/pain_ policy_july2013.pdf [accessed on 26 June 2014].

11 Nuckols, T.K., Anderson, L., Popescu, I. *et al.* (2014) Opioid prescribing: a systematic review and critical appraisal of guidelines for chronic pain. *Annals of Internal Medicine*, **160** (1), 38–47.

12 Department of Veterans Affairs and Department of Defense (2010) *Clinical practice guideline for management of opioid therapy for chronic pain* [WWW document]. URL http:// www.healthquality.va.gov/COT_312_Full-er .pdf [accessed on 31 January 2014].

13 Dunn, K.M., Saunders, K.W., Rutter, C.M. *et al.* (2010) Opioid prescriptions for chronic pain and overdose: a cohort study. *Annals of Internal Medicine*, **152** (2), 85–92.

14 Bohnert, A.S., Valenstein, M., Bair, M.J. *et al.* (2011) Association between opioid prescribing patterns and opioid overdose-related deaths. *JAMA*, **305** (13), 1315–1321.

15 Washington State Agency Medical Directors' Group (2010) *Interagency guideline on opioid dosing for chronic non-cancer pain* [WWW document]. URL http://www.agencymeddirectors .wa.gov/Files/OpioidGdline.pdf [accessed on 12 October 2015].

16 Webster, L.R., Cochella, S., Dasgupta, N. *et al.* (Jun 2011) An analysis of the root causes for opioid-related overdose deaths in the United States. *Pain Medicine*, **12** (Suppl 2), S26–35.

17 Tsao, J.C., Stein, J.A. & Dobalian, A. (2007) Pain, problem drug use history, and aberrant analgesic use behaviors in persons living with HIV. *Pain*, **133** (1–3), 128–137.

18 Hansen, L., Penko, J., Guzman, D., Bangsberg, D.R., Miaskowski, C. & Kushel, M.B. (2011) Aberrant behaviors with prescription opioids and problem drug use history in a community-based cohort of HIV-infected individuals. *Journal of Pain and Symptom Management*, **42** (6), 893–902.

19 Robinson-Papp, J., Elliott, K., Simpson, D.M. & Morgello, S. (2012) Problematic prescription opioid use in an HIV-infected cohort: the importance of universal toxicology testing. *Journal of Acquired Immune Deficiency Syndromes*, **61** (2), 187–193.

20 Passik, S.D., Kirsh, K.L., Donaghy, K.B. & Portenoy, R.K. (2006) Pain and aberrant drug-related behaviors in medically ill patients with and without histories of substance abuse. *Clinical Journal of Pain*, **22** (2), 173–181.

21 Bradley, K.A., DeBenedetti, A.F., Volk, R.J., Williams, E.C., Frank, D. & Kivlahan, D.R. (2007) AUDIT-C as a brief screen for alcohol misuse in primary care. *Alcoholism, Clinical and Experimental Research*, **31** (7), 1208–1217.

22 Skinner, H.A. (1982) The drug abuse screening test. *Addictive Behaviors*, **7** (4), 363–371.

23 Humeniuk, R., Ali, R., Babor, T.F. *et al.* (2008) Validation of the Alcohol, Smoking and Substance Involvement Screening Test (ASSIST). *Addiction*, **103** (6), 1039–1047.

24 National Institute on Drug Abuse (NIDA) (2010) Screening for drug use in medical settings [WWW document]. URL http://www

.nida.nih.gov/nidamed/screening/ [accessed on 28 May 2013].

25 Butler, S.F., Budman, S.H., Fernandez, K. & Jamison, R.N. (2004) Validation of a screener and opioid assessment measure for patients with chronic pain. *Pain*, **112** (1–2), 65–75.

26 Butler, S.F., Fernandez, K., Benoit, C., Budman, S.H. & Jamison, R.N. (2008) Validation of the revised screener and opioid assessment for patients with pain (SOAPP-R). *The Journal of Pain*, **9** (4), 360–372.

27 Knisely, J.S., Wunsch, M.J., Cropsey, K.L. & Campbell, E.D. (2008) Prescription opioid misuse index: a brief questionnaire to assess misuse. *Journal of Substance Abuse Treatment*, **35** (4), 380–386. doi:310.1016/j.jsat.2008.1002.1001. Epub 2008 Jul 1026

28 Nemes, S., Rao, P.A., Zeiler, C., Munly, K., Holtz, K.D. & Hoffman, J. (2004) Computerized screening of substance abuse problems in a primary care setting: older vs. younger adults. *American Journal of Drug and Alcohol Abuse*, **30** (3), 627–642.

29 Zeiler, C.A., Nemes, S., Holtz, K.D., Landis, Rx.D. & Hoffman, J. (2002) Responses to a drug and alcohol problem assessment for primary care by ethnicity. *The American Journal of Drug and Alcohol Abuse*, **28** (3), 513–524.

30 Webster, L.R. & Webster, R.M. (2005) Predicting aberrant behaviors in opioid-treated patients: preliminary validation of the Opioid Risk Tool. *Pain Medicine*, **6** (6), 432–442.

31 Kroenke, K., Spitzer, R.L., Williams, J.B. & Lowe, B. (2010) The patient health questionnaire somatic, anxiety, and depressive symptom scales: a systematic review. *General Hospital Psychiatry*, **32** (4), 345–359. doi:310.1016/j.genhosppsych.2010.1003.1006. Epub 2010 May 1017

32 Gourlay, D.L., Heit, H.A. & Almahrezi, A. (2005) Universal precautions in pain medicine: a rational approach to the treatment of chronic pain. *Pain Medicine*, **6** (2), 107–112.

33 Passik, S.D., Kirsh, K.L., Whitcomb, L. *et al.* (2005) Monitoring outcomes during long-term opioid therapy for noncancer pain: results with the pain assessment and documentation tool. *Journal of Opioid Management*, **1** (5), 257–266.

34 Starrels, J.L., Becker, W.C., Alford, D.P., Kapoor, A., Williams, A.R. & Turner, B.J. (2010) Systematic review: treatment agreements and urine drug testing to reduce opioid misuse in patients with chronic pain. *Annals of Internal Medicine*, **152** (11), 712–720.

35 Wiedemer, N.L., Harden, P.S., Arndt, I.O. & Gallagher, R.M. (2007) The opioid renewal clinic: a primary care, managed approach to opioid therapy in chronic pain patients at risk for substance abuse. *Pain Medicine*, **8** (7), 573–584.

36 Fagan, M.J., Chen, J.T., Diaz, J.A., Reinert, S.E. & Stein, M.D. (2008) Do internal medicine residents find pain medication agreements useful? *Clinical Journal of Pain*, **24** (1), 35–38.

37 Sullivan, M.D., Leigh, J. & Gaster, B. (2006) Brief report: training internists in shared decision making about chronic opioid treatment for noncancer pain. *Journal of General Internal Medicine*, **21** (4), 360–362.

38 Fox, A.D., Kunins, H.V. & Starrels, J.L. (2012) Which skills are associated with residents' sense of preparedness to manage chronic pain? *Journal of Opioid Management*, **8** (5), 328–336.

39 Fishman, S.M., Gallagher, R.M. & McCarberg, B.H. (2010) The opioid treatment agreement: a real-world perspective. *The American Journal of Bioethics*, **10** (11), 14–15.

40 Katz, N.P., Sherburne, S., Beach, M. *et al.* (2003) Behavioral monitoring and urine toxicology testing in patients receiving long-term opioid therapy. *Anesthesia and Analgesia*, **97** (4), 1097–1102.

41 Fleming, M.F., Balousek, S.L., Klessig, C.L., Mundt, M.P. & Brown, D.D. (2007) Substance use disorders in a primary care sample receiving daily opioid therapy. *The Journal of Pain*, **8** (7), 573–582.

42 Schuckman, H., Hazelett, S., Powell, C. & Steer, S. (2008) A validation of self-reported substance use with biochemical testing among patients presenting to the emergency department seeking treatment for backache, headache, and toothache. *Substance Use and Misuse*, **43** (5), 589–595.

43 Shults, T.F. (2009) *The Medical Review Officer Handbook*, 9th edn. Quadrangle Research, LLC, Research Triangle Park, NC.

44 Reisfield, G.M. (2007) Urine drug test interpretation: what do physicians know? *Journal of Opioid Management*, **3** (2), 80–86.

45 Starrels, J.L., Fox, A.D., Kunins, H.V. & Cunningham, C.O. (2012) They don't know what they don't know: internal medicine residents' knowledge and confidence in urine drug test interpretation for patients with chronic pain. *Journal of General Internal Medicine*, **27** (11), 1521–1527.

46 Brahm, N.C., Yeager, L.L., Fox, M.D., Farmer, K.C. & Palmer, T.A. (2010) Commonly prescribed medications and potential false-positive urine drug screens. *American Journal of Health-System Pharmacy*, **67** (16), 1344–1350.

47 Tenore, P.L. (2010) Advanced urine toxicology testing. *Journal of Addictive Diseases*, **29** (4), 436–448.

48 Heit, H.A. & Gourlay, D.L. (2004) Urine drug testing in pain medicine. *Journal of Pain and Symptom Management*, **27** (3), 260–267.

49 Prescription Drug Monitoring Program Center of Excellence at Brandeis (2013) *Briefing on PDMP effectiveness* [WWW document]. URL http://www.pdmpexcellence.org/sites/all/pdfs/briefing_PDMP_effectiveness_april_2013.pdf [accessed on 28 February 2014].

50 Reifler, L.M., Droz, D., Bailey, J.E. *et al.* (2012) Do prescription monitoring programs impact state trends in opioid abuse/misuse? *Pain Medicine*, **13** (3), 434–442.

51 Paulozzi, L.J., Kilbourne, E.M. & Desai, H.A. (2011) Prescription drug monitoring programs and death rates from drug overdose. *Pain Medicine*, **12** (5), 747–754.

52 Starrels JL, Peyser D, Fox AD, Merlin J, Arnsten JH, Cunningham CO. *HIV treatment providers' perspectives on opioid prescribing for chronic pain: the overriding concern to retain patients in care [oral abstract presentation].* Association of Medical Education and Research in Substance Abuse. Bethesda, MD.

53 Wallace LS, Keenum AJ, Roskos SE, McDaniel KS. Development and validation of a low-literacy opioid contract. *J Pain.* (2007) Oct;**8**(10):759–766.

Patient Name: _____   MR#: _____

Pain Medicine and other Controlled Substances Agreement

This agreement is for patients who are prescribed certain pain medicines called opioids and other "Controlled Substances." These medicines are sometimes called narcotics.

This agreement pertains to the following list of your medicine(s).

1 _____

2 _____

3 _____

4 _____

The purpose of this agreement is to describe how you, your physician and your treatment team will work together to make sure that your medicine is used safely and works well to help you.

You and your physician will sign the agreement to show that you both understand and agree with it. It will be saved in your medical record so that you and your treatment team can look at it again later. You will get a copy to take home.

My pain/symptoms & goals

My pain/symptoms is/are (describe): _____

_____

What (activities) do I hope to be able to do, when my pain/symptoms is/are better controlled?

Goals for me are (describe):

_____

_____

I understand the following:

☐ My pain/symptoms will probably not go completely away.

☐ My medicine may not work for me.

☐ The long term use of opioid pain medicine is controversial.

☐ It is important not to miss appointments with my physician.

☐ Treating pain/symptoms often includes physical therapy, counseling and/or other treatments.

☐ I will try additional treatments that my physician suggests.

Risks & safer use of controlled substances

Using this medicine might cause problems like:

☐ addiction

☐ allergic reactions

☐ breathing problems

☐ constipation and/or upset stomach

☐ dangerous driving and/or being charged with DUI

☐ feeling sleepy, dizzy, or confused

☐ overdose or death -- especially if taken with alcohol or other drugs, or if I take more than my doctor prescribes

☐ problems urinating and/or problems with erections

☐ worse pain or feeling sick if I stop my pain medicine suddenly

I will:

☐ only get my medicine from my physician, Dr._____, or a covering doctor at this office if my physician is not available. If any other physicians prescribe pain medicine or other controlled substances for me in an emergency, I will let my physician know as soon as possible.

☐ call my nurse, _____, between the hours of 9-5 Monday through Friday with any questions or concerns about my pain/symptoms or medications.

☐ only get the medicine(s) listed here from one pharmacy:_____ Phone number: _____

I will:

☐ be honest and open with my physician and members of my treatment team about medicines and drugs I am taking, including over the counter medications and illegal drugs.

☐ talk to my physician if I feel I need more medicine than was prescribed, but <u>I will not change it on my own or take pain medicine from other people.</u>

☐ only stop the medicine(s) listed here if my doctor and I decide this together.

☐ never give or sell any of my medicine to anyone else.

☐ always keep my medicine in a safe place AND away from children and other people who come to my home.

☐ allow my doctor to check my urine to see what medicines or drugs I am taking.

☐ bring all of my unused medicine in their pharmacy bottles to my office visits if my doctor asks me.

My physician will:

☐ work with me to find the best treatment for my pain/symptoms.

☐ be honest and open with me about my pain/symptom treatment.

☐ ask me about side effects from my medicine and treat these side effects.

☐ make sure that my medicine is refilled on time.

☐ refill my medicine during a visit.

☐ allow my nurse to refill my medicine if I don't have an scheduled appointment and I will call at least 3 days before I run out of medicine.

☐ arrange for a covering physician at the clinic to refill my medicine when my physician is not available.

☐ will not provide extra refills if my medicine or prescription is lost, stolen, destroyed, misplaced or if I run out earlier than expected.

Stopping & changing medicine

☐ **My physician will stop or change my medicine if:**
  ◦ **my goals are not being met, OR**
  ◦ **I do not follow this agreement, OR**
  ◦ **my physician thinks that my medicine may be hurting me more than it is helping me**

☐ My physician might refer me to a specialist for treatment of pain/symptoms or drug problems.

☐ If my physician believes I have stolen or forged prescriptions, sell my medicine, or if I threaten or act violently in any way, I will no longer be prescribed controlled substances from the Clinic

I have been able to ask questions about this agreement, and I understand and agree with what it says

Patient Signature: _____   Date: _____

Physician Signature: _____   Date: _____

CHAPTER 13

The "difficult patient" with HIV and chronic pain

Glenn J. Treisman and Michael R. Clark

Department of Psychiatry and Behavioral Sciences, Johns Hopkins University School of Medicine, 733 N Broadway, Baltimore, MD, USA

Introduction

The term "difficult patient" is seldom used to describe those patients with rare diagnoses or medical diseases such as cancer that are refractory to treatment. The term "difficult" is often used to describe patients whose behavior provokes a sense of frustration in their treating clinicians (Haas et al., 2004). In the HIV clinic, the typical "difficult patient" has a complex problem list that may include chronic pain, substance dependence, pain medication dependence, personality disorders, disability, and nonadherence to elements of the treatment plan. Prolonged and frustration-laced clinic visits lead to unsatisfactory outcomes for the clinician and the patient. They remain dissatisfied despite multiple interventions and heroic efforts.

In Chapter 3, we discussed strategies for communication with HIV-infected patients about chronic pain The principles we introduced, including the importance of building the provider–patient relationship, focusing on physical function, and using motivational interviewing to help patients work on relevant behavior change still apply and are echoed in this chapter. For many patients, such strategies alone are sufficient, but for some, this is not the case. The purpose of this chapter is to give providers additional insight into working with patients in whom these strategies prove challenging.

In this chapter, we discuss the complex interactions between chronic pain, personality, and behavior. We provide strategies for communication and rehabilitation of such "difficult" patients. We discuss behavioral conditioning and abnormal illness behaviors in the first section, the utility of understanding patient temperament in the second section, and the other psychiatric factors that complicate behavior in the third section. Finally, we end with a discussion of primary care-focused behavioral approaches for the "difficult patient" with chronic pain. While the strategies described in this chapter can be used for any patient with chronic pain, we pay particular attention to behaviors, personality factors, and comorbidities commonly encountered among individuals with HIV. Our examples are drawn from our experience running an inpatient multidisciplinary chronic pain program, and a chronic pain clinic that is embedded within an HIV primary care practice.

Behavior, abnormal illness behavior, and chronic pain

Definitions

Behavior
Behavior is a goal-directed activity that either increases or decreases based on the immediate response to the behavior from the environment. Thorndike first published "the law of effect"

Chronic Pain and HIV: A Practical Approach, First Edition.
Edited by Jessica S. Merlin, Peter A. Selwyn, Glenn J. Treisman and Angela G. Giovanniello.
© 2016 John Wiley & Sons, Ltd. Published 2016 by John Wiley & Sons, Ltd.

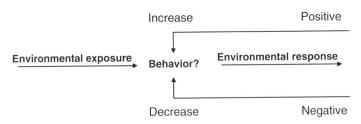

Figure 13.1 The law of effect.

in 1905 to describe this pattern of association between stimulus and response [1,2]. An overly simple representation is shown in Figure 13.1. In this diagram, the experience of a positive response from the environment will increase the likelihood of the behavior, whereas an adverse response will decrease the likelihood of the behavior. This is the essence of learning. In individuals with chronic pain, behaviors can be adaptive, such as increasing physical activity to improve pain, or maladaptive, such as limiting one's physical activity to avoid pain, or grimacing or groaning to gain attention.

A behaviorist approach applied to chronic pain helps us understand both the adaptive and maladaptive behaviors that we see can provide the basis for analyzing factors that delay recovery and amplify dysfunction. This approach can also provide a framework for a treatment plan that focuses on rehabilitation, function, quality of life, and healthy behavior [3].

Conditioning

Radical behaviorists such as Ivan Pavlov, John Watson, and B.F. Skinner developed behavioral models to explain human behavior. In the early 1900s, Pavlov described conditioning as the pairing of unrelated stimuli (such as the ringing of a tuning fork) with the presence of stimuli usually associated with a particular behavior (the presence of food is the stimuli for the behavior of salivation) [4]. Clinical examples of "classical" or "Pavlovian" conditioning include the gradual development of nausea in cancer patients when arriving at the cancer center even before the administration of chemotherapy. Many patients will spontaneously vomit on arrival to the clinic, even for visits that take place after chemotherapy has concluded. Opiate users who have experienced "cold turkey"

opiate withdrawal in a particular environment describe a similar phenomenon. Later, even if they have been opiate free for extended periods of time, they will experience withdrawal symptoms when exposed to that environment. Conditioned withdrawal can easily be produced in experimental animals using this paradigm.

Skinner later described operant conditioning as the shaping of behavior using positive or negative responses to the behavior [5]. He described four types of operant reinforcement. Positive reinforcement, where a behavior results in the delivery of something that is rewarding; negative reinforcement, where the behavior results in the removal of something unpleasant; punishment, where the behavior results in the delivery of something unpleasant; and extinction, where the behavior results in the removal or lack of delivery of something rewarding.

One of the first clinicians to apply behaviorist approaches for patients with chronic pain was William Fordyce, one of the academic leaders in Physical Medicine and Rehabilitation in the 20th century [6]. He noticed that patients who did well in rehabilitation differed from those who did poorly in terms of what they did rather than how they felt or the severity of their illness. After reading the work of Skinner, he decided to try to focus on using behavioral techniques to enhance the rehabilitative efforts of patients. He coined the term "pain behavior," which has been defined as the "any and all outputs of the individual that a reasonable observer would characterize as suggesting pain [7]." This includes verbal and visual demonstrations of pain (e.g., grimacing, groaning, and requests for assistance due to pain) and self-imposed functional restriction due to pain. These are maladaptive behaviors. Individuals with chronic

Table 13.1 Summary of operant conditioning as applied to the patient with chronic pain.

		Stimulus quality	
		Positive reinforcement	Negative reinforcement
Stimulus when behavior occurs	Deliver	Positive reinforcement Privileges Attention and praise Referral to specialists Access to tests and resources Legitimacy (behavior increases)	Punishment Restriction Informing outsiders of lack of cooperation (behavior decreases)
	Withdraw	Extinction Increasing rate of opioid taper Declining to order tests and consults Declining to provide resources Ignoring the behavior (behavior decreases)	Negative reinforcement Relief from outside criticism Removal of restriction Relief from responsibilities (behavior increases)

pain also display adaptive behaviors, such as participating in multidisciplinary therapies and working toward functional goals. Fordyce's work revealed that getting patients to display adaptive behaviors and counteracting maladaptive behaviors resulted in better outcomes, including improved overall function.

Table 13.1 summarizes the role of operant conditioning in the relationship between the provider and the patient with chronic pain. For example, when the provider notices that a patient is making even small steps toward meeting functional goals, delivery of positive reinforcement, such as attention and praise, promotes an increase in that behavior. In contrast, moaning and grimacing are maladaptive behaviors in individuals with chronic pain – they do not promote long-term function and can interfere with participation in work, school, and personal relationships. When a provider sees this type of behavior, positive reinforcement can be withdrawn, and the behavior can be ignored. This will promote extinction of the behavior. Other examples of how operant conditioning may be applied to chronic pain are provided in Table 13.1.

Abnormal illness behavior

Issy Pilowsky, a contemporary of Fordyce, used the term "abnormal illness behavior" for those behaviors that he saw in patients seeking the "sick role" despite a lack of physiological findings to support the degree of dysfunction they manifested [8]. More fundamentally, he described that these patients do not share the goal of rehabilitation and improving function with their doctor, but rather seem committed to continuing in the sick role.

Patients with abnormal illness behaviors often believe that they cannot do things that they do not feel emotionally inclined to do. As a result, they often say that they "can't" when they really mean "won't," including tasks such as attending physical therapy, engaging in psychological treatments, or tolerating medications that do not immediately relieve their discomfort. They often end up on treatments that have no pain efficacy (such as benzodiazepines) or have lost effectiveness (opiates) but do not continue treatments (even those that have been shown to be helpful to them) that are effective for the sensory component of their chronic pain.

The abnormal illness behaviors of patients with chronic pain are positively and negatively reinforced by numerous elements of their every-day existence. Common examples are shown in Table 13.2 and include disability payments and relief from expectations and criticisms of others.

In addition, commonly used pain therapies can inadvertently result in Pavlovian and operant conditioning that reinforces abnormal illness behavior. An important example is the prescription of opiates for chronic. Opiates reinforce behaviors (both pain-related behaviors and opiate-taking behaviors) through positive reinforcement (they act directly on reward pathways), negative reinforcement (they relieve ongoing discomfort and distress), and punishment (not taking opiates causes withdrawal) [16,18]. We oversaw the chronic pain care of an HIV-infected patient who described how he had been "outed" by his HIV-related illnesses at work, leading to a hostile work environment. He also struggled with rejection by his family related to having a male partner. His only real pleasures were windsailing in the summer and skiing in the winter. After a severe shoulder injury, he went to the ER where he received an injection of hydromorphone, after which he described a wonderful sense of "well-being." For a period of time, he didn't care about his family criticism, his work problems, or anything

Table 13.2 Examples of reinforcers of abnormal illness behavior.

Positive reinforcers
Opiates and benzodiazepines
Disability payments
Attention from spouses, family, doctors, and lawyers
Ability to express prohibited feelings

Negative reinforcers
Relief from requirements of work and related stress
Relief from expectations and criticism of others
Relief from depression and low self-esteem/negative
    self-worth
Relief from psychological discomfort and distress
Relief from pain and physical discomfort

Punishment
Opiate withdrawal
Benzodiazepine withdrawal

else. He was also given a note to be excused from work and told that he should be allowed to rest. He described how he remembered the note for work and the hydromorphone when he reinjured his shoulder the second time, and how he did not really "need" to go to the ER but went anyway and had a similar experience. He described how after those two experiences he began to actively seek opiates and eventually permanent disability from work. Running out of opiates after each of these experiences led him to fear withdrawal, which further fueled his desire to obtain opiates. When he was referred to the clinic, he was unemployed, without a partner, and essentially homeless. He missed the life he had before he had started opiates but was unable to imagine a life without opiates.

It is important to understand such abnormal illness behaviors in context. Although the clinician may react to the behavior as if it is a conscious effort by the patient to deceive them, patients are often unaware of the factors that condition them to behave in particular ways and feel that they "can't help it." Although the behavior the patient manifests is manipulative, it has become reflexive and feels automatic in such a way that the patient may be unaware of what they are doing, or be unable to control their behavior without clear input and direction. Cancer patients can be told the IV that they are getting is normal saline, but if they have been conditioned to vomit from repeated exposure to chemotherapy, they are unable to prevent the vomiting from occurring even if they "know" they are not getting chemotherapy.

Clinicians have been shown to prescribe opiates in response to nonverbal expressions of pain and are more likely to prescribe opiates in response to the emotional elements of pain with the result that distress is "reinforced" and increases over time [9].

Abnormal doctoring behavior

Western healthcare systems contribute to a variety of factors that reinforce the behaviors of vulnerable patients. The psychologist David Edwin has described "abnormal doctoring behavior" in much the way Issy Pilowsky described abnormal illness behavior (personal communication). Dr Edwin describes how patients and other factors inadvertently condition doctors to behave in maladaptive ways. Doctors are as susceptible to conditioning as any other organism. A variety of external forces are imposed on the medical practice that may condition doctors to inadvertently deliver care in ways that are less directed at health and more directed at other goals.

For example, in the HIV clinic, we recognize the benefit that patients can derive from getting disability and the resulting Medicare coverage. Hospitals want patients to get disability so they will have Medicare coverage, clinics want patients to have Medicare coverage so they will be paid for clinical services, and patients want to have Medicare coverage so they have access to clinical services. Although patients *can* always go back to work, they are less likely to do so once they start to receive payments for being ill. For patients with chronic pain, pressure not to work runs counter to the functional goals we ask our patients to set. David Edwin has also described how these factors reward doctors for giving patients what they request. The development of incentives around patient satisfaction, clinic efficiency, and reimbursement "push" doctors to see patients in a problem focused way, which often includes prescribing the drugs they want and completing the forms they request.

In the world of pain, perhaps the most striking example of this is the development of the visual analog pain scale and the imposed requirement to use it in medical practice [10]. Historically, a number of studies were published showing that doctors were reticent to prescribe opiates in terminal cancer patients because of reflexive concerns about opiate dependence. As was accurately pointed out by these studies, cancer pain was undertreated. In response, pain was made a "vital sign" as a result of political rather than scientific concern [11]. Reinforcing this concept, the Joint Commission on Accreditation of Healthcare Organizations adopted pain as the fifth vital sign as a quality standard and required the definition of "pain emergencies" and a response strategy for them. This type of thinking has led to a culture shift in medicine and raised the level of expectations of patients and providers alike that pain is something to be dealt with and eliminated. Due to other concurrent events (e.g., the marketing of Oxycontin as abuse-resistant, national policies

that encouraged providers to use more opioids and downplayed concerns of addiction), the response to this way of viewing pain has been to prescribe more opioids [19,20]. While opioids may reduce acute pain and may temporarily reduce chronic pain, evidence as to their ability to improve pain and function over the long term is very limited. In contrast to a purely pharmacologic approach, chronic pain typically requires a focus on chronic rehabilitation rather than a focus on suppression.

In another way of looking at this problem, our most vulnerable patients are conditioned by this paradigm to seek opioids and doctors are conditioned to prescribe them. For example, we have had many patients tell us that their pain score is above 8 and that they are therefore entitled to receive opioids due to their pain "emergency." We have also had patients who demand a specific dose and route of administration for medications. Physicians are conditioned to respond to these behaviors by prescribing opioids. Not surprisingly, clinicians have been shown to prescribe opiates in response to nonverbal expressions of pain and are more likely to prescribe opiates in response to the emotional elements of pain. This reinforces patient distress and leads to increased patient distress over time.9 While we can describe the pressures that result in increased opiate use for chronic nonmalignant pain with little data to support effectiveness for most of the types of chronic pain, this does not excuse the practice.

Table 13.3 shows some other examples of behavioral reinforcement of maladaptive behaviors for doctors and patients.

The role of personality in difficult patients

Models of personality traits

Personality or character is a set of behaviors that "characteristically" occur in response to a given stimulus [12]. Personality emerges out of the interaction between temperament (the natural affectively driven response to the stimulus) and learning (or "shaping") by the environment. The colloquialism "building character" is a

Table 13.3 Behavioral reinforcement of maladaptive behaviors for doctors and patients.

Normal doctor behavior	Abnormal doctor behavior	Reinforcer of abnormal doctor behavior	Maladaptive patient behavior reinforced
Diagnosis-directed treatment	Symptom-directed treatment	Short visits Financial efficiency	Focus on complaints
Rational strategic therapy for rehabilitation	Allowing patient to choose medications (opiates and benzodiazepines)	Patient "autonomy" Patient "satisfaction" and fear of complaints	Increasing medication dependence Using medication to cope
A single coordinating primary physician who communicates with consultants and controls treatment	Allowing patients to receive care from multiple noncommunicating sources	No reimbursement for time spent communicating Multiple barriers to physician communication (e.g., HIPPA)	Patients increasingly choosing doctors directed at comfort rather than rehabilitation "Splitting" of clinicians
Thorough formulation and individualized treatment planning	Using algorithms for treatment	Fear of criticism Increasing bureaucratic regulation of medical care with guidelines becoming "recipes"	Identification of themselves as a "patient" and increasing the sick role
Comprehensive assessment of the type of pain quality, location, mitigating and exacerbating features	Pain as a vital sign and linear assessment of pain severity	Increasing bureaucratic regulation of efficient medical care with required "measures" that oversimplify cases	Amplification of pain complaints and escalating need for narcotics to meet the target number on a visual analog scale

reasonably accurate description of the process of refining the behaviors that emerge from temperament to produce more successful and effective behaviors, as opposed to those that are counterproductive. We define temperament as a measurable human endowment or dimension, whereas we define personality as the developed style of interacting with the world that is a combination of temperament and learning or shaping. While different psychologists have measured temperament in different ways, we have found the dimensions described by Hans Eysenck are particularly applicable to the HIV clinic described more extensively in the book "The Psychiatry of AIDS [13,14]."

The model we use describes two dimensions of temperament, the introversion–extraversion axis and the stability–instability axis (Figure 13.2). In the figure, y-axis shows the frequency of a trait in the population and the x-axis shows the extreme of introversion at one end to that of extraversion at the other. The trait of introversion encompasses consequence avoidance, a focus on the future, and placing importance on function, whereas extraversion manifests as reward seeking a focus on now (the present), and assigns importance to feeling. The average person is in the center of the curve and has a temperament that has a balance of traits. People with an average temperament are able to function in most environments but are not "specialized" to excel in any particular environment. People with extreme endowments of introversion or extraversion are highly specialized, being extremely well suited to particular environments or tasks but poorly suited to others.

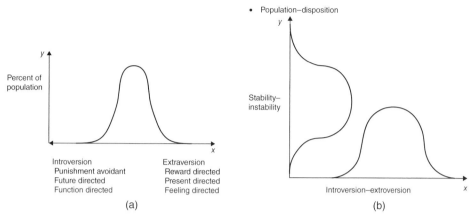

Figure 13.2 (a) A simplified diagram of the introversion–extraversion dimension. (b) Interaction between traits of stability–instability and introversion–extraversion.

Introverted styles are good for careful, detail-oriented, consequence-avoiding, and future-directed tasks, such as going to school, studying for tests, and evaluating situations requiring difficult decisions. Most physicians are introverted. They spend years studying for tests to avoid failing and going to school delaying gratification to obtain a professional status, checking patients' laboratory studies to avoid bad outcomes, and analyzing medication side effects to avoid toxicity. Salespeople, politicians, and entertainers tend to be extroverts. These individuals are charismatic, emotionally intense and dramatic, now-focused, and have a "get-it-done" attitude that allows them to galvanize people and complete projects.

In figure 13.2(b), the stability-instability dimension is displayed as orthogonal to the introversion-extraversion dimension. People with prominent instability (sometimes referred to as neuroticism) are emotionally reactive, exhibit a large emotional response to a given emotional stimulus, have the capacity for very intense emotions, and have variable or unpredictable emotional responses to stimuli. Stable people have modest, even muted emotional response to stimuli, a modest capacity for emotions, and a predictable emotional response to a given stimulus.

Extroverted patients try to solve problems immediately by trying to "feel better." In medical settings, they often seek out medical solutions that blunt pain at the cost of function and future capacity because of their nature. If they are also unstable, they act impulsively and find discomfort catastrophic. This brings an intense emotional pressure to the clinic because they "need" to feel better. In the setting of a heart attack or other true emergency, this might be an effective response, but in the face of a chronic disease such as HIV, or a chronic condition such as chronic pain, this style of response is ultimately ineffective and even destructive. Based on their style, they pressure doctors to give them opioids or benzodiazepines, and help them apply for disability, while declining rehabilitative interventions and long-term solutions that require patience and effort. The majority of difficult patients with personality disorders are unstable extroverts or "Cluster B" patients as described in the Diagnostic and Statistical Manual (DSM) of psychiatry [15].

DSM personality clusters

The DSM-V uses the term Cluster B (borderline, narcissistic, histrionic, or antisocial) personality disorders for those patients with heavy endowments of extraversion and instability. The subgroups overlap but share an unstable, reward-driven, now-focused, feeling oriented style. Cluster B patients all tend to have an unstable personality structure and are prone to negative, labile emotions. This quantitative dimension allows us to avoid pejorative terms like those above that "pathologize" personality styles while not recognizing their utility or strength. These patients are resilient to change in the environment, emotionally connected and reactive, and have charismatic capacity to emotionally manipulate others. These characteristics are often found in actors, politicians, rock stars, and CEOs of corporations.

Persons with strong, quick emotions who are more consequence avoidant have been called obsessive–compulsive, dependent, or avoidant. They fall within Cluster C, or unstable introverts. These patients tend to be challenging primary care and outpatient cases, but they are less common in the HIV clinic. When they do seek medical care, they are difficult because of their ambivalence about treatment and their obsessional styles that make it hard to get them to make decisions. These patients may end up with low T cells because they have been too ambivalent to act on problems until they become a crisis. They can frustrate clinicians with their back-and-forth style of medication taking and treatment decisions.

We also see Cluster A patients with schizoid, schizotypal, or paranoid personalities who tend not to be care seeking but can become infected with HIV and therefore are driven to come to clinic. They can be problematic in HIV care settings because of their reticence to accept care and/or actively avoiding care. They are best engaged to accept HIV care provided that they can intellectually understand the need for treatment. Also, because they are often introverted, clinicians have an easier time relating to their concerns and can persuade them to accept treatment.

Personality and behavior

Patients with these vulnerable personalities and temperaments soon realize that their ability to get what they want varies from shift to shift, from staff member to staff member, and from hospital to hospital. Unfortunately, for reward-seeking people, such an intermittent reinforcement schedule positively reinforces and therefore increases problematic behavior. In other words, if a patient is relatively insensitive to consequences and highly motivated to obtain a dose of intravenous opioid, she may visit multiple emergency rooms or pit staff against each other until she finally obtains her reward, a dose of medication. Although the providing team may try to talk to the patient about her inappropriate behavior, the message is clear to the patient: Increasingly problematic behavior will eventually bring about a reward.

A specific example is a 28-year-old female with a history of opioid and cocaine dependence who came to the clinic as a walk-in with suicidal ideation along with a very superficial cut on her wrist that did not require more than a simple dressing. She complained that "I was feeling real bad and I missed my methadone appointment and then I got to wanting to kill myself." On further questioning, she revealed that she missed her scheduled methadone appointment because she went out to use cocaine. It is easy to see how her extroverted and emotionally unstable temperament makes her impulsively try to solve her problem by disrupting the clinic. She has received methadone under these circumstances before to keep from having to call a formal psychiatric consult or send her to the emergency department. She even intimates that if she gets her methadone, she knows her suicidal feelings will probably resolve. It is easy to see in this example how the personality of the patient has played a role in making the patient's behavior ever more difficult.

The complicating role of other comorbid conditions in difficult patients

Several other psychiatric issues conspire to make patients more "difficult." These include disease states such as schizophrenia, bipolar disorder, and major depression as well as addictions and adverse life experiences. Cognitive impairment may also make assessing and communicating with patients more challenging. A comprehensive discussion of all of these disorders is beyond the scope of this chapter but it is important to note the role these diseases play in our interactions with patients.

Behaviorally based approaches to "difficult" patients with chronic pain

We know each other through behavior. We develop internal models of people to predict their likely behavioral responses to circumstances, and then test and refine those models with repeated experiences. Changing the way patients feel and think in reaction to their circumstances may change their behavior, but similarly, changing their behavior will change their feelings and thinking. Ultimately, behaviors become nearly automatic as they are shaped and reinforced by repetition and rehearsal. It is often difficult to change how patients feel if their temperaments are extreme or if their experiences have programmed them to behave in particular ways.

The complex nature of the interactions between temperament, life experience, episodes of mental illness, and years of classical and operant conditioning make for an overwhelmingly complex picture for many of our patients. Cognitive behavioral therapy uses this model and can help patients make profound changes that improve their quality of life and function. Focusing on behavior rather than feelings offers a more effective approach to rehabilitate patients who fail to respond to the usual pharmacologic and nonpharmacologic approaches to chronic pain treatment (see Chapter X).

We have a series of steps we follow to work with all chronic pain patients that we have outlined below. We have found these steps to be particularly important and useful in the care of the "difficult" patient. This simplistic rubric can be used by the primary care provider, and augmented by the care of a psychologist and other chronic pain specialists, if available, when problems arise.

Evaluation

All patients need a comprehensive evaluation for their chronic pain, and their medical and psychological conditions. The evaluation should include a thorough medical history including all available medical records, a careful physical examination including both neurological and mental state evaluation, and appropriate laboratory and radiological assessment. Anomalous findings should be worked up with appropriate consultation.

Diagnosis, treatment plan, and role induction

As described in Chapter 3 (Communication with Patients about Chronic Pain), most clinicians are working toward engaging the patient from the moment they start to evaluate them. We often discuss some elements of diagnosis and treatment during our evaluation. We find that it is useful to formally discuss the diagnosis and treatment plan at the end of the interview, particularly in patients who may have difficulty cooperating or engaging. We discuss the full formulation of the patient, including our belief about the nature of their pain, exacerbating physical and psychiatric factors, and our goals for treatment. With chronic nonmalignant pain, our goals are usually function, quality of life, and longevity (as opposed to comfort, passivity, and helplessness).

In lay terms, we discuss pain amplification syndromes, central sensitization, opiate-mediated hyperalgesia, and other mechanisms of chronic pain that patients often have not considered. We also discuss ongoing nervous system adaptation and the need for graded activation for the readjustment of the nervous system to increasing function. We point out that our goal is not the elimination of pain per se (although we certainly hope for that) but rather a gradual decrease in pain with a gradual increase in function. Techniques such as motivational interviewing (see Chapter 3) and cognitive behavioral therapy play an important role in this part of the treatment. While psychologists and psychiatrists are specifically trained in these approaches, primary care providers can participate in formal motivational interviewing training and learn cognitive behavioral approaches from their behavioralist colleagues.

In our diagnostic formulation, we often talk about the fact that pain has two parts, a somatosensory component and a distress component, and how we can affect both of these elements separately. We also discuss the nature of the person, acknowledging their frustration with an uncaring "system" that ignores their distress. We also point out when someone is "generously endowed" with feelings and emotions as described above, and that this endowment complicates their treatment and makes them tend to follow their feelings rather than their thinking. We discuss depression if appropriate and discuss how it can complicate pain as well.

As a part of this conversation, we describe the role of the doctor–patient relationship and the problems with that relationship. It is essentially one of unequal power and unfair by its very nature. The patient is ill and suffering, and we are not. We also describe that this means that the doctor must act in the patient's best interest in terms of health care, even if it means saying no to what the patient requests. This can be a challenge to explain, but it is critical that patients know we will advocate for their best interests (although not necessarily their stated interests). We explain how pain, addiction, depression, and desperation can impair autonomy, and that the relationship is one where a doctor "takes care of the patient" using judgment and a careful balance of the risks and benefits of the varying options for treatment.

After a careful discussion of what we intend to provide, including the limits of what we will provide, and what we expect of the patient, the patient must then decide if they will accept the treatment plan. We discuss the possibility that we are diagnostically wrong, that treatment may not work, that we may lack adequate skills to tackle the problem, but that this is the best we can offer. We tell patients that we will always be prepared to reassess our diagnostic formulation in case we are not succeeding according to the plan we have made. Unless acutely ill in a manner that needs immediate intervention, the patient is able to decline to enter into a treatment relationship or accept. There is always some other treatment choice, and we acknowledge this during this part of the conversation.

Personality features, past experiences, conditioned behavior, and suffering often make it hard for patients to live up to their commitment. Patience, encouragement, and support combined with firm limits must be applied over time

for success with these patients. Reiteration of what is wrong, why we are doing, what we are doing, and most importantly, constant pointing out of progress and improvement are essential to success. Patients who live in the "now" can be 95% improved, but will be as distressed about the 5% that remains as they were to begin with. Most of these patients respond well to positive reinforcement utilizing personalized attention, and enthusiastic encouragement.

Treat comorbid conditions

Make certain that the treatment plan provides for treatment of depression, personality features with cognitive behavioral theories, addictions, and medical comorbidities. It is important that someone is coordinating and monitoring the progress of the patient across all the areas of treatment, and to make sure the patient has not "split" the treatment team, getting one clinician to do something that is contrary to the treatment plan. This often means getting all the clinicians in the same room to discuss the plan of care.

Assessment of progress

As we just noted, it is essential to constantly remind our patients of their progress, but it is also essential to monitor the progress of treatment to make sure nothing is going wrong. Patients may be getting opiates from other sources, they may be less than forthcoming about their issues, and we might be wrong. Always consider that you may have missed something when treatment seems to stall.

Goals of treatment

We often take patients completely off opiates, but sometimes it can be useful for them to remain on a stable dose. This allows us to insist on progress, as the opiates are there to aid their recovery, not to make them comfortable while they remain debilitated. We set firm goals of a certain number of hours per day and week of "structured activity" with a requirement that patients make a time schedule and when possible, bring a collateral informant to validate their progress.

The behaviorally based treatment plan

With all patients, an outline of the behavioral goals is critical to success. "These are the things you will need to do to get better." Physical therapy, group therapy, mastery of individual exercises such as relaxation and biofeedback, and ongoing education are burdensome for patients but essential. We outline the expected schedule for our patients to give them structure and to increase their activity at a graded pace. As we note, generous encouragement will be required for most patients, and positive reinforcement is better than criticism for extraverts. Constant amendment to the plan is reasonable, provided the patients are doing their part. Many patients will provide decreasing progress for increasing praise, but praising success allows the clinician to overcome this obstacle. The occasional "I am sorry, you have not done any of the things you agreed to do, so we don't have anything to discuss about your chronic pain until you can make some progress" is a useful intervention. During this, advocacy for the patient in terms of getting them resources and trying to improve their regimen of medication for maximum benefit is a good form of positive reinforcement.

It isn't working, now what?

Clinicians tend to be harsh judges of their care and blame themselves for treatment failure. Similarly, patients often hold their providers responsible for their lack of cooperation and progress. This set of circumstances is a setup for frustration and failure. If patients repeatedly are unable to follow the treatment plan (they do not take the medications, cannot get to PT, cannot make it to their clinic appointments, forget that they have agreed to only obtain opiates from one clinic, and continue to seek other doctors who will provide treatments and tests that are not appropriate) it may be that some other doctor will be more successful, more convincing, or at least more compliant. We owe our patients the opportunity to get better and to try other options for care if they are unable to benefit from our interventions.

Patients do not follow the treatment recommendations for several reasons. One reason is that they disagree with the diagnosis. This is certainly a reasonable position and most of us are happy to explain our diagnostic reasoning and decision-making, and if the patients are still unconvinced, send them for a second opinion. A second reason is that patients disagree with the treatment. If they simply do not agree, this problem is identical to the one we have already discussed. For example, a patient may insist on a drug that is new to the market or is more convenient but has more risk for them specifically than another drug (such as might be seen with the choice between warfarin and dabigatran in a patient with a fall risk). Alternatively, the patient may have a specific goal, such as obtaining medications that are reinforcing such as opiates and benzodiazepines, that the clinician may feel are not indicated or are problematic. These issues often result in the patient feeling angry and unsatisfied with the treatment regardless of the reasonableness of the explanation for the clinical decision. The patient needs to decide if they wish to accept treatment as recommended or seek treatment elsewhere. A third reason is that the patient is unable to follow the treatment plan, sometimes due to limitations in resources or cognition. This needs further evaluation and planning by the treatment team.

Patient preference and patient satisfaction

It is reasonable to ask the question here: why not give the patient what they ask for? If they want to take dabigatran as an alternative to warfarin and have been informed of the risks, why not let them make the decision? Might we not be conflicted by our wish to save money and therefore may be conflicted in our decision-making process? Perhaps avoiding the blood draws is a reasonable choice despite the person having a risk for falls. If patients feel like they are better on benzodiazepines and opioids to manage their pain, why not provide them?

In the current environment of resource conservation, patient satisfaction, and consumer-focused treatment, we are all pressed to simply comply with the patient's wishes. The looming threat of multidrug-resistant bacteria, epidemic prescription opiate use, and the explosion of disability claims are consequences of our practice. We have a responsibility to practice medicine in ways that minimize risk and maximize benefit, even if it means saying "no" to patient requests and to the pressures from the healthcare system. Administrators see that patients on disability get Medicare benefits but do not see the tragic deterioration in function that patients undergo when they are paid to be sick instead of being supported in their efforts to get well. Work in our field becomes unrewarding when the goal is to appease administrators and patients instead of getting people well, leading to physician burnout, cynicism, and hopelessness.

An equally important element to saying "no" to patients is therapeutic optimism. Allowing patients access to comfort-directed treatments in lieu of restorative treatments is therapeutically nihilistic. It says in effect that we do not think we can get you better so we will make you comfortable. Saying "no" to the treatment demanded by the patient suggests that you think your treatment will help and get the person better. While patients may not like hearing "no," they are aware of the therapeutic optimism in saying "no" and trying to get them better.

The alternative to giving patients what they want is to simply refer them to other care. Having explained a diagnostic formulation and reasonable treatment plan, the patient who is uncooperative deserves the opportunity to seek alternative care. Other clinicians may be able to persuade them to see the reasons for your approach or may simply give the patient what they want. If you are correct in your appraisal, they will get worse in this scenario and may eventually return to your care ready for the help you offer. If they get better with someone else, this is a positive outcome. Telling patients you are happy to have them back if they decide that they wish to follow your prescription is a form of both patient advocacy and therapeutic optimism.

Summary

Chronic pain patients labeled as "difficult" in the HIV clinic are usually distinguished by their lack of cooperation with treatment. They may be unable to cooperate; a situation where mental illness, cognitive limitations or other vulnerabilities make it impossible for them; or they may be unwilling to cooperate due to their vulnerabilities.

In any case, a careful comprehensive evaluation including assessment of their pain, their psychiatric comorbidities, and their physical illness is the crucial first step. A diagnostic formulation of their illness must include the way in which the various elements of their condition exacerbate each other. Comorbid mental illness complicating when present needs treatment for the patient to be able to successfully recover from their chronic pain. Such patients benefit from a behaviorally based rehabilitation strategy to reduce illness behaviors and pain behaviors, and to focus on improving function, quality of life, and longevity.

References

1 Catania, A.C. (1999) Thorndike's legacy: learning, selection, and the law of effect. *Journal of Experimental Analysis of Behavior*, **72**, 425–428.

2 Thorndike, E.L. (1927) The law of effect. *American Journal of Psychology*, **39**, 212–222.

3 Keefe, F.J., Dunsmore, J. & Burnett, R. (1992) Behavioral and cognitive-behavioral approaches to chronic pain: recent advances and future directions. *Journal of Consulting and Clinical Psychology*, **60** (4), 528–536.

4 Pavlov, I.P. (1927) *Conditioned Reflexes: An Investigation of the Physiological Activity of the Cerebral Cortex (translated by G.V. Anrep)*. Oxford University Press, London.

5 Skinner, B.F. (1938) *The Behavior of Organisms: An Experimental Analysis*. Appleton-Century, Oxford, England, 457 pp.

6 Fordyce, W.E. (1976) *Behavioral methods for chronic pain and illness*. St. Louis, MO. Mosby.

7 Loeser J.D., Fordyce W.E. (1983) Chronic pain. In: J.E. C'arr, H.A. Dengerink (eds). *Behavioral Science in the Practice of Medicine*, Elsevier, Amsterdam.

8 Pilowsky, I. (1969) Abnormal illness behavior. *British Journal of Medical Psychology*, **42**, 347–351.

9 Turk, D.C. & Okifuji, A. (1997) What factors affect physicians' decisions to prescribe opioids

for chronic noncancer pain patients? *Clinical Journal of Pain,* **13**, 330–336.

10 Carlsson, A.M. (1983) Assessment of chronic pain. I. Aspects of the reliability and validity of the visual analogue scale. *Pain,* **16**, 87–101.

11 Walid, M.S., Donahue, S.N., Darmohray, D.M., Hyer, L.A. & Robinson, J.S. (2008) The fifth vital sign – what does it mean? *Pain Practice*, **8**, 417–422.

12 Allport, G.W. (1937) *Personality: A Psychological Interpretation*. England, Holt, Oxford, 588 pp.

13 Eysenck, H.J. (1991) Dimensions of personality: 16 or 5 or 3? Criteria for a taxonomic paradigm. *Personality and Individual Differences*, **12**, 773–790.

14 Treisman, G.J. & Angelino, A.F. (2004) *The Psychiatry of AIDS: A Guide to Diagnosis and Treatment*. Johns Hopkins University Press, Baltimore, 244 pp.

15 American Psychiatric Association (2013) *Diagnostic and Statistical Manual of Mental Disorders,* 5th edn. American Psychiatric Press Inc., Washington, DC.

16 Treisman, G.J., Clark, M.R.. (2011) Chronic Pain and Addictions; A behaviorist perspective. *Adv Psychosom Med*. **30**: 8–21.

17 Gardner, E.L. (2011) Addiction and brain reward and antireward pathways. *Advances in Psychosomatic Medicine*, **30**, 22–60.

18 Haas, L.J., Leiser, J.P., Magill, M.K. & Sanyer, O.N. Management of the difficult patient. *Am Fam Physician*. (2005) Nov 15;**72**(10):2063–2068.

19 Manchikanti, L., Helm, S., Fellows, B. *et al.* (2012) Opioid epidemic in the United States. *Pain Physician*, **15** (3 Suppl), ES-9–38.

20 Marcus, D.A. (2000) Treatment of nonmalignant chronic pain. *American Family Physician*, **61** (5), 1331–1338.

CHAPTER 14

HIV-related pain in low- and middle-income countries with reference to sub-Saharan Africa

Richard Harding[1], Irene J. Higginson[1] and Liz Gwyther[2]

[1] Department of Palliative Care, Policy, & Rehabilitation, Cicely Saunders Institute, King's College London, London, United Kingdom
[2] School of Public Health and Family Medicine, University of Cape Town, Chair, World Hospice and Palliative Care Alliance, Cape Town, South Africa

Epidemiology of HIV in low-resource regions

The most recent estimates from UNAIDS demonstrate that the greatest burden of HIV disease falls on low- and middle-income countries [1]. The greatest HIV prevalence continues to be in sub-Saharan Africa, where generalized epidemics are common and formal health resources and services are weakest. UNAIDS estimates that during 2012, there were 25 million people living with HIV, 1.6 million new infections, and 1.2 million HIV-related deaths. The UNAIDS 2012 data also report that South Africa has 6.1 million people living with HIV infection and 240,000 HIV-related deaths (the highest burden of any country in the world). Therefore, in this chapter, we focus on sub-Saharan Africa as it has the greatest burden of HIV disease and the largest body of research evidence among low- and middle-income countries.

The concept of pain

The concept of "total pain" is useful when trying to define, assess, and manage pain among people living with HIV disease. HIV is clearly understood as impacting on the physical, psychological, social, and spiritual domains of an infected person's life. "Total pain" was proposed as a way of understanding the subjective nature of pain and guides clinical assessment and care to pay attention to all domains of need in order to adequately manage pain [2]. This model of "total pain" has been successfully used to systematically review the needs of HIV patients, including physical pain, psychological distress, social, and existential problems [3]. This multidimensional approach to measuring patient outcomes is incorporated in the African Palliative Care Association's (APCA) African Palliative Outcome Scale (POS) – a brief tool that measures all four dimensions of "total pain" in line with the WHO definition [4,5].

The concept of "total pain" was developed by Cicely Saunders in Western Europe and has been adopted globally. However, assessing "total pain" needs is very different without the background of a well-resourced welfare system. Therefore, when addressing "total pain" needs in a low- or middle-income country, other familywide needs such as food security, housing, travel to care, and planning orphan needs are also likely to be sources of pain. The range of needs of African patients with advanced HIV or cancer has been well described and includes pain relief, counseling, and financial assistance for basic needs such as food, shelter, and school

Chronic Pain and HIV: A Practical Approach, First Edition.
Edited by Jessica S. Merlin, Peter A. Selwyn, Glenn J. Treisman and Angela G. Giovanniello.
© 2016 John Wiley & Sons, Ltd. Published 2016 by John Wiley & Sons, Ltd.

fees for their children [6]. Interestingly, a comparative study found that the emotional pain of facing death was the prime concern of Scottish patients and their carers, whereas physical pain and financial worries dominated the lives of Kenyan patients and their carers [7]. The concept of total pain has been well articulated by HIV patients living in East Africa, in a research paper titled *"My dreams are shuttered down and it hurts a lot* [8]*."* This study of 189 in-depth interviews described the components of total pain experienced by patients and families affected by HIV in Africa and as observed by their formal healthcare providers. Patients explained that they did not routinely report their pain to their clinicians as they felt it was not of interest during their care appointments, and staff reported their difficulties in accessing analgesia to control pain. Pain is exacerbated by stigma, poverty, and worry. A study to determine what constitutes quality of life in advanced HIV or cancer patients found that relationships, feeling at peace, meaning in life, and being active were all ranked as more important than physical comfort; therefore, understanding what matters to the patient is essential when planning care to optimize quality of life [9].

The data supporting a concept of "total pain" underline the importance of person-centered multidimensional structured and regular assessment in order to understand the origins, manifestations, and likely effective management of pain in its broadest sense, especially where social needs are great and economic resources few.

Prevalence and correlates of pain

While much pain advocacy in Africa and other low- and middle-income settings has focused on the provision of effective pain relief in advanced disease, a study of the needs of 438 newly diagnosed HIV patients in East Africa found that 19.4% scored on the worst half of the response scale for pain experienced in the previous 3 days (independent of CD4 count or ART eligibility) [10]. Pain and symptoms were associated with worse physical function and worse poverty. A further systematic review of the evidence found that pain prevalence within 6 months of diagnosis was reported to be 69–76% in studies of inpatients (69% in severe pain) and outpatients (76% of AIDS patients reporting pain) [3]. Data from Uganda revealed a pain 7-day-period prevalence of 51.3% among HIV outpatient attendees [11], and again pain was the most common symptom with a 7-day-period prevalence of 76% at the time of diagnosis, with over half of these (56%) reporting severe pain [12]. The associated distress was highest (i.e., worst five response levels on a range of five points of a Likert Scale, labeled "Quite a bit" or "Very much") among 20.2% of the sample. Pain was the seventh most prevalent physical symptom and the first most distressing. Overall physical symptom burden (including pain) was greater for women later WHO clinical stage, lower CD4 count, and worse physical performance score. No association was found for current ART use. Among HIV patients receiving palliative care in South Africa and Uganda, pain had a greater burden than the other patient-oriented items on POS of symptoms, worry, sharing feelings, feeling life worthwhile, feeling at peace, or receiving enough information [13]. A further two-country study of HIV palliative care patients in sub-Saharan Africa found pain to have the highest 7-day-period prevalence at 82.6%, and the second most burdensome (35.3% scoring the worst intensity scores) after hunger. Among ambulatory outpatients in Uganda, 47% reported 7-day-period prevalence of pain, and 27% reported severe pain [14]. Importantly, increased pain intensity was associated with poorer quality of life. The number of patients likely to require pain relief in hospital settings has also been measured, with a census of all inpatients at a national referral hospital in Uganda finding that 28% of inpatients were diagnosed with HIV infection, and 52% scored on the worst half on the self-report pain intensity scale [15].

For patients specifically on ART, a South African study found pain to be the third most prevalence symptom (53% 7-day-period prevalence) and the seventh most burdensome (29.1% with worst responses on the pain score) [16]. The patient-reported burden was worse for those longer on treatment [17].

Public and patient preferences for pain relief

Several population-based surveys are being conducted in sub-Saharan Africa to determine the preferences and priorities of the public if they were to be faced with serious illness. Interestingly, when prioritizing their greatest concerns in advanced disease, respondents surveyed in Kenya ranked "Having pain and discomfort relieved" third after "Keeping a positive attitude" and "Making sure friends and relatives are not worried and distressed [18]." However, when asked to rank the most concerning symptom or problem, pain was ranked as first by a majority (28.4%) over other problems such as being a burden to others (second), psychological distress (third), and breathlessness (fourth). When this survey was replicated in Namibia, as in Kenya respondents ranked "Having pain and discomfort relieved" third after "Keeping a positive attitude," and "Making sure friends and relatives are not worried and distressed," and pain was also ranked first out of most concerning symptoms or problems (26.1%) [19]. These data contrast to the same survey conducted in seven European countries, where "Keeping a positive attitude" and "Having and pain and discomfort relieved" were joint first priority (36%) [20]. This comparison reveals the difference in care planning and priorities between collectivist and individualistic societies and that treatment plans in sub-Saharan Africa must include the family's concerns.

Measurement of pain

A systematic review found that the lack of locally developed and validated outcome measures was responsible for the absence of evidence of relief of problems among people with HIV, including pain relief [21]. In response to this, we consulted HIV care providers in Africa who pointed to the need for tools to measure care outcomes [22], consulted with healthcare professionals to determine the optimal tool features [23], developed a tool across eight countries in Africa [24], and subjected it to full validation [25]. This tool is now embedded into quality standards and quality guidance across Africa.

Subsequent factor analysis of the tool known as the African Palliative Care Association (APCA) African Palliative Outcome Scale (POS) has demonstrated that a factor exists that combines the three pain symptoms and worry item to construct a factor that is termed "physical and psychological [26]." Given the importance of a sense of peace (described above) as a core construct in quality of life for people with advanced disease, we have advanced measurement of spiritual well-being to form a component of outcome measurement alongside pain, symptoms, and psychological well-being [27].

The measurement of pain among people with HIV in sub-Saharan Africa has been greatly enhanced by the development and validation of the African Palliative Care Association African Palliative Outcome Scale (APCA African POS). The POS family of tools is brief and simple, and measures the severity of problems and concerns among people with life-limiting or life-threatening conditions (www.pos-pal.org). The POS provides full support free online resources, and the APCA POS is widely implemented across Africa to direct care, audit services, train and educate, allocate resources, and conduct research [28]. It has been fully validated [25], and it can be analyzed by item (including pain) and by factors [29]. It offers a novel scoring system, which has been validated showing that scoring using hands and fingers provides good sensitivity and specificity when measuring pain [30]. In addition to cross-sectional studies [31,32], it has been used in longitudinal audit [33] and as an outcome measure in an HIV pain trial in Malawi [34]. The pain item in POS has been identified by users in Africa and Europe as one of the most useful in the tool [35]. The essential spiritual dimension to the experience of disease progression and especially pain has been identified among second-generation African–Caribbean British cancer patients [36]. Within the APCA African POS, African practitioners report pain as being the most important item within the 10 items, with 55% of respondents ranking it as the most important item [37].

A subsequent systematic review of palliative care for children has found a similar absence of a tool to specifically measure outcomes for children in Africa [38], and so the pediatric POS is now under validation [39].

Drug availability

The WHO pain ladder [40] clearly demonstrates the necessity of nonopioids, weak opioids, and strong opioids plus adjuvants. The WHO strategy for palliative care integration into public health systems states that policy and drug availability are key [40], and much effort has been placed on opioid availability. Within Africa, Hospice Africa Uganda has served as a model country in terms of being the first African country to have palliative care in its National Health Plan [41], the first to enable trained nurses to prescribe opioids and the first to undertake a rollout programme to provide opioids throughout health districts [42]. Further evaluation of the WHO public health strategy to expand opioid use in Zambia has found advocacy and funding strategies that center on the WHO model have increased the reliable supply of analgesics, advocacy with the Ministry of Health has improved the policy environment, and healthcare professionals feel more confident in delivering pain relief [43].

However, data have revealed that within 120 HIV care facilities across two countries in East Africa (Uganda and Kenya), only 7% of facility pharmacies stocked morphine, drug availability was generally worse in health centers and home-based care settings compared to hospitals, and that stockouts were frequent [44]. Even nonopioid analgesics had been subject to a stockout in the previous 6 months in almost half the facilities (47%).

Pain management and advocacy

Studies to determine the effectiveness of pain relief strategies for people living with HIV in low- and middle-income countries are few, with most evidence historically emerging from high-income settings and pre-ART. The study designs have been mainly observational. In Tanzania, integration of palliative care to manage pain and other symptoms for all patients attending with HIV disease (irrespective of disease stage) has shown to be highly effective in improving patient-reported outcomes [45]. Audit studies have embedded continuous quality improvement into services providing advanced care and have demonstrated that locally determined pain control targets can be set and achieved [33]. Beyond sub-Saharan Africa, a further comparative observational study in Vietnam found that a palliative care intervention improved pain management practice and patient satisfaction among HIV patients [46].

Resources

There are a number of key, free of charge, and open access clinical resources for HIV pain relief that have been produced by and for African settings. The guidance is largely a product of the National/pan-African Palliative Care Associations, who have been responsible for promoting pain and symptom relief from the point of diagnosis, alongside treatment, and into advanced disease stages in line with WHO and UNAIDS guidance.

Health Resources and Services Administration (HRSA)

A clinical guide to supportive and palliative care for HIV/AIDS in sub-Saharan Africa: http://www.hospiceafrica.or.ug/index.php/blue-book/category/3-blue-book

Hospice Palliative Care Association of South Africa (HPCA): http://www.hpca.co.za/category/clinical-guidelines.html

African Palliative Care Association (APCA), core competencies including pain relief http://www.africanpalliativecare.org/images/stories/pdf/Core_Competency.pdf

African Palliative Care Association (APCA), core curriculum including pain relief: http://www.africanpalliativecare.org/images/stories/pdf/Palliative_Care_Core_Curriculum.pdf

Quality standards including pain relief: http://
www.africanpalliativecare.org/images/
stories/pdf/APCA_Standards.pdf

Guidelines for POS use: http://www.african
palliativecare.org/images/stories/pdf/POS_
Guidelines.pdf

Pocket guide to pain management: http://www
.africanpalliativecare.org/images/stories/
pdf/POS_Guidelines.pdf

Guide to opioid use for pain relief: http://www
.africanpalliativecare.org/images/stories/
pdf/using_opiods.pdf

Hospice Africa Uganda (HAU)/Palliative Care
Association of Uganda (PCAU), pain and
symptom control in the cancer and/or
AIDS patient in Uganda and other African
countries: http://www.hospiceafrica.or.ug/
images/attachements/blue%20book%
20english.pdf

Palliative Outcome Scale (POS): www.pos-pal
.org

References

1 UNAIDS. (2013) UNAIDS report on the global
HIV epidemic 2012.

2 Saunders, C. (1978) *The Management of Terminal Malignant Disease*, 1st edn. Edward Arnold,
London.

3 Simms, V.M., Higginson, I.J. & Harding, R.
(2011) What palliative care-related problems
do patients experience at HIV diagnosis? A
systematic review of the evidence. *Journal of
Pain and Symptom Management*.

4 Powell, R.A., Downing, J., Harding, R.,
Mwangi-Powell, F. & Connor, S. (2007)
Development of the APCA African Palliative
Outcome Scale. *Journal of Pain and Symptom
Management*, **33** (2), 229–232.

5 Harding, R., Selman, L., Agupio, G. *et al.* (2010)
Validation of a core outcome measure for palliative care in Africa: the APCA African Palliative Outcome Scale. *Health and Quality of Life
Outcomes*, **8**, 10.

6 Kikule, E. (2003) A good death in Uganda: survey of needs for palliative care for terminally
ill people in urban areas. *BMJ*, **327** (7408),
192–194.

7 Murray, S.A., Grant, E., Grant, A. & Kendall,
M. (2003) Dying from cancer in developed and
developing countries: lessons from two qualitative interview studies of patients and their
carers. *BMJ*, **326** (7385), 368–371.

8 Selman, L., Simms, V., Penfold, S. *et al.* (2013)
My dreams are shuttered down and it hurts
lots – a qualitative study of palliative care
needs and their management by HIV outpatient services in Kenya and Uganda. *BMC
Palliative Care*, **12** (1), 35.

9 Selman, L.E., Higginson, I.J., Agupio, G. *et al.*
(2011) Quality of life among patients receiving
palliative care in South Africa and Uganda: a
multi-centred study. *Health and Quality of Life
Outcomes*, **9** (1), 21.

10 Simms V, Gikaara N, Munene G, Atieno M,
Kataike J, Nsubuga C, *et al.* (2013) Multidimensional patient-reported problems within
two weeks of HIV diagnosis in East Africa: a
multicentre observational study. *PLoS One*, **8**
(2), e57203.

11 Namisango, E., Powell, R.A., Atuhaire, L.,
Katabira, E.T., Mwangi-Powell, F. & Harding,
R. (2013) Is symptom burden associated with
treatment status and disease stage among
adult HIV outpatients in East Africa? *Journal of
Palliative Medicine*.

12 Wakeham, K., Harding, R., Bamukama-
Namakoola, D. *et al.* (2010) Symptom burden
in HIV-infected adults at time of HIV diagnosis
in rural Uganda. *Journal of Palliative Medicine*,
13 (4), 375–380.

13 Harding, R., Selman, L., Agupio, G. *et al.* (2012)
Intensity and correlates of multidimensional
problems in HIV patients receiving integrated
palliative care in sub-Saharan Africa. *Sexually
Transmitted Infections*, **88** (8), 607–611.

14 Namisango, E., Harding, R., Atuhaire, L. *et al.*
(2012) Pain among ambulatory HIV/AIDS
patients: multicenter study of prevalence,
intensity, associated factors, and effect. *The
Journal of Pain*, **13** (7), 704–713.

15 Lewington, A.J., Namukwaya, E., Limoges, J.,
Leng, M. & Harding, R. (2012) Provision of
palliative care for life-limiting disease in a low
income country national hospital setting: how
much is needed? *BMJ Support Palliative Care.*,
2, 140–144.

16 Farrant, L., Gwyther, L., Dinat, N., Mmoledi,
K., Hatta, N. & Harding, R. (2012) The prevalence and burden of pain and other symptoms
among South Africans attending highly active

antiretroviral therapy (HAART) clinics. *South African Medical Journal*, **102** (6), 499–500.

17 Farrant, L., Gwyther, L., Dinat, N., Mmoledi, K., Hatta, N. & Harding, R. (2014) Maintaining wellbeing for South Africans receiving ART: the burden of pain and symptoms is greater with longer ART exposure. *South African Medical Journal*, **104** (2), 119–123.

18 Downing, J., Gomes, B., Gikaara, N. *et al.* (2014) Public preferences and priorities for end-of-life care in Kenya: a population-based street survey. *BMC Palliative Care*, **13** (1), 4.

19 Powell, R.A., Namisango, E., Gikaara, N. *et al.* (2013) Public priorities and preferences for end-of-life care in Namibia. *Journal of Pain and Symptom Management*.

20 Higginson, I.J., Gomes, B., Calanzani, N. *et al.* (2014) Priorities for treatment, care and information if faced with serious illness: a comparative population-based survey in seven European countries. *Palliative Medicine*, **28** (2), 101–110.

21 Harding, R. & Higginson, I.J. (2005) Palliative care in sub-Saharan Africa. *Lancet*, **365** (9475), 1971–1977.

22 Harding, R., Stewart, K., Marconi, K., O'Neill, J. & Higginson, I. (2003) Current HIV/AIDS end-of-life care in sub-Saharan Africa: a survey of models, services, challenges and priorities. *BMC Public Health*, **3**.

23 Harding, R., Dinat, N. & Mpanga, S.L. (2007) Measuring and improving palliative care in South Africa: multiprofessional clinical perspectives on development and application of appropriate outcome tools. *Progress in Palliative Care*, **15** (2), 55–59.

24 Powell, R.A., Downing, J., Harding, R., Mwangi-Powell, F. & Connor, S. (2007) Apca. Development of the APCA African Palliative Outcome Scale. *Journal of Pain and Symptom Management*, **33** (2), 229–232.

25 Harding, R., Selman, L., Agupio, G. *et al.* (2010) Validation of a core outcome measure for palliative care in Africa: the APCA African Palliative Outcome Scale. *Health and Quality of Life Outcomes*, **8**, 10.

26 Harding, R., Selman, L., Simms, V.M. *et al.* (2013) How to analyze palliative care outcome data for patients in Sub-Saharan Africa: an international, multicenter, factor analytic examination of the APCA African POS. *Journal of Pain and Symptom Management*, **45** (4), 746–752.

27 Selman, L., Harding, R., Higginson, I., Gysels, M., Speck, P. & Encompass-Collaborative (2011) Spiritual wellbeing in sub-Saharan Africa: the meaning and prevalence of 'feeling at peace'. *BMJ Support Palliative Care*, **1** (Suppl 1), A22.

28 Defilippi, K. & Downing, J. (2013) Feedback from African palliative care practitioners on the use of the APCA POS. *International Journal of Palliative Nursing*, **19** (12), 577–581.

29 Harding R, Selman L, Simms V, Penfold S, Agupio G, Dinat N, *et al.* (2012) How to analyse palliative care outcome data for patients in sub-Saharan Africa: an international multi-centred factor analytic examination of the APCA African POS. *Journal of Pain and Symptom Management*, In Press.

30 Blum, D., Selman, L.E., Agupio, G. *et al.* (2014) Self-report measurement of pain & symptoms in palliative care patients: a comparison of verbal, visual and hand scoring methods in Sub-Saharan Africa. *Health and Quality of Life Outcomes*, **12** (1), 118.

31 Harding, R., Selman, L., Agupio, G. *et al.* (2012) Prevalence, burden, and correlates of physical and psychological symptoms among HIV palliative care patients in sub-Saharan Africa: an international multicenter study. *Journal of Pain and Symptom Management*, **44** (1), 1–9.

32 Harding, R., Simms, V., Penfold, S. *et al.* (2014) Quality of life and wellbeing among HIV outpatients in East Africa: a multicentre observational study. *BMC Infectious Diseases*, **14** (1), 613.

33 Harding, R., Gwyther, L., Mwangi-Powell, F., Powell, R.A. & Dinat, N. (2010) How can we improve palliative care patient outcomes in low- and middle-income countries? Successful outcomes research in sub-Saharan Africa. *Journal of Pain and Symptom Management*, **40** (1), 23–26.

34 Nkhoma, K., Seymour, J. & Arthur, A. (2013) An educational intervention to reduce pain and improve pain management for Malawian people living with HIV/AIDS and their family carers: study protocol for a randomised controlled trial. *Trials*, **14**, 216.

35 Higginson, I.J., Simon, S.T., Benalia, H. *et al.* (2012) Republished: which questions of two commonly used multidimensional palliative

care patient reported outcome measures are most useful? Results from the European and African PRISMA survey. *Postgraduate Medical Journal*, **88** (1042), 451–457.

36 Koffman, J., Morgan, M., Edmonds, P., Speck, P. & Higginson, I.J. (2008) Cultural meanings of pain: a qualitative study of Black Caribbean and White British patients with advanced cancer. *Palliative Medicine*, **22** (4), 350–359.

37 Higginson, I.J., Simon, S.T., Benalia, H. *et al.* (2012) Republished: which questions of two commonly used multidimensional palliative care patient reported outcome measures are most useful? Results from the European and African PRISMA survey. *Postgraduate Medical Journal*, **88** (1042), 451–457.

38 Harding, R., Albertyn, R., Sherr, L. & Gwyther, L. (2013) Pediatric palliative care in Sub-Saharan Africa: a systematic review of the evidence for care models, interventions, and outcomes. *Journal of Pain and Symptom Management*.

39 Downing J, Atieno M, Powell RA, Ali Z, Marston J, Meiring M, *et al.* (2012) Development of a palliative care outcome measure for children in sub-Saharan Africa: findings from early phase instrument development. *European Journal of Palliative Care*, In Press.

40 World Health Organization (1996) *Cancer Pain Relief: With a Guide to Opioid Availability*. WHO, Geneva.

41 Merriman, A. & Harding, R. (2010) Pain control in the African context: the Ugandan introduction of affordable morphine to relieve suffering at the end of life. *Philosophy, Ethics, and Humanities in Medicine*, **5**, 10.

42 Logie, D.E. & Harding, R. (2005) An evaluation of a morphine public health programme for cancer and AIDS pain relief in Sub-Saharan Africa. *BMC Public Health*, **5**, 82.

43 Logie, D.E. & Harding, R. (2012) An evaluation of a public health advocacy strategy to enhance palliative care provision in Zambia. *BMJ Supportive and Palliative Care*, **2** (4), 276.

44 Harding, R., Simms, V., Penfold, S. *et al.* (2013) Availability of essential drugs for managing HIV-related pain and symptoms within 120 PEPFAR-funded health facilities in East Africa: a cross-sectional survey with onsite verification. *Palliative Medicine*.

45 Harding, R., Simms, V., Alexander, C. *et al.* (2012) Can palliative care integrated within HIV outpatient settings improve pain and symptom control in a low-income country? A prospective, longitudinal, controlled intervention evaluation. *AIDS Care*.

46 Green, K., Tuan, T., Hoang, T.V., Trang, N.N., Ha, N.T. & Hung, N.D. (2010) Integrating palliative care into HIV outpatient clinical settings: preliminary findings from an intervention study in Vietnam. *Journal of Pain and Symptom Management*, **40** (1), 31–34.

CHAPTER 15

Pain at the end of life in individuals with AIDS

Alen Voskanian

David Geffen School of Medicine, University of California, Los Angeles, VITAS Healthcare, Los Angeles, CA, USA

Introduction

Pain is underrecognized and undertreated in as many as 60–85% of HIV patients in the developed world [1]. Although patients with cancer often experience pain at the end of life, patients with other nonmalignant terminal illnesses such as AIDS also suffer from pain during the end-of-life period. Patients in the last hours and days of life often have uncontrolled physical pain in addition to significant emotional, spiritual, and social distress [2]. Dr Cicely Saunders conceptualized pain associated with the dying process as "total pain" consisting of physical pain, emotional pain, interpersonal conflict, and nonacceptance of one's own dying [2]. Total pain management is extremely important in patients dying from AIDS since they often tend to be younger in age and have significant suffering related to interpersonal and emotional issues. Therefore, not only physical pain management but also total pain management is critical at the end of life in patients with HIV [3,4].

This section addresses management of pain in the last hours and days of life. The most relevant ethical issues related to pain management at the end of life will also be discussed.

Prevalence

Ninety-three percent of patients dying from HIV/AIDS recorded pain at the end of life [5]. The pain prevalence has decreased over the last decade due to antiretroviral therapy. Uncontrolled pain at the end of life is highly distressing [6]. Uncontrolled pain also leads to decline in functioning and quality of life. As patients approach death, their pain characteristics change, thereby requiring ongoing modification and adjustment of medications.

Mortality rates

Based on the World Health Organization, 1.5 million people died of AIDS-related illnesses worldwide in 2013 [7]. Based on data from the Centers for Disease Control and Prevention, as estimated 13,834 people with an AIDS diagnosis died in 2011 [8]. The recorded deaths are not exclusively caused by AIDS and can be due to any other causes. The Antiretroviral Therapy Cohort Collaboration examined specific causes of mortality in HIV-infected patients in Europe and North America from 1996 to 2006. They analyzed 1876 patients who had died and were able to assign a definitive cause in 85% (1597) of deaths; 49.5% (792) were AIDS related, followed by non-AIDS malignancies in 11.8% (189), non-AIDS infections in 82% (131), violence and/or drug-related cause in 7.7% (124), liver disease in 7% (113), and cardiovascular disease in 6.5% (103) [9].

This highlights the fact that the cause of mortality in patients with HIV infection is changing. Patients with HIV who are dying from other causes such as cardiovascular disease will have pain symptoms that might present differently and will require different interventions. Therefore, pain management in patients with HIV at the end of life can be complicated due to the presence of multiple comorbidities.

Barriers to effective pain management

There are multiple barriers for effective pain management at the end of life. These barriers fall under three main categories:

1 Clinician barriers
2 Patient barriers
3 Regulatory barriers.

Clinician barriers include inadequate pain assessment and reassessment. The end-of-life period is very dynamic and pain levels fluctuate. Therefore, pain needs to be reassessed frequently. Other clinician-related barriers include inadequate education and unfound biases within the healthcare providers. Studies have demonstrated that minority status, older age, history of substance abuse, and female gender are associated with a higher likelihood of undertreatment of pain. Sixty-five percent of minority patients did not receive guideline-recommended analgesic prescriptions compared with 50% of nonminority patients [10,11]. Given that a large number of patients dying from HIV/AIDS are minorities, this barrier can lead to significant undermanagement of pain. Other clinician barriers include the fear of hastening death with opioids as well as concerns regarding potential substance abuse or addiction [12].

Patient barriers include reluctance to report pain, desire to please clinicians, fear of addiction, and issues related to cost and copayments for medications. Furthermore, patients might believe that acceptance and reporting of pain might be equivalent to giving up and denial of pain might be used as a psychological coping mechanism.

Regulatory barriers include constraints by federal and state regulatory bodies to insure safe prescribing of opioids. A recent increase in prescribed opioid-related deaths has increased the amount of scrutiny and monitoring by regulatory bodies to insure safety, and this in turn has led to challenges in delivering opioids to dying patients in a timely manner. While the increased scrutiny is not aimed at terminally ill patients, the overall environment has created misconceptions and some prescribers have become hesitant to prescribe opioids even when necessary in terminally ill patients.

Total pain management

Physical pain management at the end of life only addresses one dimension. In addition to treating physical pain, emotional, psychosocial, and spiritual issues need to be discussed and addressed. Pain can optimally be managed when all of the dimensions have been addressed. In patients with HIV/AIDS, there are often many unresolved psychosocial issues that get heightened at the end of life. The stigma associated with HIV can severely influence those infected with the virus and they might not disclose the diagnosis to their loved ones or family members. This might lead to social isolation and lost connections with family members. Clinicians can play a large role in assisting patients and families with the disclosure process by addressing fears and dispelling myths [13].

HIV disease often affects younger patients, and this creates unique challenges that need to be addressed at the end of life. Psychological issues such as depression, anxiety, and fear are common symptoms in patients with AIDS. The best way to address total pain is by using an interdisciplinary approach containing social workers, chaplains, nurses, and physicians.

Pain assessment

Pain management at the end of life needs to start with a thorough and complete pain assessment. Complete pain assessment is discussed in detail in other chapters of this book.

At the end of life, it is important to remember that the underlying pathophysiology of pain will change as the patient approaches death. Furthermore, the ability to communicate about pain might become compromised and this will require using different tools for assessing pain.

The most important point is to always remember that pain needs to be reassessed frequently in order to achieve pain control. Behavioral measures such as vocalization, moaning, facial grimacing, and breathing patterns are often used to assess pain when patients are unable to communicate. Furthermore, caregivers and family members should always be included for pain assessment. The information provided by surrogates can be helpful in identifying the existence of the pain but might not accurately reflect the severity. Based on a study in hospitalized patients with advanced illness, surrogates were able to identify the existence of pain 73% of the time but estimated the severity only 53% of the time [14].

Medication history

Knowledge of all the medications that the patient is currently taking or has taken in the past is crucial. First, there are multiple drug interactions between antiretroviral medications and opioids. Furthermore, understanding what medications have been effective in the past for managing pain can be helpful in deciding the most appropriate medication. In addition to prescribed medications, the history should include over-the-counter medications, herbal medications such as marijuana, and also recreational drug use.

Pharmacotherapy

At the end of life, pain management is achieved by using three distinct classes of analgesic medications. First are nonopioid analgesic medications. This group consists of nonsteroidal anti-inflammatory drugs and acetaminophen. The second group consists of opioids. Some of the opioids in this group are combined with nonopioids such as hydrocodone with acetaminophen and some are opioids alone such as morphine. The last group consists of adjuvant medications such as glucocorticoids, anticonvulsants, and antidepressants. These medications have been described in the previous chapters of this book. In this section, issues that are relevant to analgesic medications at the end of life will be discussed.

At the end of life, the main challenge related to pain management is finding a balance between minimizing pain and suffering and minimizing side effects. Furthermore, as patients become less conscious and lose the ability to swallow, alternative routes for administering pain medications need to be utilized.

Short-acting oral or sublingual opioids are often used for pain management at the end of life. Liquid morphine concentrate is the prototypical agent. Immediate release morphine is rapidly absorbed by the gastrointestinal tract and achieves peak plasma concentration within 15–30 min after administration. The starting dose for oral morphine for most dying patients who are opioid naive is 5 mg orally. This dose is repeated as needed usually every 2–4 h.

For patients who have been on opioid agonists or a combination analgesic, the starting dose of oral opioid should be determined based on an equianalgesic dose of the prior medications. It is very important to pay attention to all of the medications that the patient is taking (such as antiretroviral medications) because the opioid levels will need to be adjusted based on the inhibitory or stimulatory effects of other medications (Tables 15.1 and 15.2).

Routes

The oral route is generally the most preferred route for administration of pain medications. Other routes of administration include transdermal, oral transmucosal, rectal, gastrostomy tube, subcutaneous, intravenous, intramuscular, vaginal, epidural, and intrathecal. It is preferable to use the least invasive routes first.

Oral pain medications can help in achieving pain control in up to 90% of patients [16]. Orally administered medications provide great value by being convenient and safe while being cost-effective. Oral medications also empower patients and caregivers to be actively involved in the care.

Opioids can be provided based on need (p.r.n.), based on a regular schedule around the clock, or in combination of p.r.n. and around

Table 15.1 Commonly used opioids at the end of life.

Medication	Availability	Equianalgesic (mg) dose	Usual initial dose for adult	Comment
Morphine	Tablet (IR-SR), elixir, suppository, parenteral (IV, IT, SQ, IM)	30 orally (po)	5–15 po q 4 h	Gold standard, avoid in renal failure
		10 IV/SQ/IM	2–5 IV/SQ q 2–4 h	
Hydromorphone	Tablet (ER), suppository, parenteral (IV,IT, SQ, IM)	7.5 po	2–4 po every 3–4 h	Seven times more potent per mg than morphine
		1.5 IV/SQ/IM	0.3–1 IV/SQ/IM q 3–4 h	Avoid in renal failure
Methadone	Tablet, liquid, parenteral (SQ, IM, IV), can be used rectally	See Table 15.2 for an example	2.5–10 po q 4–8 h	Appears to be safe in renal failure
			1.25–5 IV/SQ/IM q 4–8 h	Long half-life and complex equianalgesic dosing

Table 15.2 An example of methadone dosing protocol [15].

Oral morphine equivalent daily dose (mg/day)	Conversion ratio (oral Morphine: oral Methadone)
<30	2–1
30–99	4–1
100–299	8–1
300–499	12–1
500–999	15–1
≥1000	20–1 or greater

the clock. The preferred method for managing pain in patients who have a longer time to live is to provide a long-acting opioid around the clock with shorter acting breakthrough pain medications to be provided p.r.n.

During the active dying process, various factors such as diminished blood perfusion, dehydration, and multiorgan failure might lead to a decrease in metabolism of opioids, and long-acting opioids may accumulate excessively. Because of this, pain medications need to be adjusted at the end of life and possibly switched to shorter acting medications that can be given as needed based on frequent pain assessment.

Buccal and sublingual routes are non-invasive alternative routes of analgesic administration. Fentanyl is lipophilic and has substantial absorption across the lipid membranes of the buccal and sublingual mucosa. There are various types of oral transmucosal fentanyl formulations discussed in the earlier chapters. Most of the other opioids are hydrophilic and have limited absorption across the lipid membranes. Despite this fact, oral opioids are often used at the end of life in the hospice and palliative care setting because these medications are absorbed by trickling down the gastrointestinal tract.

Transdermal administration of fentanyl patch is another noninvasive alternative for administration of opioids. A transdermal fentanyl patch is not recommended for opioid naïve patients because it has a long half-life and also a long time for analgesic onset. After administering the first patch, pain should be managed by alternative opioids for the first 24 h until the fentanyl blood levels reach the therapeutic range. Each patch provides analgesia for about 72 h.

The rectal route can also be used as an alternative for administration of opioids. Blood levels of morphine after rectal administration are about the same as after oral ingestion due to rectal blood flow bypassing the liver and first pass metabolism. The rectal administration of medications can be uncomfortable for the patient and caregiver due to physical constrains. Morphine, hydromorphone, methadone, oxycodone, codeine, and tramadol can be administered rectally [17].

A gastrostomy tube can be used if one is already in place and is functional. Most of the oral medications that are available in liquid form, and some of the tablets can be crushed and administered via the gastrostomy tube. Long-acting formulation of opioids should not be crushed.

Parenteral analgesia should be used when other routes are not available or if the pain is severe and uncontrolled. Subcutaneous infusion is often used in hospice settings, and it is a great alternative for patients without venous access. When venous access is available, intravenous route is preferred. When patients can no longer take medications orally at the end of life, total daily dose of opioids can be calculated and easily converted into a single drug, with basal and breakthrough dosing based on equianalgesic table.

Discontinuation of antiretroviral therapy and drug–drug interactions

The evidence base for interaction between methadone and antiretroviral medications is underdeveloped as most of the evidence is based on case reports and often in patients receiving methadone maintenance treatment [18]. When the patient's pain is being managed with methadone and the patient is also taking antiretroviral medications, it is important to pay close attention to drug–drug interactions,

especially if antiretroviral medications are being discontinued at the end of life. Some of the antiretroviral medications such as abacavir can increase methadone clearance. Therefore, when discontinuing these medications, it is important to monitor for signs of higher methadone levels. Table 15.3 summarizes potential interactions between methadone and some of the commonly used antiretroviral medications [19,20].

Neurotoxicity

Opioid-induced neurotoxicity (OIN) is a potential side effect of opioids and can occur at the end of life. Awareness and early recognition of OIN is very important for minimizing harm and suffering. OIN is characterized by severe pain, tremors, seizures, confusion, and hallucinations. Patients who are on high doses of opioids and have decreased renal clearance have a higher risk for developing OIN. Increased opioid metabolite levels lead to neuroexcitatory and antianalgesic adverse effects. The challenge is that as the pain level increases, healthcare providers tend to increase the level of opioids. This in turn leads to higher opioid metabolite levels, which in turn leads to more neurotoxicity. This is a paradoxical situation where increasing doses of opioids lead to pain exacerbation. Upregulation of excitatory N-methyl-d-aspartate (NMDA) receptors in the dorsal horn neurons are responsible for the neurotoxicity [21].

OIN can be diagnosed when rapidly escalating doses of opioids fail to control pain and paradoxically make pain worse [22]. Allodynia is defined as unexplained pain from stimuli that normally does not cause pain. For example, gently touching the patient or contact with clothing might lead to severe pain. Allodynia tends to occur with OIN. Generalized neuroexcitation can lead to agitation, myoclonus, delirium, and seizures.

Treatment of OIN involves opioid rotation, efforts to reduce the opioid dose, and using an adjuvant analgesic such as ketamine [23]. Ketamine is being used more frequently in management of OIN due to its NMDA receptor antagonism. Furthermore, ketamine

Table 15.3   Interactions of commonly used antiretrovirals with methadone [19].

Antiretroviral	Effect on ARV level	Effect on methadone level	Management for starting ARV when patient is on methadone	Management for discontinuing ARV when patient is on Methadone and ARV
Abacavir (ABC)	Not significant	Increases methadone clearance by 22%	Starting ABC can lead to withdrawal and require increasing the dose	Discontinuing ABC can lead to higher methadone level and require decreasing the dose
Darunavir (DRV)	Not studied	May decrease methadone effects	Starting DRV can lead to withdrawal and require increasing the dose	Discontinuing DRV can lead to higher methadone level and require decreasing the dose
Lopinavir/ritonavir (LPV/r)	Not significant	Decreased methadone effects	Starting LPV/r can lead to withdrawal and require increasing the dose	Discontinuing LPV/r can lead to higher Methadone level and require decreasing the dose
Efavirenz (EFV)	Not significant	Decreased methadone effects	Starting EFV can lead to withdrawal and require increasing the dose	Discontinuing EFV can lead to higher methadone level and require decreasing the dose
Nevirapine (NVP)	Not significant	Decreased methadone effects	Starting NVP can lead to withdrawal and require increasing the dose	Discontinuing NVP can lead to higher methadone level and require decreasing the dose
Lamivudine (3TC)	Not significant	Not significant	No dose adjustment necessary	No dose adjustment necessary
Tenofovir (TDF)	Not studied	Not significant	No dose adjustment necessary	No dose adjustment necessary
Zidovudine (AZT)	Not significant	Not significant	No dose adjustment necessary	No dose adjustment necessary
Etravirine (ETR)	Not significant	Not significant	No dose adjustment necessary	No dose adjustment necessary
Atazanavir (ATV)	Not significant	Not significant	No dose adjustment necessary	No dose adjustment necessary
Dolutegravir	Not significant	Not significant	No dose adjustment necessary	No dose adjustment necessary
Elvitegravir/ cobicistat	Not significant	Not significant	No dose adjustment necessary	No dose adjustment necessary
Fosamprenavir (FPV)	Not significant	Not significant	No dose adjustment necessary	No dose adjustment necessary

has sedative, amnestic, and analgesic properties. Methadone is a weak NMDA antagonist and may be effective in managing OIN in some patients [24–26].

Palliative sedation for uncontrollable pain

Palliative sedation involves using specific sedative medications to relieve intolerable suffering from refractory symptoms such as pain. This procedure involves reducing patient's consciousness [27]. Palliative sedation is used when alternative therapies for relieving symptoms have not been effective or have caused unacceptable side effects, and when the goal is to relive the symptom but not to hasten death [28].

Ethical issues

Management of pain and suffering at the end of life is a balancing act. Every intervention has the potential pros and cons that need to be fully evaluated. For example, opioids are very effective for managing pain but also lead to constipation. When pain is severe and unrelenting, higher doses of opioids might be needed for pain management. The principle of double effect is a set of ethical guidelines that is used when an action performed for a specific goal, for example, prescribing opioids for managing pain at the end of life, might cause an undesirable effect such as shortening someone's life. This action would be ethically justifiable if the following are true:

- The nature of the act is good or morally natural.
- The agent intends the good effect and not the bad.
- The good effect outweighs the bad effect [29].

Summary

Pain management at the end of life is critical for reducing suffering in patients with HIV. HIV providers should develop skills and knowledge

for providing comfort and palliating symptoms at the end of life. Providing the right medications at the right time and via the right route will reduce pain and minimize suffering.

References

1 Larue, F., Fontaine, A., Colleau, S.M. (1997) Underestimation and undertreatment of pain in HIV disease: multicentre study. *BMJ*, **314** (7073), 23–28 [PubMed ID: 9001475].

2 Saunders, C.M. (1976) The challenge of terminal care. In: Symington T, Carter RL, (eds). *Scientific Foundations of Oncology*. London, England: Heinemann, 673–679.

3 Breitbart, W., Rosenfeld, B.D., Passik, S.D., McDonald, M.V., Thaler, H. & Portenoy, R.K. (1996) The undertreatment of pain in ambulatory AIDS patients. *Pain*, **65** (2-3), 243–249.[PubMed ID: 8826513]

4 Singer, E.J., Zorilla, C., Fahy-Chandon, B., Chi, S., Syndulko, K. & Tourtellotte, W.W. (1993) Painful symptoms reported by ambulatory HIV-infected men in a longitudinal study. *Pain*, **54** (1), 15–19.[PubMed ID: 8378098]

5 Kimball, L.R. & McCormick, W.C. (1996) The pharmacologic management of pain and discomfort in persons with AIDS near the end of life: use of opioid analgesia in the hospice setting. *Journal of Pain and Symptom Management*, **11** (2), 88.

6 Vogl, D., Rosenfeld, B., Breitbart, W. *et al.* (1999) Symptom prevalence, characteristics, and distress in AIDS outpatients. *Journal of Pain and Symptom Management*, **18** (4), 253.

7 "HIV/AIDS." WHO. N.p., n.d. Web. 06 Feb. 2015. <http://www.who.int/gho/hiv/en/>.

8 Centers for Disease Control and Prevention. Centers for Disease Control and Prevention, 25 Nov. 2014. Web. 02 Feb. 2015. <http://www.cdc.gov/hiv/statistics/basics/ataglance.html>.

9 Antiretroviral Therapy Cohort Collaboration. "Causes of death in HIV-1 – infected patients treated with antiretroviral therapy, 1996–2006: collaborative analysis of 13 HIV cohort studies." *Clinical Infectious Diseases* **50**.10 (2010): 1387–1396.

10 Cleeland, C.S., Gonin, R., Hatfield, A.K. *et al.* (1994) Pain and its treatment in outpatients with metastatic cancer. *New England Journal of Medicine*, **330** (9), 592.

11 Cleeland, C.S., Gonin, R., Baez, L., Loehrer, P. & Pandya, K.J. (1997) Pain and treatment of pain in minority patients with cancer. The Eastern Cooperative Oncology Group Minority Outpatient Pain Study. *Annals of Internal Medicine*, **127** (9), 813–816.

12 Breitbart, W., Kaim, M. & Rosenfeld, B. (1999) Clinicians' perceptions of barriers to pain management in AIDS. *Journal of Pain and Symptom Management*, **18**, 203–212.

13 Dew, M.A., Becker, J.T., Sanchez, J. *et al.* (1997) Prevalence and predictors of depressive, anxiety and substance use disorders in HIV-infected and uninfected men: a longitudinal evaluation. *Psychological Medicine*, **27** (2), 395–409.

14 Desbiens, N.A. & Mueller-Rizner, N. (2000) How well do surrogates assess the pain of seriously ill patients? *Critical Care Medicine*, **28**, 1347.

15 Fisch, M.J. & Cleeland, C.S. (2003) Managing cancer pain. In: Skeel, R.T. (ed), *Handbook of Cancer Chemotherapy*, 6th edn. Lippincott Williams & Wilkins, Philadelphia, PA, p. 663.

16 Jacox, A., Carr, D.B. & Payne, R. (1994) New clinical-practice guidelines for the management of pain in patients with cancer. *New England Journal of Medicine*, **330**, 651–655.

17 Samala R.V., Davis M.P. (2012) *Use of rectal meds for palliative care patients. Fast facts and concepts* [WWW document].URL http://www.eperc.mcw.edu/EPERC/FastFactsIndex/ff_257.htm. ©2012 EPERC.

18 Weschules, Douglas J., Kevin T. Bain, Steven Richeimer. Actual and potential drug interactions associated with methadone. *Pain Medicine* **9**(3) (2008): 315–344. Print.

19 David, E. (2012) Substance abuse in HIV populations. In: *AAHIVM Fundamentals of HIV Medicine*, 2012 edn. Vol. **507**. American Academy of HIV Medicine, Washington, DC.

20 Comprehensive, Up-to-date Information on HIV/AIDS Treatment, Prevention, and Policy from the University of California San Francisco. Interactions with Methadone, 2006: N.p., n.d. Web. 07 Feb. 2015. <http://hivinsite.ucsf.edu/insite?page=ar-00-02&post=8¶m=42#66>.

21 Compton P. (2008) *The OIH paradox: can opioids make pain worse? Pain treatment topics* [WWW document]. URL http://pain-topics.org/pdf/Compton-OIH-Paradox.pdf [accessed on 24 October 2011].

22 Chu, L.F., Angst, M.S. & Clark, D. (2008) Opioid-induced hyperalgesia in humans: molecular mechanisms and clinical considerations. *Clinical Journal of Pain*, **24**, 479–496.

23 Mitra, S. (2008) Opioid-induced hyperalgesia: pathophysiology and clinical implications. *Journal of Opioid Management*, **4**, 123–130.

24 Pasero, C., Quinn, T.E., Portenoy, R.K. *et al.* (2011) Opioid analgesics. In: Pasero, C. & McCaffery, M. (eds), *Pain Assessment and Pharmacologic Management*. Mosby/Elsevier, St. Louis, MO, pp. 277–622.

25 Chu, L.F., Clark, D. & Angst, M.S. (2009) Molecular basis and clinical implications of opioid tolerance and opioid-induced hyperalgesia. In: Sinatra, R.S., de Leon-Casasola, O.A., Ginsberg, B. & Viscusi, E.R. (eds), *Acute Pain Management*. Cambridge University Press, Cambridge, NY, pp. 114–143.

26 Ramaasubbu, C. & Gupta, A. (2011) Pharmacological treatment of opioid-induced hyperalgesia: a review of the evidence. *Journal of Pain & Palliative Care Pharmacotherapy*, **25**, 219–230.

27 De Graeff, A. & Dean, M. (2007) Palliative sedation therapy in the last weeks of life: a literature review and recommendations for standards. *Journal of Palliative Medicine*, **10** (1), 67–85.

28 Lo, B. & Rubernfeld, G. (2005) Palliative sedation in dying patients: "we turn to it when everything else hasn't worked". *JAMA*, **294**, 1810–1816.

29 T. A. Cavanaugh, *Double-Effect Reasoning: Doing Good and Avoiding Evil*, p.36, Oxford: Clarendon Press.

CHAPTER 16

Disparities and barriers in management of chronic pain among vulnerable populations with HIV infection

Catherine Deamant[1] and Susan Nathan[2]

[1] Division of General Internal Medicine and Primary Care, Cook County Health and Hospitals System, Chicago, IL, USA

[2] Department of Internal Medicine, Division of Geriatrics, Section of Palliative Medicine, Rush University Medical Center, Chicago, IL, USA

Introduction

Disparities in health care have long been recognized as a significant problem within the healthcare system. There are well-recognized and studied disparities and barriers to identifying and treating pain in non-Caucasian populations and women. Vulnerable populations are groups that are not well integrated into the healthcare system because of ethnic, cultural, economic, geographic, or health characteristics. Vulnerable populations are at increased risk for health disparities and face unique barriers to care. Commonly cited examples of vulnerable populations include racial and ethnic minorities, the rural and urban poor, incarcerated people, immigrants, older or younger adults, people with different sexual orientations, and people with disabilities or multiple chronic conditions [1]. Disparities or barriers in pain management and relief are more severe in vulnerable populations. Providing effective and culturally competent care to these populations requires intentionality around recognizing at-risk populations and identifying effective strategies for pain assessment and management.

Prevalence of HIV infection in vulnerable populations

Men who have sex with men (MSM) remain the group most heavily affected by HIV in the United States, Canada, and the United Kingdom; [2,3] other vulnerable populations also disproportionately impacted by HIV/AIDS include African–American and Hispanic men and women [4,5]. Young, African–American, MSM now account for more new infections than any other subgroup by age, race/ethnicity, and gender/sexual orientation category. Transgender people are also heavily affected by HIV with 28% of transgender women testing positive for HIV in 2008 [6]. Foreign-born Africans and Hispanics are also disproportionately affected by HIV infection compared to the general US population [7–9]. HIV-infected populations are also more likely to experience homelessness, incarceration, and injection drug use [10].

Pain experience in HIV-infected vulnerable populations

Pain is a common symptom in patients living with HIV/AIDS, and vulnerable populations have reported a high prevalence of pain and greater severity of pain.

Pain rates may be higher in patients of lower socioeconomic status. In a recent systematic review of palliative care–related problems in patients with HIV infection, the reports of pain in prospective observational studies ranged from 11% to 62% in high-income countries, ranged from 31% to 53% in middle-income

Chronic Pain and HIV: A Practical Approach, First Edition.
Edited by Jessica S. Merlin, Peter A. Selwyn, Glenn J. Treisman and Angela G. Giovanniello.
© 2016 John Wiley & Sons, Ltd. Published 2016 by John Wiley & Sons, Ltd.

countries, and were 76% among low-income countries [11].

In one study of 296 indigent adults with HIV infection who were homeless or marginally housed, 90% reported pain that was classified as chronic pain (>6months duration) and 64.8% reported daily pain. Those with more severe pain reported poorer quality of life, both in physical and psychological domains. Patient attribution to the cause of pain included HIV/AIDS related (disease or side effects of medications) in 60.4%, physical assault in 21.5%, and living conditions in 34.1%. Female gender and having less formal education were associated with more severe pain in this already vulnerable cohort [12]. In another study of HIV-infected patients with a history of intravenous drug use in Canada, those who had experienced homelessness were more likely to have self-medicated for pain [13].

In addition, women and ethnic minorities reported significantly higher levels of pain intensity than men and Caucasian patients [14]. Yet, in a longitudinal study of HIV-infected women receiving highly active antiretroviral therapy (HAART), Caucasian women reported a higher prevalence of symptoms, including pain, compared to other race/ethnicities. Despite a difference in prevalence of pain between Caucasian women and other race/ethnicities, this study did not evaluate whether there were differences in the intensity of pain nor the impact on function or quality of life. Older aged people had a higher likelihood of pain-related symptoms [15]. HIV-infected patients with posttraumatic stress disorder (PTSD) reported having significantly higher pain intensity and greater pain-related interference in performing activities of daily living and affective areas of functioning compared to HIV-infected patients without PTSD [16]. Notably, HIV-infected men and women have higher trauma rates and subsequent PTSD than uninfected individuals [17,18]. HIV-positive immigrants may be at a greater risk of developing depression due to additional stressors such as language and citizenship barriers [19].

Among HIV-infected patients in the post-HAART era, histories of psychiatric illness and patients with a history of intravenous drug use were more likely to report the pain as moderate or severe [20]. The association of pain

prevalence, severity, and response to treatment in HIV-infected patients with a history of psychiatric illness and with history of aberrant drug use is covered in Chapters 7 and 8.

Disparities and barriers in chronic pain and implications for pain assessment and management

Health disparities are defined "as observed clinically and statistically significant differences in health outcomes or healthcare use between socially distinct vulnerable and less vulnerable populations that are not explained by the effects of selection bias [21]." While evidence for disparities in pain recognition and management in vulnerable populations with HIV/AIDS in the current HIV treatment era is limited, there is applicable evidence for pain disparities by race and ethnicity in the general population. Consistent data has emerged showing marked disparities in access to and use of effective pain treatment across racial and ethnic groups. In general, African–Americans with chronic, non-malignant pain report increased pain severity, higher disability level, more symptoms consistent with depression and PTSD, and poorer quality of life compared to Caucasians [22].

Factors that influence disparities can be divided into three main categories: provider factors, patient factors, and healthcare system factors [23,24].

Provider factors
Underestimation and undertreatment of pain
In the general population, providers are more likely to underestimate and undertreat pain in African–Americans and Hispanics anrd are less likely to prescribe analgesics, both opioids and nonopioids [25]. These differences in analgesic prescribing have been described across settings (emergency department, postoperative care, ambulatory care, and nursing homes) [22] and across types of pain (i.e., acute, malignant, chronic, and nonmalignant) [26]. Providers of patients with HIV infection also are less likely to recognize patient's symptom burden,

including pain. This underrecognition may impact on a patient's quality of life, as well as on hospitalization and mortality [27].

Lack of trust

Primary care providers caring for indigent HIV-infected patients overestimated patient misuse of opioids, used race as a predictor of misuse, and were found to be less trusting of non-Caucasian patients [28]. Most of the medical literature on trust [29] focuses on patient trust in the clinician. Trust is defined as a firm belief in the reliability, truth, ability, or strength of something or someone. However, mutual trust in the provider–patient relationship, including the provider's trust of the patient, can influence the clinician's behavior, positively or negatively affecting his or her management of patients with chronic pain.

One study evaluated a measure of physician trust with patients with HIV infection with chronic, nonmalignant pain on opioids. Six themes for patient behaviors engendering trust by the provider include the following: provide accurate and complete information, adhere to the agreed upon treatment plan, actively participate in his or her care, respect the physician, not manipulate for secondary gain, and remain committed to the relationship [30].

Available evidence indicates that minority patients are not more likely than non-Caucasian patients to misuse prescription medications [31–33]. Misuse was most accurately predicted by patient history of alcohol abuse or illicit substance use, which is not more prevalent among all minorities compared to Caucasians [28,34]. Despite this, studies have shown that providers judge non-Caucasian patients to have a higher risk for prescription opioid misuse compared to Caucasian patients [34–36].

Healthcare providers of HIV-infected patients report low confidence and satisfaction levels in treating chronic pain. Lack of confidence in caring for patients with perceived aberrant drug-related behaviors with chronic pain may be reflected by emotion-laden language in the medical record [37]. In one study, lower provider confidence was associated with no direct clinical experience treating HIV-infected patients for opioid addiction. In addition, providers attitudes toward comfort in

diagnosis and treating chronic pain and comfort in prescribing opioid analgesics, in general, and in patients with a history of substance use was also associated with lower confidence. Higher confidence in recognizing abuse of opioid medications in HIV-infected patients was correlated with prior training in addiction medicine or addiction psychiatry and having prescribed buprenorphine for opioid dependence [38].

Provider uncertainty on how to best manage chronic pain in HIV-infected patients, especially with prior or active illicit substance use, can contribute to disparities in treatment [39]. Providers who only selectively screen for substance abuse, perform urine toxicology screening or discuss medication diversion with patients who they suspect of aberrant behavior, rather than applying routine practice of clinical guidelines, may miss abuse. These providers may further stigmatize patients and further contribute to provider-patient mistrust [38].

Patient factors: Chronic pain, like other chronic diseases, is influenced by physical, cognitive, and emotional factors. The subjective nature of chronic pain can have significant cultural, spiritual, and other meanings that influence a person's pain experience. The biopsychosocial model provides a multidimensional framework for understanding and recognizing the complex and dynamic interactions of the biological, psychological, sociocultural, and economic factors in the patient's experience of chronic pain. (Figure 16.1) [40,41]

Biopsychosocial model for chronic pain

A biopsychosocial framework for chronic pain in HIV has been proposed that identifies factors that may contribute to pain in patients with HIV, including biological factors, such as HIV-related neuropathy, osteonecrosis, psychiatric illnesses (depression and anxiety), and substance abuse; psychological factors of anger, fear, and trauma, and social factors, including stigmatization and environmental stressors (housing). These factors can influence healthcare-related outcomes, including medication adherence, retention in HIV primary care, quality of life, and healthcare utilization [42].

Psychological and cultural factors also influence pain perceptions. Despite higher reports of symptoms consistent with depression and

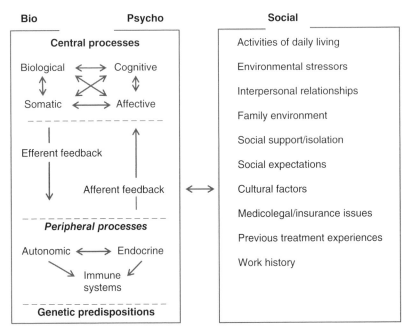

Figure 16.1 A conceptual model of the biopsychosocial interactive processes involved in health and illness. From Ref. 41. ©2004 by the American Psychological Association.

PTSD, African–Americans are less likely to seek mental health services than Caucasians. The lack of mental health care may influence their psychological and social well-being as they relate to chronic pain [26,36]. Women who report a history of intimate partner violence, regardless of race or ethnicity, are more likely to report chronic pain [43] and less likely to describe coping skills [26].

Among foreign-born patients, acculturation influences increased or decreased risk of reporting pain based on the prevalence of pain syndromes in the native country. In one study, acculturation in Hispanic immigrants, based on English proficiency, was associated with an increased risk of reporting chronic back and neck problems [44].

For patients with limited English proficiency, linguistic differences in describing pain may be a barrier to appropriate care and can contribute to disparities in assessing and managing pain. In addition, both patients with limited English and those proficient in English can have limited health literacy. Health literacy is defined as "the degree to which an individual has the capacity to obtain, communicate, process and understand basic health information and services to make appropriate decisions [45]." Health literacy is closely tied to socioeconomic status and education. Low health literacy in patients with HIV infection can significantly affect their knowledge of HIV and pain, as well as their problem-solving skills and their adherence to medication or other treatment recommendations [46].

Patients' attitudes and beliefs about pain and their coping strategies influence psychosocial and physical function and use of healthcare services. Patients who identified pain as being disabling, uncontrollable, and medically curable were less likely to be employed, less functional, and likelier to report distress than patients who demonstrated more self-reliant attitudes toward pain [47]. Psychological health is an important consideration in the management of HIV. Depression (covered in Chapter 8) may be a factor in decreased ability to cope with pain.

In one study, African–Americans with chronic nonmalignant pain compared to Caucasians reported worse pain management scores and lower quality of life. Perceived discrimination and hopelessness were implicated as explanatory factors for these disparities [48].

Finally, the uneven prevalence of depression in some groups may be an independent patient-level factor affecting disparities in pain. Unique stressors, due to language, immigration, and documentation status barriers, may put HIV-infected immigrants at greater risk of developing depression. Immigrants with HIV infection in Canada reported higher rates of stress and depression compared to the native-born population [49]. Immigrants with undocumented status may fear seeking health care because they are marginalized, fear deportation, or are unfamiliar with how to navigate the healthcare system. They also may avoid seeking care because they have prioritized seeking food and shelter over health concerns [50]. Any or all of these factors may negatively influence the ability to adhere to complex medication regimens, refill prescriptions, and incorporate nonpharmacologic strategies as part of comprehensive pain management.

Healthcare system factors
Remuneration
Reimbursement policies do not support the time required for comprehensive pain assessments, care coordination, and multidisciplinary care or for planning and implementing patient education initiatives.

Access
Other causes of disparities in pain management are lack of access to patient education materials in different languages and for various literacy levels, interdisciplinary practice or integrated care models, behavioral health, and rehabilitative services. Clinical services focused on disease-specific categories, such as HIV disease, may not have readily available specialty services, such as pain specialists or addiction specialists to meet patients' multiple needs [51].

Strategies to improve pain assessment and management for vulnerable populations

HIV/AIDS in the pre-HAART era had high mortality rates and often involved opioid therapy for managing symptoms at the end of life. Now, HIV/AIDS has become a chronic disease, with a near-normal life expectancy, and over time will have anticipated changes in physical health, psychological well-being, and social relationships. Chronic pain, whether due to the underlying condition of HIV, to its complications, or to other health conditions, can be thought of as its own comorbid chronic disease. As such, it requires a prescribed treatment plan, including strategies for self-management and coping with emotional and psychological distress and impact on role and function (see Chapter 10 and 12, Section on Nonpharmacologic Strategies) [52]. A rational approach to effective pain assessment and management and strategies for working with HIV-infected patients with chronic pain is needed (Table 16.1).

Provider level interventions
Standardization
Routine use of standardized symptom assessments, including pain, and guidelines within healthcare systems may reduce physician bias in perception of patient's pain [53]. The Brief Pain Inventory is a self-administered questionnaire that has been validated across a variety of languages, cultures, and illnesses, and addresses both pain severity and functional impact of pain [54].

There are several risk assessment tools that can help risk stratify patients being considered for opioid management of pain [55]. Questionnaires such as the Screener and Opioid Assessment for Patients with Pain-Revised (SOAPP-R), (self-administered by the patient) [56] and the Opioid Risk Tool (ORT), (administered by the clinician) [57] are both validated tools for substance abuse risk assessment in patients with chronic nonmalignant pain. In light of the chronic disease management model for HIV care and chronic pain, the limited evidence for the use of chronic opioid therapy and potential harm from opioids needs to be recognized by providers. When opioid therapy is considered appropriate, then providers should apply opioid therapy guidelines in a standardized manner for all patients, with descriptive, evidence-based approaches to identify and monitor for aberrant

Table 16.1 Strategies to reduce disparities in pain assessment and management.

Factors	Strategies [51,55,61,62]
Provider	• Self-awareness of unconscious biases and applies bias-reducing strategies focused on intentional behavioral change, such as individuating and perspective taking • Use standard pain assessment tool and evidence-based protocols and guidelines • Use risk assessment tool to risk stratify patients when considering use of opioids • Explore the physical, psychological, social, and functional impact of chronic pain in the individual patient • Use a collaborative care model in caring for patients with chronic pain • Guide, coach, and support patient self-management strategies
Patient	• Self-management techniques to improve function and quality of life emphasizing participation in daily activities • Develop problem-solving skills • Encourage lifestyle changes (strengthening exercises, physical activity, proper lifting, and adequate sleep) • Enhance self-efficacy believing one has control over chronic pain • Identify realistic goals and action plan • Practice cognitive behavioral strategies to build coping skills, think in new ways, relaxation techniques, and reduce pain catastrophizing
System	• Ensure use of bilingual healthcare professionals or medically trained interpreters for all health encounters • Set system-wide standards of care and quality metrics regarding pain assessment and management • Provide interdisciplinary, multimodal integrated services, including physical and psychological support focused on patients' needs • Conduct multimedia, public health education with attention to culture, literacy, and language

drug-related behaviors [58], side effects, as well as improvements in functional domains around pain with the given treatment plan.

Providers should recognize potential variables, economic or cultural, that may affect appropriate implementation of recommendations.

Trust building

Key elements to building a trusting relationship between provider and patient include active listening and exploration of concerns, whole person assessment, and engaging the patient in the decision-making process. As communication is a core element to building trust, providers must ensure that medically trained interpreters are utilized for healthcare encounters when needed. Strategies for building trust include encouraging exploration of patient concern and responding with validation of expressed concern, less verbal dominance by provider, and receiving more input by patient in the psychosocial and lifestyle aspects, allowing the patient to ask questions and then provide clear answers [59].

The five behaviors that were most strongly associated with trust with the provider were as follows: (1) being comforting and caring, (2) demonstrating competency, (3) encouraging and answering questions, (4) explaining what they were doing, and (5) referring to a specialist if needed [60].

Healthcare professionals must be aware that bias, even when unintended, influences medical decision-making and may contribute to disparities in the management of chronic pain. Second, they must identify strategies for behavioral change to reduce this unconscious bias. Two behavioral strategies used to reduce bias in medical decision-making are *individuating*, whereby the provider focuses on specific information about an individual and not on their social category (race, ethnicity, or gender), and *perspective-taking*, whereby the provider consciously attempts to imagine another person's perspective [61].

Patient-level interventions:
Self-management
As in other chronic disease models, self-management programs are essential to the care plan. Key components to self-management programs include educating the patient about their condition, engaging the patient in developing active problem-solving skills, and supporting patients in identifying achievable goals and actions [62]. Cognitive behavioral strategies help patients build coping skills by addressing beliefs and feelings to develop new ways of thinking about their pain and learn other techniques [42] such as relaxation or mindfulness-based stress reduction. Promoting self-efficacy – the belief that one can have some control over one's pain – has been shown to improve physical and psychological functioning and pain tolerance [51]. In one qualitative study of HIV-infected patients, the patients recognized the bidirectional relationship between mood and pain and the importance of addressing the psychological aspects of pain [63].

Incorporation of cognitive behavioral therapy (CBT) into primary care clinics for HIV-infected patients serving minority populations has proven to be feasible and acceptable. In one 12-week CBT intervention in a primary care setting, non-Caucasian HIV-positive patients reported greater improvements in pain-related anxiety, pain-related functioning and greater response to treatment compared to Caucasian participants. Of note, in this "real-world" study in clinical practice, patients did not attend all the sessions and were provided a manual for self-study. Attendance at the treatment sessions focused on progressive muscle relaxation and cognitive reconceptualization proved to be statistically significant in explaining improvement in psychological pain related to functioning. Given barriers to transportation, unstable housing and need for childcare, simple brief coaching and instruction may prove to be a useful initial intervention in a primary care setting, combined with self-help workbooks and exercises for self-learning [64].

Community health workers or patient navigators can provide cultural leverage by focusing on strategies to improve the health of racial and ethnic minority groups through culturally tailored interventions, which present information using a group's own values and practices. One such model provided a culturally targeted HIV/AIDS health literacy toolkit for dissemination of HIV/AIDS health information using teach-back methods [65]. Integrating health education about chronic pain in already existing HIV-tailored interventions can address misconceptions, identify behaviors to reduce or prevent pain, facilitate health decision-making, and enhance patient–provider communication, as well as reduce strain in low-resource settings.

System-level interventions
Multidisciplinary and multimodality approach to care
Within health systems, healthcare leaders should ensure availability of bilingual staff, access to an interdisciplinary team that may include mid-level providers, psychologists for nonpharmacologic, behavioral strategies, addiction specialists, complementary and alternative medicine specialists, physical or occupational therapists, and physical medicine and rehabilitation specialists. As integrated treatment models for care of HIV-infected patients have demonstrated effectiveness for addressing substance use disorders [66], similar approaches should be developed and evaluated for addressing pain [67]. Develop or make available low literacy, linguistically appropriate educational materials about the nature of pain, self-management strategies to prevent, cope and reduce pain, and the various pain management options, as well as opioid treatment agreements for patients with low literacy.

One study of vulnerable patients, who were predominantly African-American, low socioeconomic status and low literacy levels, demonstrated that CBT was feasible, efficacious and acceptable. Patients participating in this study showed significant improvement in depressive symptoms; reduced catastrophizing; some improvement in pain intensity; and moderate reduction in pain interference [68]. Material was adapted from an evidence-based chronic pain CBT protocol with attention to limiting the concepts presented at each session; revising the written materials to ensure use of simple terms; removing jargon; using large fonts and bolding for emphasis; diagrams and other visuals;

sentences that were simple, direct, and in active voice; readability at fifth grade level [69].

When provided at the site of care, computer technology can be useful as an assessment and intervention tool. One such tool, audio computer-assisted self-interviewing (ACASI), has been used effectively to assess self-reported health risk behaviors in HIV-infected women and patients with low-level literacy [70]. ACASI modules focusing on pain beliefs, symptom burden, and quality of life may serve as an additional educational tool in the clinic setting and can be conducted in multiple languages.

Large public outreach efforts, such as the efforts to discourage smoking and promote cancer prevention, have proven successful in modifying health behaviors. These efforts can serve as models for public education initiatives about pain and its management. Australia and Scotland have conducted public health education campaigns on low back pain, effecting health beliefs with some measure of success. Suggested outreach tools included multimedia efforts (television, radio, and advertisements), leaflets, signage, fact sheets, and videos [51].

Conclusion

Disparities in the assessment and management of chronic pain can negatively effect the care of racial and ethnic minorities and women. These disparities are influenced by factors at multiple levels. Primary care providers caring for these vulnerable populations with HIV infection and chronic pain must utilize a multimodal approach to overcome these disparities.

References

1 Aday, L. (2001) *At Risk in America: The Health and Health Care Needs of Vulnerable Populations in the United States*, 2nd edn. Jossey-Bass, San Francisco, CA.

2 Brown A.E., Hughes G., Nardone A., Gill O.N., Delpech V.C., *et al. HIV in the United Kingdom 2014 report: data to end December 2013* [WWW document]. Public Health England, London. URL https://www.gov.uk/government/ uploads/system/uploads/attachment_data/ file/377194/2014_PHE_HIV_annual_report_ 19_11_2014.pdf [accessed on 20 February 2015].

3 *At a glance – HIV and AIDS in Canada: surveillance report to December 31, 2012* [WWW document]. URL http://www.phac-aspc.gc.ca/aids-sida/ publication/survreport/2012/dec/index-eng .php [accessed on 20 February 2015].

4 Aziz, M. & Smith, K. (2011) Challenges and successes in linking HIV-infected women to care in the United States. *Clinical Infectious Diseases*, **52**, S231–37.

5 Espinoza, L., Hall, H., Campsmith, M. *et al.* (2005) Trends in HIV/AIDS diagnoses-33 states, 2001–2004. *Morbidity and Mortality Weekly Report*, **54**, 1149–1153.

6 Herbst, J., Jacobs, E., Finlayson, T. *et al.* (2008) Estimating HIV prevalence and risk behaviors of transgender persons in the United States: a systematic review. *AIDS and Behavior*, **12** (1), 1–17.

7 Blanas, D.A., Nichols, K., Bekele, M. *et al.* (2013) HIV/AIDS Among African-born Residents in the United States. *Journal of Immigrant and Minority Health*, **15**, 718–724.

8 Centers for Disease Control and Prevention. (2013) Monitoring selected national HIV prevention and care objectives by using HIV surveillance data – United States and 6 dependent areas – 2011. *HIV surveillance supplemental report* 2013 [WWW document]; **18** (5). URL http://www.cdc.gov/hiv/library/ reports/surveillance/ [accessed on 14 June 2014].

9 Centers for Disease Control and Prevention. (2012) Estimated HIV incidence in the United States, 2007–2010. *HIV surveillance supplemental report* 2012 [WWW document]; **17** (4). http://www.cdc.gov/hiv/pdf/statistics_hssr_ vol_17_no_4.pdf [accessed on 20 February 2015].

10 Robertson, M.J., Clark, R.A., Charlebois, E.D. *et al.* (2011) HIV seroprevalence among homeless and marginally housed adults in San Francisco. *American Journal of Public Health*, **94** (7), 1207–1217.

11 Simms, V., Higginson, I. & Harding, R. (2011) What palliative care-related problems do patients experience at HIV diagnosis? A systematic review of the evidence. *Journal*

of Pain and Symptom Management, **42**, 734–753.

12 Miakowski, C., Penko, J.M., Guzman, D., Mattson, J.E., Bangsberg, D.R. & Kushel, M.B. (2011) Occurrence and characteristics of chronic pain in a community-based cohort of indigent adults living with HIV infection. *The Journal of Pain*, **12** (9), 1004–1016.

13 Voon, P., Callon, C., Nguyen, P. *et al.* (2014) Self-management of pain among people who inject drugs in Vancouver. *Pain Management*, **4** (1), 27–35.

14 Breitbart, W., McDonald, M., Rosenfeld, B. *et al.* (1996) Pain in ambulatory AIDS patients. I: Pain characteristics and medical correlates. *Pain*, **68**, 315–321.

15 Silverberg, M., Jacobson, L., French, A. *et al.* (2009) Age and racial/ethnic differences in the prevalence of reported symptoms in human immunodeficiency virus-infected persons on antiretroviral therapy. *Journal of Pain and Symptom Management*, **38** (2), 197–207.

16 Smith, M., Egert, J., Winkel, G. & Jacobson, J. (2002) The impact of PTSD on pain experience in persons with HIV/AIDS. *Pain*, **98**, 9–17.

17 Kimerling, R., Calhoun, K., Forehand, R. *et al.* (1999) Traumatic stress in HIV-infected women. *AIDS Education and Prevention*, **11**, 321–330.

18 Kalichman, S., Sikkema, K., DiFonzo, K. *et al.* (2002) Emotional adjustment in survivors of sexual assault living with HIV/AIDS. *Journal of Traumatic Stress Disorders & Treatment*, **15**, 289–296.

19 Asian Community AIDS Services (2004) *Intersecting sexuality, gender, race and citizenship: mental health issues faced by immigrants and refugees living with HIV/AIDS* [WWW document]. URL http://www.hivimmigration.ca/wp-content/uploads/2011/07/IRPHA-mental-Health-Lit-review-2004.pdf [accessed on 20 February 2015]. Asian Community AIDS Services, Toronto, ON.

20 Merlin, J.S., Cen, L., Praestgaard, A. *et al.* (2012) Pain and physical and psychological symptoms in ambulatory HIV patients in the current treatment era. *Journal of Pain and Symptom Management*, **43** (3), 638–645.

21 Kilbourne, A.M., Switzer, G., Hyman, K. *et al.* (2006) Advancing health disparities research within the health care system: a conceptual

framework. *American Journal of Public Health*, **96**, 2113–2121.

22 Anderson, K.O., Green, C.R. & Payne, R. (2009) Racial and ethnic disparities in pain: causes and consequences of unequal care. *The Journal of Pain*, **10** (12), 1187–1204.

23 Cintron, A. & Morrison, S. (2006) Pain and ethnicity in the United States: a systematic review. *Journal of Palliative Medicine*, **9**, 1454–1473.

24 Agency for Healthcare Research and Quality, Rockville M.D. (2012) *National Healthcare Disparities Report. June 2013* [WWW document]. URL http://www.ahrq.gov/research/findings/nhqrdr/nhdr12/2012nhdr.pdf [accessed on 20 February 2015].

25 Smedley, B., Stith, A., Nelson, A. (eds). (2002) *Unequal Treatment: Confronting Racial and Ethnic Disparities in Health Care*. National Academy Press. Washington, DC.

26 Green, C., Anderson, K., Baker, T. *et al.* (2003) The unequal burden of pain: confronting racial and ethnic disparities in pain. *Pain Medicine*, **4** (3), 277–294.

27 Edelman, E.J., Gordon, K. & Justice, A.C. (2011) Patient and provider-reported symptoms in the post-cART era. *AIDS and Behavior*, **15** (4), 853–861.

28 Vijayaraghavan, M., Penko, J., Guzman, D. *et al.* (2010) Primary care providers' judgments of opioid analgesic misuse in a community-based cohort of HIV-infected indigent adults. *Journal of General Internal Medicine*, **26** (4), 412–418.

29 Pearson, S.D. & Raeke, L.H. (2000) Patients' trust in physicians: many theories, few measures, and little data. *Journal of General Internal Medicine*, **15**, (7), 509–513.

30 Thom, D.H., Wong, S.T., Guzman, D. *et al.* (2011) Physician trust in the patient: development and validation of a new measure. *Annals of Family Medicine*, **9** (2), 148–154.

31 Ives, T., Chelminski, P., Hammett-Stabler, C. *et al.* (2006) Predictors of opioid misuse in patients with chronic pain: a prospective cohort study. *BMC Health Services Research*, **6**, 46.

32 Edlund, M., Steffick, D., Hudson, T. *et al.* (2007) Risk factors for clinically recognized opioid abuse and dependence among veterans using opioids for chronic non-cancer pain. *Pain*, **129** (3), 355–362.

33 Cicero, T., Inciardi, J. & Munoz, A. (2005) Trends in abuse of Oxycontin and other opioid analgesics in the United States: 2002-2004. *The Journal of Pain*, **6**, 662–672.

34 Moskowitz, D., Thom, D., Guzman, D. *et al.* (2011) Is primary care providers' trust in socially marginalized patients affected by race? *Journal of General Internal Medicine*, **26** (8), 846–851.

35 Burgess, D., Crowley-Matoka, M., Phelan, S. *et al.* (2008) Patient race and physicians' decisions to prescribe opioids for chronic low back pain. *Social Science and Medicine*, **67** (11), 1852–1860.

36 Van Ryn, M. & Burke, J. (2000) The effect of patient race and socio-economic status on physicians' perceptions of patients. *Social Science and Medicine*, **50** (6), 813–828.

37 Merlin, J.S., Turan, J.M., Herbey, I. *et al.* (2014) Aberrant drug-related behaviors: a qualitative analysis of medical record documentation in patients referred to an HIV/chronic pain clinic. *Pain Medicine*, **15**, 1724–1733.

38 Lum, P.J., Little, S., Botsko, M. *et al.* (2011) Opioid-prescribing practices and provider confidence recognizing opioid analgesic abuse in HIV primary care settings. *Journal of Acquired Immune Deficiency Syndromes*, **56**, S91–S97.

39 Vijayaraghavan, M., Penko, J., Guzman, D. *et al.* (2012) Primary care providers' views on chronic pain management among high-risk patients in safety net settings. *Pain Medicine*, **13** (9), 1141–1148.

40 Gatchel, R.J., Peng, Y.B., Peters, M.L. *et al.* (2007) The biopsychosocial approach to chronic pain: scientific advances and future directions. *Psychological Bulletin*, **133** (4), 581–624.

41 Gatchel, R.J. (2004) Comorbidity of chronic mental and physical health conditions: the biopsychosocial perspective. *American Psychologist*, **59**, 792–805.

42 Merlin, J.S., Zinski, A., Norton, W.E. *et al.* (2014) A conceptual framework for understanding chronic pain in patients with HIV. *Pain Practice*, **14** (3), 207–216.

43 Coker, A.L., Smith, P.H., Bethea, L. *et al.* (2000) Physical health consequences of physical and psychological intimate partner violence. *Archives of Family Medicine*, **9**, 451–457.

44 Bui, Q., Doescher, M., Takeuchi, D. *et al.* (2011) Immigration, acculturation and chronic back and neck problems among Latino-Americans. *Journal of Immigrant and Minority Health*, **13**, 194–201.

45 Nielsen-Bohlman, L., Panzer, A.M. & Kindig, D.A. (eds) (2004) *Health Literacy: A Prescription to End Confusion*. National Academy of Sciences, Washington DC, pp. 31–58.

46 Warwrzyniak, A.J., Ownby, R.L., McCoy, K. *et al.* (2013) Health literacy: impact on the health of HIV-infected individuals. *Current HIV/AIDS Reports*, **10**, 295–304.

47 Tait, R.C. & Chibnall, J.T. (1998) Attitude profiles and clinical status in patients with chronic pain. *Pain*, **78**, 49–57.

48 Ezenwa, M.O. & Fleming, M.F. (2012) Racial disparities in pain management in Primary Care. *Journal of Health Disparities Research and Practice*, **5** (3), 12–26.

49 Noh, M., Rueda, S., Bekle, T. *et al.* (2012) Depressive symptoms, stress and resources among adult immigrants living with HIV. *Journal of Immigrant and Minority Health*, **14**, 405–412.

50 Garland, J.M., Andrade, A.S. & Page, K.R. (2010) Unique aspects of the care of HIV-positive Latino patients living in the United States. *Current HIV/AIDS Reports*, **7**, 107–116.

51 IOM (Institute of Medicine) (2011) *Relieving Pain in America: A Blueprint forTransforming Prevention, Care, Education, and Research*. The National Academies Press, Washington, DC.

52 Marcus, K.S., Kerns, R.D., Rosenfeld, B. & Breitbart, W. (2000) HIV/AIDS-related pain as a chronic pain condition: implications of a biopsychosocial model for comprehensive assessment and effective management. *Pain Medicine*, **1** (3), 260–273.

53 Justice, A.C., Holmes, W., Gifford, A.L. *et al.* (2001) Development and validation of a self-completed HIV symptom index. *Journal of Clinical Epidemiology*, **54**, S77–S90.

54 Cleeland, C.S. & Ryan, K.M. (1994) Pain assessment: global use of the Brief Pain Inventory. *Annals of the Academy of Medicine, Singapore*, **23** (2), 129–138.

55 Moore, T.M., Jones, T., Browder, J.H. *et al.* (2009) A comparison of common screening methods for predicting aberrant behavior among patients receiving opioids for

chronic pain management. *Pain Medicine*, **10**, 1426–1433.

56 Butler, S.F., Fernandez, K., Benoit, C., Budman, S.H. & Jamison, R.N. (2008) Validation of the revised screener and opioid assessment for patients with pain (SOAPP-R). *The Journal of Pain*, **9** (4), 360–372.

57 Webster, L.R. & Webster, R.M. (2005) Predicting aberrant behaviors in opioid-treated patients: preliminary validation of the opioid risk tool. *Pain Medicine*, **6** (6), 432–442.

58 Gaither, J.R., Goulet, J.L., Becker, W.C. *et al.* (2014) Guideline-concordant management of opioid therapy among human immunodeficiency virus (HIV)-infected and uninfected veterans. *The Journal of Pain*, **15** (11), 1130–1140.

59 Fiscella, K., Meldrum, S., Franks, P. *et al.* (2004) Patient trust: is it related to patient-centered behavior of primary care physicians? *Medical Care*, **42**, 1049–1055.

60 Thom, D.M. (2001) Physician behaviors that predict patient trust. *Journal of Family Practice*, **50** (4), 323–328.

61 Chapman, E.N., Kaatz, A. & Carnes, M. (2013) Physicians and implicit bias: how doctors may unwittingly perpetuate health care disparities. *Journal of General Internal Medicine*, **28** (11), 1504–1510.

62 Bodenheimer, T., Lorig, K., Holman, H. *et al.* (2002) Patient self-management of chronic disease in primary care. *JAMA*, **288**, 2469–2475.

63 Merlin, J.S., Walcott, M., Ritchie, C., *et al.* (2014) 'Two pains together': patient perspectives on psychological aspects of chronic pain while living with HIV. *PLoS One*, **9** (11), e111765.

64 Cucciare, M.A., Sorrell, J.T. & Trafton, J.A. (2009) Predicting response to cognitive-behavioral therapy in a sample of HIV-positive patients with chronic pain. *Journal of Behavioral Medicine*, **32**, 340–348.

65 Rikard, R.V., Thompson, M.S., Head, R. *et al.* (2012) Problem posing and cultural tailoring: developing an HIV/AIDS health literacy toolkit with the African American community. *Health Promotion Practice*, **13** (5), 626–636.

66 Chaudhry, A.A., Botsko, M., Weiss, L. *et al.* (2011) Participant characteristics and HIV risk behaviors among individuals entering integrated buprenorphine/naloxone and HIV care. *Journal of Acquired Immune Deficiency Syndromes*, **56**, S14–S21.

67 Perry, B.A., Westfall, A.O., Molony, E. *et al.* (2013) Characteristics of an ambulatory palliative care clinic for HIV-infected patients. *Journal of Palliative Medicine*, **16** (8), 934–937.

68 Thorn, B.E., Day, M.A., Burns, J. *et al.* (2011) Randomized trial of group cognitive-behavioral therapy compared to a pain education control for low literacy rural people with chronic pain. *Pain*, **152** (12), 2710–2720.

69 Kuhajda, M.C., Thorn, B.E., Gaskins, S.W., Day, M.A. & Cabbil, C.M. (2011) Literacy and cultural adaptations for cognitive behavioral therapy in a rural pain population. *Translational Behavioral Medicine*, **1**, 216–223.

70 Estes, L.J., Lloyd, L.E., Teti, M., *et al.* (2010) Perceptions of audio computer-assisted self-interviewing (ACASI) among women in an HIV-positive prevention program. *PLoS One*, **5** (2), e9149.

Index

Chronic Pain and HIV: A Practical Approach, First Edition.
Edited by Jessica S. Merlin, Peter A. Selwyn, Glenn J. Treisman and Angela G. Giovanniello.
© 2016 John Wiley & Sons, Ltd. Published 2016 by John Wiley & Sons, Ltd.